Introduction to
HUMAN ANATOMY AND PHYSIOLOGY

Eldra Pearl Solomon, Ph.D.

W.B. SAUNDERS COMPANY
A Division of Harcourt Brace & Company
Philadelphia London Toronto Montreal Sydney Tokyo

A Division of
Harcourt Brace & Company

The Curtis Center
Independence Square West
Philadelphia, Pennsylvania 19106

Library of Congress Cataloging-in-Publication Data

Solomon, Eldra Pearl.
Introduction to human anatomy and physiology / Eldra Pearl
Solomon.
p.   cm.
Includes index.

ISBN 0-7216-3966-6

1. Human physiology.   2. Human anatomy.   I. Title.
[DNLM: 1. Anatomy.   2. Physiology.   QS 4 S689i]
QP34.5.S682   1992
612—dc20
DNLM/DLC   91-46850

Editor: Michael J. Brown
Designer: Bill Donnelly
Cover Designer: Paul Fry
Production Manager: Peter Faber
Manuscript Editor: Allison Esposito
Illustration Specialist: Peg Shaw

Introduction to Human Anatomy and Physiology   ISBN 0-7216-3966-6

Preface

*I*ntroduction *To Human Anatomy and Physiology* focuses on the human body as a living, functioning organism. A principal goal in preparing this book has been to share a sense of excitement about the body's elegant design and function. The emphasis is on how tissues, organs, and body systems work together to carry on complex activities such as taking a step, eating, and responding to stress. As each of the body's many parts is described, its interaction with other structures and its role in the organism are discussed.

Because people learn best when they can relate what they are studying to familiar issues, problems, and experience, this book uses examples that are easily recognized. Suntan and sunburn help explain melanin and pigment cells. Normal body functioning is made clearer by showing what happens when its balance is upset by diabetes mellitus.

LEARNING AIDS
In addition to the conversational tone of the text, numerous aids facilitate learning:

1. A chapter outline at the beginning of each chapter provides the student with an overview of the material covered in the chapter.

2. Learning objectives tell the student how to demonstrate mastery of the material covered in the chapter.

3. Headings within each chapter introduce the key idea in the information that follows.

4. Numerous tables, many of them illustrated, summarize and organize material presented in the text.

5. Carefully drawn illustrations support ideas covered in the text.

6. The sequence summaries within the text are used to simplify information presented in paragraph form. For example, paragraphs describing a sequence of blood flow are followed by a sequence summary that recaps the sequence of flow.

7. The chapter summary in outline form at the end of each chapter provides quick review of the material presented.

8. Post Tests following each chapter provide an opportunity to evaluate mastery of material in the chapter; answers are provided at the end of each chapter.

9. Review questions focus on important concepts and applications.

10. New terms are boldfaced, permitting easy identification as well as emphasis, and their phonetic pronunciations are given in parenthesis.

11. In this edition, a separate glossary is provided, facilitating rapid finding of definitions of terms.

SUPPLEMENTS
To further facilitate learning and teaching, a supplement package has been carefully designed. *Study Guide for Introduction to Anatomy and Physiology,* written for students, highlights concepts in the text and provides testing exercises and answers, and *Test Bank to Accompany Understanding Human Anatomy and Physiology,* written for instructors, provides two tests for each chapter.

Dedication

For Kathleen

A distinguished educator,
skilled boat captain,
and superb friend

Acknowledgments

The author wishes to acknowledge the support and valuable input received from family, friends, editors, students, and colleagues. I especially thank Amy Solomon and Belicia Efros for their help in editing, Mical Solomon for keeping the word processors functioning, and Kathleen M. Heide for critically reading selected portions of the manuscript and for providing encouragement.

I greatly appreciate the support of Michael J. Brown, Editor-in-Chief of Nursing Books at W. B. Saunders. In our more than ten years of working together, Michael has become a valued colleague and friend. I thank the Production Manager, Peter Faber, who guided the project through the process of production, the designer, Paul Fry, and the Illustration Coordinator, Peg Shaw. I also thank Cass Stamato, Administrative Assistant, who expertly facilitated resolution of many questions and problems. All of these dedicated professionals and many others at W. B. Saunders provided the skills needed to produce *Introduction to Human Anatomy and Physiology*. I thank them for their help and support throughout this project.

I am grateful to the professors who took the time to read the manuscript and provide valuable suggestions for improving it. Their input has contributed greatly to this final product. Among those who provided this assistance are Mary Sanders, R.N., of Erwin Technical Center in Tampa; Barbara Talik, R.N., B.S.N., M.Ed., of Northwest Technical Institute in Springdale, AR; and Carolyn Walker, R.N., B.S., of Herkimer County B.O.C.E.S. (Board of Cooperative Educational Services) in Herkimer, NY.

Contents

One

INTRODUCING THE HUMAN BODY...1

Two

CELLS AND TISSUES..**25**

Three

THE SKIN..**41**

Four

THE SKELETAL SYSTEM...**47**

Five

THE MUSCULAR SYSTEM...**77**

Six

THE CENTRAL NERVOUS SYSTEM..**91**

Seven

THE PERIPHERAL NERVOUS SYSTEM..**109**

Eight

THE SENSE ORGANS..**119**

Nine

ENDOCRINE CONTROL...**131**

Ten

THE CIRCULATORY SYSTEM: BLOOD...**147**

Eleven

THE CIRCULATORY SYSTEM: THE HEART..**159**

Twelve

CIRCULATION OF BLOOD AND LYMPH...**169**

Thirteen

THE BODY'S DEFENSE MECHANISMS **189**

Fourteen

THE RESPIRATORY SYSTEM.. **199**

Fifteen

THE DIGESTIVE SYSTEM... **209**

Sixteen

THE URINARY SYSTEM.. **229**

Seventeen

REGULATION OF FLUIDS AND ELECTROLYTES **241**

Eighteen

REPRODUCTION.. **247**

Appendix A

DISSECTING TERMS: Common Prefixes, Suffixes, and Word Roots.......................... **265**

Appendix B

THE METRIC SYSTEM **269**

GLOSSARY.. **271**

INDEX **297**

One

INTRODUCING THE HUMAN BODY

CHAPTER OUTLINE

    I. The body has several levels of organization
    II. The body is composed of inorganic compounds and organic compounds
    III. The body systems work together to maintain life
    IV. Metabolism is essential to maintenance, growth, and repair of the body
    V. Homeostatic mechanisms maintain an appropriate internal environment
    VI. The body has a basic plan
        A. Directions in the body are relative
        B. The body has three main planes
        C. We can identify specific body regions
        D. There are two main body cavities
        E. It is important to view the body as a whole

LEARNING OBJECTIVES

After you have studied this chapter, you should be able to:

1. Define anatomy and physiology.
2. List in sequence the levels of biological organization in the human body, starting with the simplest (the chemical level: atoms and molecules) and ending with the most complex (the organism).
3. Describe the ten principal organ systems.
4. Define metabolism and contrast anabolism and catabolism.
5. Define homeostasis and describe it as a basic mechanism of human physiology, giving examples.
6. Describe the anatomical position of the human body.
7. Define and use properly the principal orientational terms employed in human anatomy.
8. Recognize sagittal, transverse, and frontal sections of the body and of body structures.
9. Define and locate the principal regions and cavities of the body.

This book is an introduction to **anatomy** (uh-**nat′**-uh-me), the science of body structure, and to **physiology** (fiz-ee-**ol′**-uh-jee), the study of body function. The anatomy and physiology of the body are closely related. Each body part is marvelously adapted for carrying out its specific job. For example, the stomach has muscular walls constructed for churning and breaking down food. Its lining produces substances that break down food chemically. As you study the human body look for the relationships between the structure and function of the body parts you are studying. Notice how the size, shape, and structure of each part is related to the job it performs.

THE BODY HAS SEVERAL LEVELS OF ORGANIZATION

The body is highly organized. Its simplest level of organization is the **chemical level** (Fig. 1–1). All

TABLE 1–1
Elements that make up the human body

NAME	CHEMICAL SYMBOL	APPROXIMATE COMPOSITION BY MASS (%)	IMPORTANCE OR FUNCTION
Oxygen	O	65	Required for cellular respiration; present in most organic compounds; component of water
Carbon	C	18	Backbone of organic molecules
Hydrogen	H	10	Present in most organic compounds; component of water
Nitrogen	N	3	Component of all proteins and nucleic acids.
Calcium	Ca	1.5	Structural component of bones and teeth; important in muscle contraction, conduction of nerve impulses, and blood clotting
Phosphorus	P	1	Component of nucleic acids; structural component of bone; important in energy transfer
Potassium	K	0.4	Principal positive ion within cells; important in nerve function; affects muscle contraction
Sulfur	S	0.3	Component of most proteins.
Sodium	Na	0.2	Principal positive ion in interstitial (tissue) fluid; important in fluid balance; essential for conduction of nerve impulses
Magnesium	Mg	0.1	Needed in blood and other body tissues
Chlorine	Cl	0.1	Principal negative ion of interstitial fluid; important in fluid balance; component of sodium chloride
Iron	Fe	Trace amount	Component of hemoglobin and myoglobin; component of certain enzymes
Iodine	I	Trace amount	Component of thyroid hormones

Other elements found in very small amounts in the body include manganese (Mn), copper (Cu), zinc (Zn), cobalt (Co), fluorine (F), molybdenum (Mo), selenium (Se), and a few others. They are called trace elements.

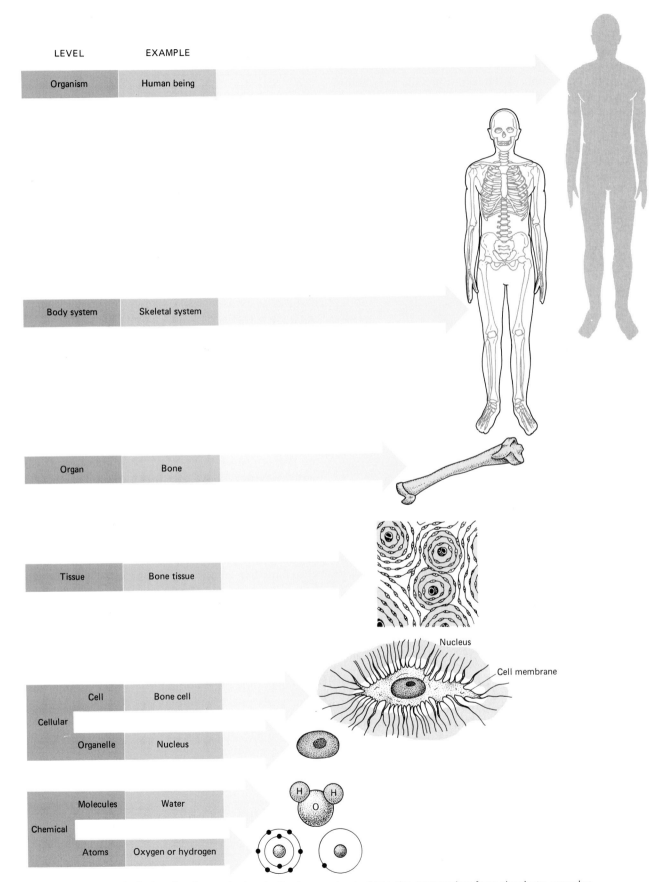

LEVEL	EXAMPLE
Organism	Human being
Body system	Skeletal system
Organ	Bone
Tissue	Bone tissue
Cellular — Cell	Bone cell
Cellular — Organelle	Nucleus
Chemical — Molecules	Water
Chemical — Atoms	Oxygen or hydrogen

Nucleus

Cell membrane

FIGURE 1–1 Levels of organization in the human body. Note the progression from simple to complex.

matter is composed of **chemical elements,** pure chemical substances such as iron, calcium, or oxygen. About 98% of the body is composed of only six elements—oxygen, carbon, hydrogen, nitrogen, calcium, and phosphorus. Table 1–1 lists the most abundant elements that make up the human body and explains why each is important.

An **atom** is the smallest amount of a **chemical element** that has the characteristic properties of that element. An electrically charged atom is called an **ion** (**eye'**-ahn). For example, an electrically charged hydrogen atom is called a hydrogen ion.

Different kinds of atoms can combine chemically forming **molecules. A chemical compound** is a molecule that consists of two or more different elements combined in a fixed proportion. Water is a chemical compound consisting of two atoms of hydrogen chemically combined with one atom of oxygen.

The next level of organization above the chemical level is the **cellular level.** In living things, atoms and molecules associate in specific ways to form **cells,** the building blocks of the body. The human body is composed of about 100 trillion cells of many types, such as blood cells and muscle cells. Although cells vary in size and shape according to their function, most are so small that they can be seen only with a microscope. Each cell consists of specialized cell parts called **organelles** (or-gah-**nells'**). One organelle, the nucleus, serves as the information and control center of the cell. Several other kinds of organelles scattered throughout the cell perform specific functions such as manufacturing needed substances or breaking down fuel molecules to provide energy.

The next highest level of organization after the cellular level is the **tissue level. A tissue** is a group of closely associated cells specialized to perform particular functions. The four main types of tissue in the body are muscle tissue, nervous tissue, connective tissue, and epithelial tissue. Tissues will be discussed in Chapter 2.

Tissues are organized into **organs,** such as the brain, stomach, or heart. Although the heart consists mainly of muscle tissue, it is covered by epithelial tissue and also contains connective and nervous tissue.

A group of tissues and organs that work together to perform specific functions makes up a **body system,** or organ system. The circulatory system, for example, consists of the heart, blood vessels, blood, lymph structures, and several other organs. Working together with great precision and complexity, the body systems make up the living **organism** (**or'**-guh-nizm)—that is, you yourself.

THE BODY IS COMPOSED OF INORGANIC COMPOUNDS AND ORGANIC COMPOUNDS

The body is made up of atoms, and life processes depend on the organization and interaction of these chemical units. Chemical compounds can be classified in two broad groups—inorganic and organic. **Inorganic compounds** are relatively small, simple compounds such as water, salts, simple acids (such as hydrochloric acid), and simple bases (such as ammonia). These substances are required for water balance and for many cell activities such as transporting materials through cell membranes.

Organic compounds are large, complex compounds containing carbon. They are the chemical building blocks (structural components) of the body and also serve as fuel molecules that provide energy for body activities. Organic compounds also regulate and participate in thousands of chemical reactions necessary for life. Four important groups of organic compounds are carbohydrates, lipids, proteins, and nucleic acids.

Carbohydrates (kar"-bow-**hi'**-drates) are sugars and starches. They are used by the body as fuel molecules and to store energy. **Lipids** include neutral fats, compounds that store energy. Other lipids are components of cell membranes. The steroids are another type of lipid; several hormones, including male and female sex hormones, are steroids.

Some **proteins** (**pro'**-teens) serve as **enzymes** (**en'**-zymes), catalysts that regulate chemical reactions. Proteins are important components of cells and tissues. The kinds and amounts of proteins in a cell determine to a large extent what a cell looks like and how it functions. For example, muscle cells have proteins that are responsible for their appearance and their ability to contract. Proteins are large, complex molecules composed of subunits called **amino acids.**

Nucleic acids (new-**klee'**-ik), like proteins, are large, complex compounds. Two very important nucleic acids are **DNA** (deoxyribonucleic acid) and **RNA** (ribonucleic acid). DNA makes up the genes, the hereditary material; it contains the instructions for making all the proteins needed by the cell. RNA is important in the process of manufacturing proteins.

THE BODY SYSTEMS WORK TOGETHER TO MAINTAIN LIFE

Each body system contributes to the dynamic, carefully balanced state of the body. Table 1–2 sum-

TABLE 1–2

The body systems

SYSTEM	COMPONENTS	FUNCTIONS
Integumentary	Skin, hair, nails, sweat glands	Covers and protects body
Skeletal	Bones, cartilage, ligaments	Supports body, protects; muscles attach to bones; provides calcium storage; blood cell formation
Muscular	Skeletal muscle, cardiac muscle, smooth muscle	Moves parts of skeleton, locomotion; pumps blood; aids movement of internal materials
Nervous	Nerves and sense organs, brain and spinal cord	Receives stimuli from external and internal environment, conducts impulses, integrates activities of other systems
Endocrine	Pituitary, adrenal, thyroid, and other ductless glands	Regulates body chemistry and many body functions
Circulatory	Heart, blood vessels, blood; lymph and lymph structures	Transports materials from one part of body to another; defends body against disease
Respiratory	Lungs and air passageways	Exchanges gases between blood and external environment
Digestive	Mouth, esophagus, stomach, intestines, liver, pancreas	Ingests and digests foods, absorbs them into blood
Urinary	Kidney, bladder, and associated ducts	Excretes metabolic wastes; removes substances present in excess from blood
Reproductive	Testes, ovaries, and associated structures	Reproduction; provides for continuation of species

marizes and Figure 1–2 illustrates the ten main systems of the human body.

METABOLISM IS ESSENTIAL TO MAINTENANCE, GROWTH, AND REPAIR OF THE BODY

All the chemical processes that take place within the body are referred to as its **metabolism.** Two phases of metabolism are catabolism and anabolism. **Catabolism,** the breaking-down phase of metabolism, provides the energy needed to carry on life processes (Fig. 1–3). For example, catabolism provides the energy needed for transmitting nerve impulses and for muscle contraction. Cells obtain energy from food molecules by a complex series of catabolic chemical reactions referred to as **cellular respiration.** During this process certain nutrients are used as fuel. They are slowly broken down, and the energy

released is packaged within a special energy-storage molecule called **ATP (adenosine triphosphate).** Cellular respiration requires oxygen, as well as nutrients.

Anabolism is the building, or synthetic, phase of metabolism. In anabolism, energy is used to produce the chemical substances and parts needed for growth, maintenance, and repair of the body. The raw materials used to manufacture chemical substances and body parts are nutrients from food.

HOMEOSTATIC MECHANISMS MAINTAIN AN APPROPRIATE INTERNAL ENVIRONMENT

Metabolic activities occur continuously in every living cell and they must be carefully regulated to maintain a constant internal environment, or steady state, for the body. The steady state of the body must
Text continued on page 10

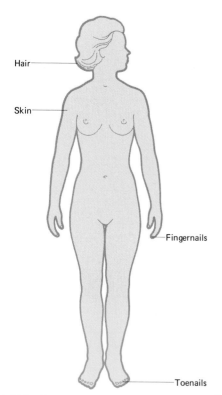

Hair

Skin

Fingernails

Toenails

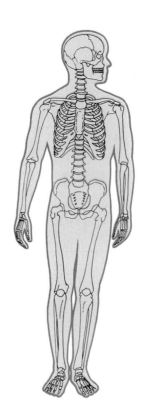

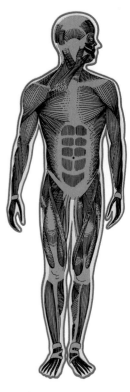

(a) The integumentary system consists of the skin and the structures derived from it. The integumentary system protects the body, helps to regulate body temperature, and receives information about touch, pressure, pain, and temperature.

(b) The skeletal system consists of bones and cartilage. This system helps to support and protect the body.

(c) The muscular system consists of the large skeletal muscles that enable us to move, the cardiac muscle of the heart, and the smooth muscle of the internal organs.

FIGURE 1–2 The principal systems of the human body.

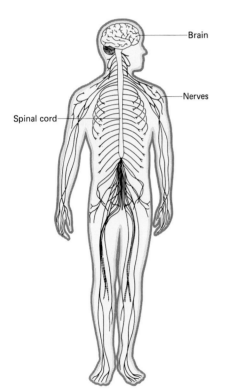

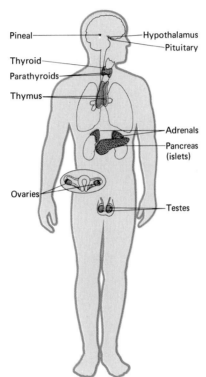

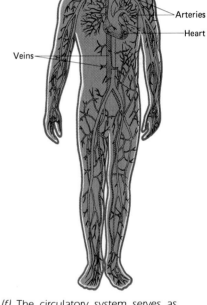

(d) The nervous system consists of the brain, spinal cord, sense organs, and nerves. The nervous system regulates other body systems.

(e) The endocrine system consists of the glands and tissues that release chemical messengers called hormones. The endocrine system works with the nervous system in regulating metabolic activities.

(f) The circulatory system serves as the transportation system of the body. The heart and blood vessels are part of this system.

FIGURE 1–2 *Continued*

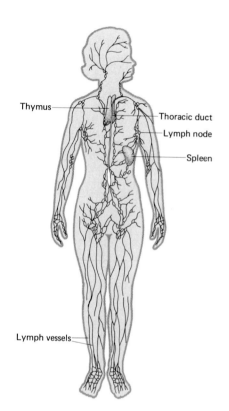

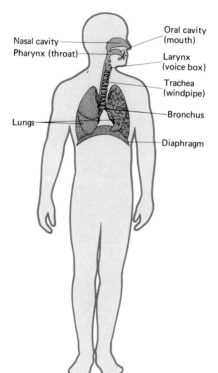

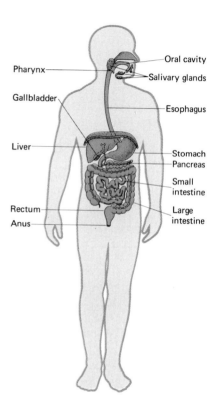

(g) The lymphatic system is a subsystem of the circulatory system. This system defends the body against disease.

(h) The respiratory system consists of the lungs and air passageways. This system supplies oxygen to the blood and rids the body of carbon dioxide.

(i) The digestive system consists of the digestive tract and glands that secrete digestive juices into the digestive tract. This system breaks down food and eliminates wastes.

FIGURE 1–2 *Continued*

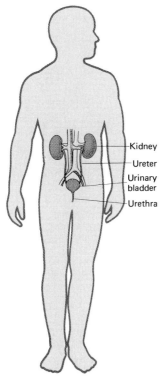

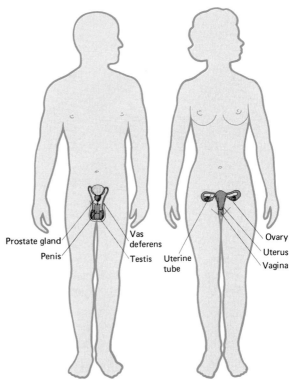

(j) The urinary system is the main excretory system. The kidneys remove wastes and excess materials from the blood and produce urine. This system helps to regulate blood chemistry.

(k) Male and female reproductive systems. Each reproductive system consists of gonads and associated structures. The male reproductive system produces and delivers sperm. The female reproductive system produces ova (eggs) and incubates the developing offspring. The reproductive system maintains sexual characteristics and reproduces the species.

FIGURE 1–2 Continued

FIGURE 1–3 Metabolism. Catabolism, the breaking-down phase of metabolism, provides the energy for anabolism, the phase of metabolism in which molecules, cells, and tissues are manufactured.

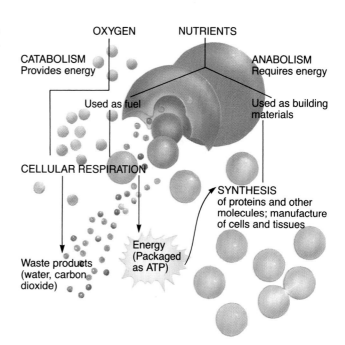

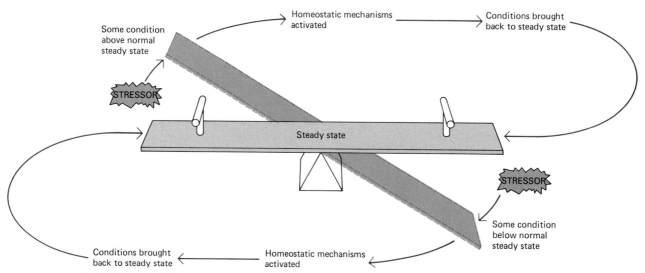

FIGURE 1-4 *Homeostasis is the process of maintaining steady states. Stressful stimuli, called stressors, disrupt homeostasis. In the body, any deviation from the steady state is regarded as stress. Stress activates homeostatic mechanisms that bring conditions back toward the steady state.*

be maintained even when conditions change in the external environment. Temperature within the body must be maintained within narrow limits, and an appropriate concentration of nutrients, oxygen and other gases, and various chemical compounds must be maintained at all times.

The automatic tendency to maintain a relatively constant internal environment is called **homeostasis** (ho″-me-oh-**stay′**-sis). The mechanisms designed to maintain the steady state are **homeostatic mechanisms** (Fig. 1–4). A stressor is a stimulus that disrupts homeostasis and causes stress in the body. When homeostatic mechanisms are unable to compensate for stress and to restore the steady state, stress may lead to a malfunction, which can cause disease or even death.

How do homeostatic mechanisms work? They are feedback systems like the thermostat in your furnace or air conditioning system. A feedback system consists of a cycle of events. Information about a change (for example, a change in temperature) is fed back into the system so that the regulator (the thermostat) can control the process (temperature regulation). When temperature increases too much, the thermostat shuts off the furnace. In this way the temperature is kept at the desired steady state.

In this type of feedback system, the response of the regulator *counteracts* the inappropriate change, thus restoring the steady state. This is a **negative feedback system,** because the response of the regulator is to reverse the stimulus. Most homeostatic mechanisms in the body are negative feedback systems. When some condition varies too far from the steady state (either too high or too low), a control

system uses negative feedback to bring the condition back to the steady state. Body temperature, regulation of sugar (glucose) level in the blood, and many other metabolic processes are regulated by negative feedback.

The body has a few **positive feedback** systems. In these systems the variation from the steady state sets off a series of events that intensify the changes. A positive feedback cycle operates in the delivery of a baby. As the head of the baby pushes against the opening of the uterus (cervix), a reflex action causes the uterus to contract. The contraction forces the baby's head against the cervix again, resulting in another contraction, and the positive feedback cycle is repeated again and again until the baby is delivered.

THE BODY HAS A BASIC PLAN

The body consists of right and left halves that are mirror images; that is, it has **bilateral symmetry.** Two other important features are the **cranium** (**kray′**-nee-um), or brain case, and the backbone, or **vertebral column.** These structures characterize us as vertebrates. Humans are also mammals and so have hair, mammary (milk) glands, and four limbs, each with five digits bearing nails.

DIRECTIONS IN THE BODY ARE RELATIVE

In order to identify the structures of the body it is useful to learn some basic terms and directions.

Directional terms in human anatomy are relative, somewhat like directional terms in geography. Thus you could say that New York City is north of Washington, D.C., but south of Boston or that Chicago is west of Philadelphia but east of San Francisco. Bear this in mind as you learn the anatomical directional terms. These terms are applied to the body when it is in the **anatomical position,** which means that the body is standing erect, eyes looking forward, arms at the sides, and palms and toes directed forward (Fig. 1–5).

1. **Superior/Inferior.** The "North Pole" of the human body is the top of the head, its superior point. Its "South Pole" is represented by the soles of the feet, its most inferior part (Fig. 1–5). Thus the heart is superior to the stomach because it is closer to the head. The heart is inferior to the brain. The stomach is inferior to the heart. The terms **cephalic** (seh-**fal'**-ik) and **craniad** (toward the skull) are sometimes used instead of the word superior. The term **caudad** (toward the tail) is sometimes used instead of the word inferior.

2. **Anterior/Posterior.** The front (belly) surface of the body is anterior, or **ventral.** The stomach is anterior to the vertebral column. The back surface of the body is posterior, or **dorsal.** The vertebral column is posterior to the stomach.

3. **Medial/Lateral.** The body axis is an imaginary line extending from the center of the top of the head to the groin. This main superior-inferior body axis is medial, going right through the midline of the body. A structure is said to be medial if it is closer to

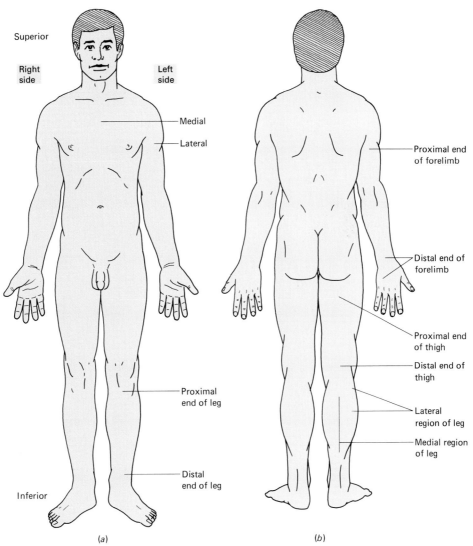

FIGURE 1–5 The body in the anatomical position and some directional terms. The body is erect, eyes forward, arms at the sides, and palms and toes directed forward. (a) Anterior view. (b) Posterior view.

the midline of the body than to another structure. The navel is medial to the hip bone. A structure is lateral if it is toward one side of the body. Thus the hip bone is lateral to the navel.

4. **Proximal/Distal.** When a structure is closer to the body midline or point of attachment to the trunk, it is described as proximal. This term is used especially in locating limb structures. Thus the wrist is proximal to the fingers. Distal means farther from the midline or point of attachment to the trunk. The fingers are distal to the wrist.

5. **Superficial/Deep.** Structures located toward the surface of the body are superficial. Blood vessels in the skin are superficial to those lying beneath in the muscle. Structures located farther inward (away from the body surface) are deep. Blood vessels in the muscle are deep to those in the skin.

THE BODY HAS THREE MAIN PLANES

In studying anatomy as well as in clinical practice it is often helpful to view internal structures by cutting the body into sections, or slices. Such cuts are made along body planes, imaginary flat surfaces that divide the body into parts (Fig. 1–6).

1. **Sagittal (sadj'-i-tul) plane.** A sagittal plane divides the body into right and left parts. A midsagittal (or median) plane passes through the body axis and divides the body into two (almost) mirror-image halves.

2. **Transverse (cross) plane.** This plane is at right angles to the body axis. It divides the body into superior and inferior parts.

3. **Frontal (coronal) plane.** This plane divides the body into anterior and posterior parts.

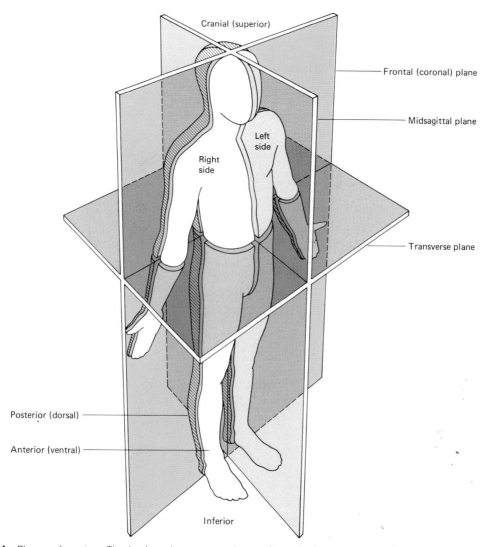

FIGURE 1–6 Planes of section. The body or its parts can be cut in sagittal, transverse, or frontal sections.

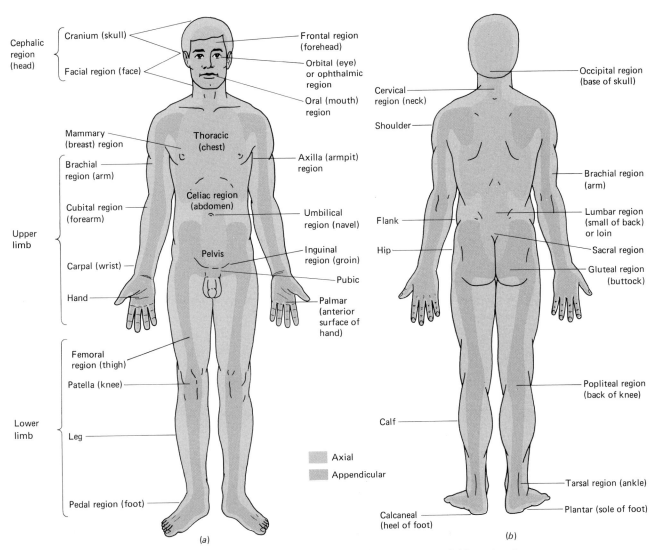

Cephalic region (head)
- Cranium (skull)
- Facial region (face)

Frontal region (forehead)
Orbital (eye) or ophthalmic region
Oral (mouth) region

Mammary (breast) region
Brachial region (arm)
Cubital region (forearm)

Thoracic (chest)
Celiac region (abdomen)

Axilla (armpit) region
Umbilical region (navel)

Upper limb

Carpal (wrist)
Hand

Pelvis

Inguinal region (groin)
Pubic
Palmar (anterior surface of hand)

Femoral region (thigh)
Patella (knee)

Lower limb

Leg

Pedal region (foot)

(a)

Cervical region (neck)
Shoulder

Occipital region (base of skull)

Flank
Hip

Brachial region (arm)
Lumbar region (small of back) or loin
Sacral region
Gluteal region (buttock)

Popliteal region (back of knee)

Calf

Axial
Appendicular

Tarsal region (ankle)
Plantar (sole of foot)

Calcaneal (heel of foot)

(b)

FIGURE 1–7   Some specific regions of the body. (a) Anterior view. (b) Posterior view.

WE CAN IDENTIFY SPECIFIC BODY REGIONS

The body can be subdivided into an **axial** portion, consisting of head, neck, and trunk, and an **appendicular** (ap-pen-**dik′**-u-lar) portion, consisting of the limbs. The trunk, or **torso,** consists of the thorax, abdomen, and pelvis (Fig. 1–7).

Some of the terms used to indicate specific body regions or structures follow.

Region	Part of the body referred to
Abdominal	Portion of trunk below the diaphragm
Arm	Technically, the part of the upper limb between the shoulder and the elbow, as distinguished from the forearm. (Popularly, the term arm refers to the entire upper limb.)
Axillary (**ak′**-sih-lar-ee)	Armpit area
Brachial (**bray′**-kee-al)	Arm
Buccal (**buk′**-al)	Inner surfaces of the cheeks
Carpal (**kar′**-pal)	Wrist
Celiac (**see′**-lee-ak)	Abdomen
Cephalic	Head

Cervical	Neck	Leg	Lower limb; especially the part from the knee to the foot
Costal (**kos′**-tal)	Ribs	Lumbar	Loin, the region of the lower back and side, between the lowest rib and the pelvis
Cranial	Skull		
Cubital	Elbow or forearm	Mammary	Breasts
Cutaneous (ku-**tay′**-nee-us)	Skin	Occipital (ok-**sip′**-ih-tal	Back of the head
Femoral (**fem′**-or-al)	Thigh; the part of the lower extremity between the hip and the knee	Ophthalmic (of-**thal′**-mik)	eyes
		Oral	Mouth
Forearm	Upper extremity between the elbow and the wrist	Orbital	Bony cavity containing the eyeball
Frontal	Forehead	Palmar	Palm
Gluteal (**gloo′**-tee-al)	Buttock	Patellar	Knee
		Pectoral (**pek′**-tow-ral)	Chest
Groin	Depressed region between the abdomen and the thigh	Pedal	Foot
Inguinal (**ing′**-gwih-nal)	Groin	Pelvic	Pelvis, the bony ring that

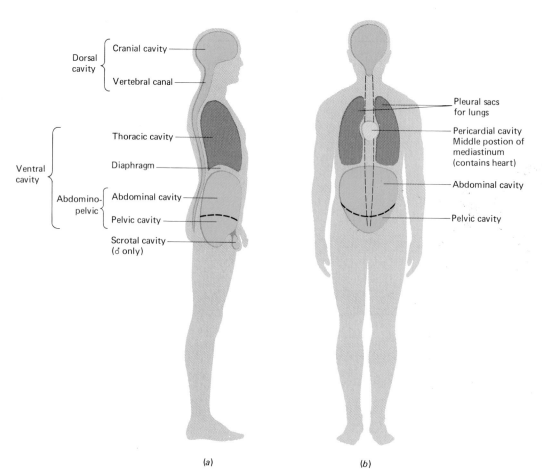

(a)   (b)

FIGURE 1–8 Principal cavities of the human body. (a) Lateral view of the body showing dorsal and ventral cavities and some of their subdivisions. (b) Anterior view, showing subdivisions of the ventral cavity.

	girdles the lower portion of the trunk
Perineal (per″-ih-**nee**′-al)	Between the anus and the pubic arch; includes the region of the external reproductive structures
Plantar	Sole of the foot
Popliteal (pop-**lit**′-ee-al)	Behind the knee
Sacral	Base of spine
Tarsal	Ankle
Thoracic	Chest, the part of the trunk below the neck and above the diaphragm
Umbilical	Navel, depressed scar marking the site of entry of the umbilical cord in the fetus

THERE ARE TWO MAIN BODY CAVITIES

The spaces within the body, called **body cavities,** contain the internal organs, or **viscera** (**vis**′-ur-uh). The two principal body cavities are the **dorsal cavity** and the **ventral cavity** (Fig. 1–8). The bony dorsal cavity is located near the dorsal (posterior) body surface. The dorsal cavity is subdivided into the **cranial cavity,** which holds the brain, and the **vertebral** (or **spinal**) **canal,** which contains the spinal cord. The ventral cavity is located near the ventral (anterior) body surface. It is subdivided into the **thoracic** (or **chest**) **cavity** and the **abdominopelvic cavity** (ab-dom″-ih-no-**pel**′-vik).

The thoracic and abdominopelvic cavities are separated by a broad muscle, the **diaphragm** (**die**′-uh-fram), which forms the floor of the thoracic cav-

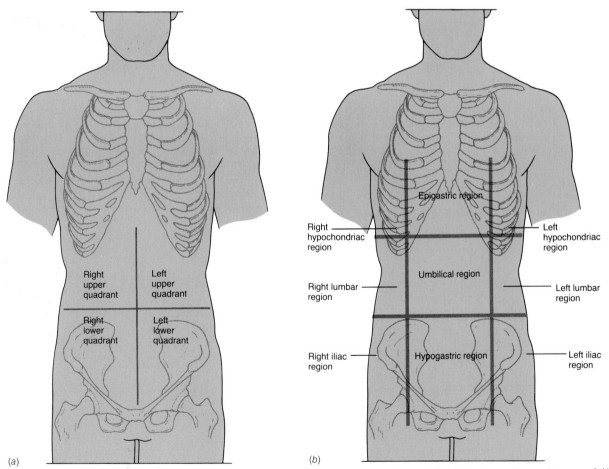

(a)

(b)

FIGURE 1–9 The abdominopelvic cavity can be divided into regions that can be used clinically to locate internal organs. *(a)* In one system, the abdominopelvic cavity is divided into four quadrants by drawing imaginary transverse and sagittal lines through the umbilicus (navel). *(b)* In a second system, the abdominopelvic cavity is divided into nine regions using two transverse and two sagittal planes.

ity. Divisions of the thoracic cavity are the **pleural sacs,** each containing a lung, and the **mediastinum** (me″-dee-as-**tie′**-num) between them. Within the mediastinum lies the heart, thymus gland, and parts of the esophagus and trachea. The heart is surrounded by yet another cavity, the **pericardial** (per″-ee-**kar′**-dee-al) **cavity.**

The upper portion of the abdominopelvic cavity is the **abdominal cavity,** which contains the stomach, small intestine, much of the large intestine, liver, pancreas, spleen, kidneys, and ureters. Although not

separated by any kind of wall, the lower portion of the abdominopelvic cavity is the **pelvic cavity,** which holds the urinary bladder, part of the large intestine, and in the female, the reproductive organs. In males, the pelvic cavity has a small outpocket called the scrotal cavity, which contains the testes.

To simplify the task of identifying internal organs or locating pain, health professionals often divide the abdominopelvic cavity into four quadrants: right upper, right lower, left lower, and left upper (Fig. 1–9(a)). These quadrants are established by a midsagit-

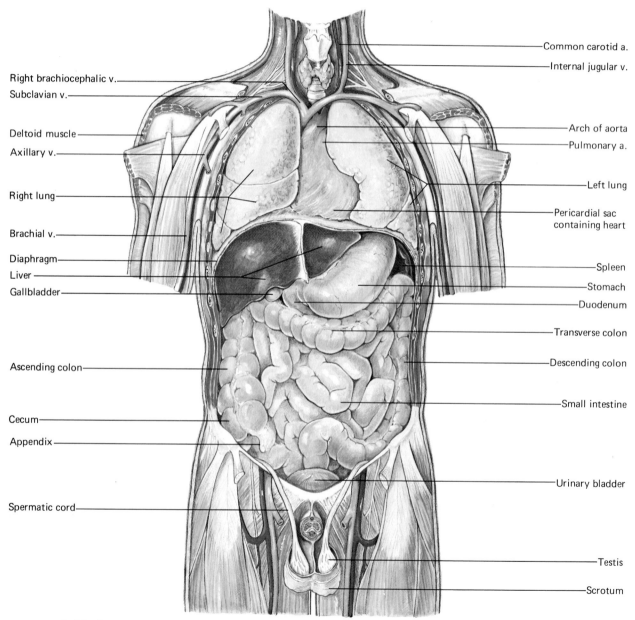

FIGURE 1–10 Anterior view of the body with skin and most of the muscles removed. The rib cage and the fatty membrane that hangs down from the stomach have also been removed. (a., artery; v., vein.) Many of the structures shown here and in Figures 1–11 through 1–14 will be discussed in later chapters.

tal and a transverse plane that pass through the umbilicus. Another system divides the abdominopelvic cavity into nine regions using two transverse and two sagittal planes. These nine regions of the abdomen are indicated in Figure 1–9(*b*).

IT IS IMPORTANT TO VIEW THE BODY AS A WHOLE

In this chapter you have been introduced to the organization of the body and its systems. You have

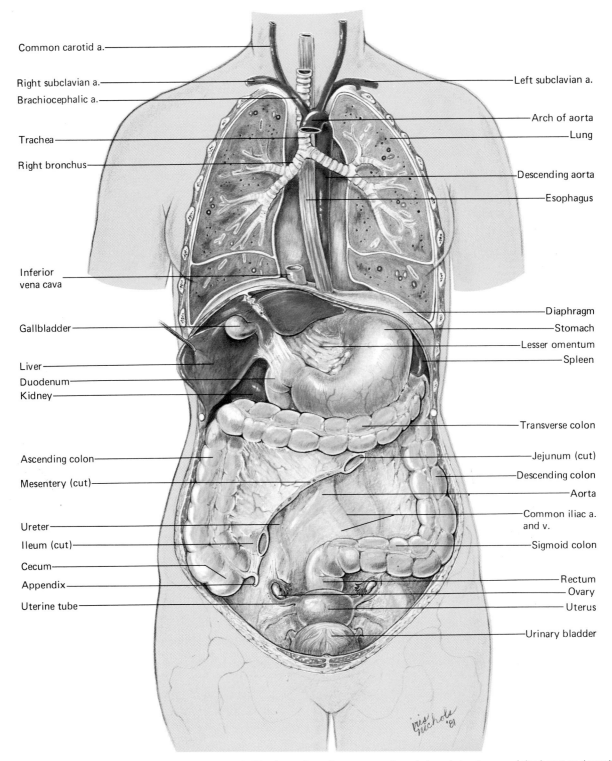

Common carotid a.
Right subclavian a.
Brachiocephalic a.
Trachea
Right bronchus
Inferior vena cava
Gallbladder
Liver
Duodenum
Kidney
Ascending colon
Mesentery (cut)
Ureter
Ileum (cut)
Cecum
Appendix
Uterine tube

Left subclavian a.
Arch of aorta
Lung
Descending aorta
Esophagus
Diaphragm
Stomach
Lesser omentum
Spleen
Transverse colon
Jejunum (cut)
Descending colon
Aorta
Common iliac a. and v.
Sigmoid colon
Rectum
Ovary
Uterus
Urinary bladder

FIGURE 1–11 Deeper anterior view of the body. The lungs have been cut to show internal structure, and the heart and small intestine have been removed.

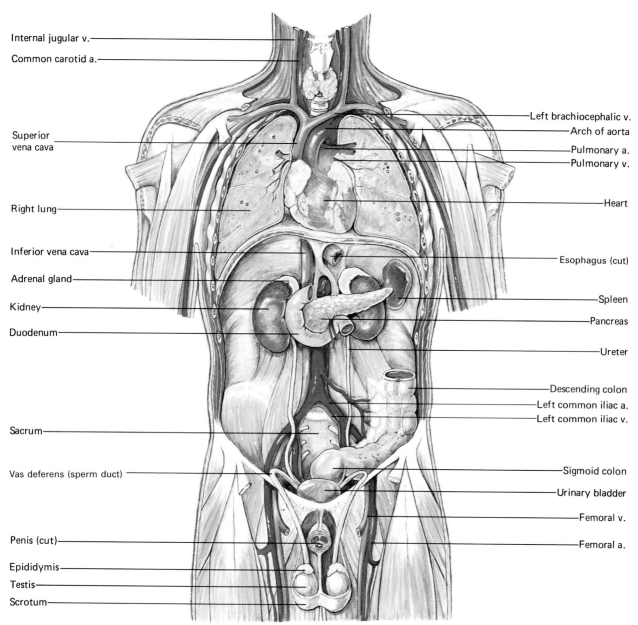

Internal jugular v.

Common carotid a.

Superior
vena cava

Right lung

Inferior vena cava

Adrenal gland

Kidney

Duodenum

Sacrum

Vas deferens (sperm duct)

Penis (cut)

Epididymis

Testis

Scrotum

Left brachiocephalic v.

Arch of aorta

Pulmonary a.

Pulmonary v.

Heart

Esophagus (cut)

Spleen

Pancreas

Ureter

Descending colon

Left common iliac a.

Left common iliac v.

Sigmoid colon

Urinary bladder

Femoral v.

Femoral a.

FIGURE 1–12 Deep anterior view of the body. The stomach, small intestine, and most of the large intestine have been removed. The kidneys, pancreas, and other deep structures are visible.

examined the principal regions and cavities of the body and have learned to follow anatomical directions and to visualize body planes and sections. Now you can begin to integrate all these bits of knowledge and view the body as a whole, functioning organism.

In Figure 1–10 all the parts have been put back together so that you can study them in relation to one another and to the body as an integrated, functioning organism. Anterior structures have been pro-

gressively removed in Figures 1–11 and 1–12 so that you can study the relationship of the deeper organs. Figure 1–13 is a posterior view.

A different perspective is provided in Figure 1–14. There transverse sections through the head, mediastinum, and abdomen give you the opportunity to study the relationships between anterior and posterior structures within each of these body regions.

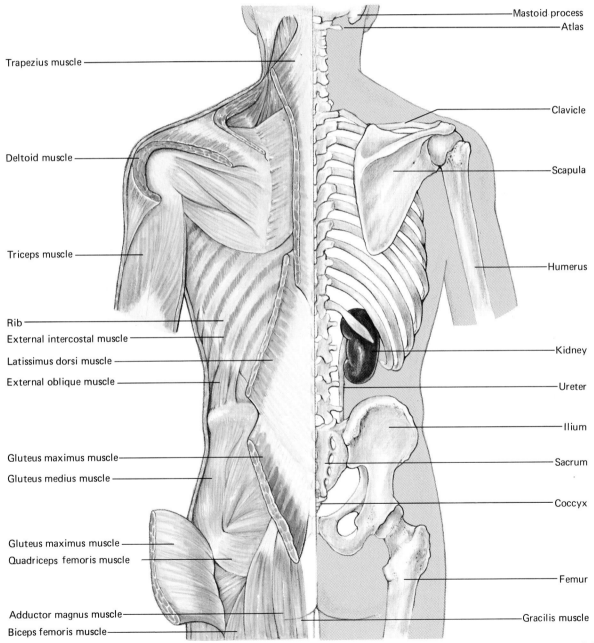

FIGURE 1–13 Posterior view of the body. Muscles have been removed to show the skeletal structures and position of the kidneys.

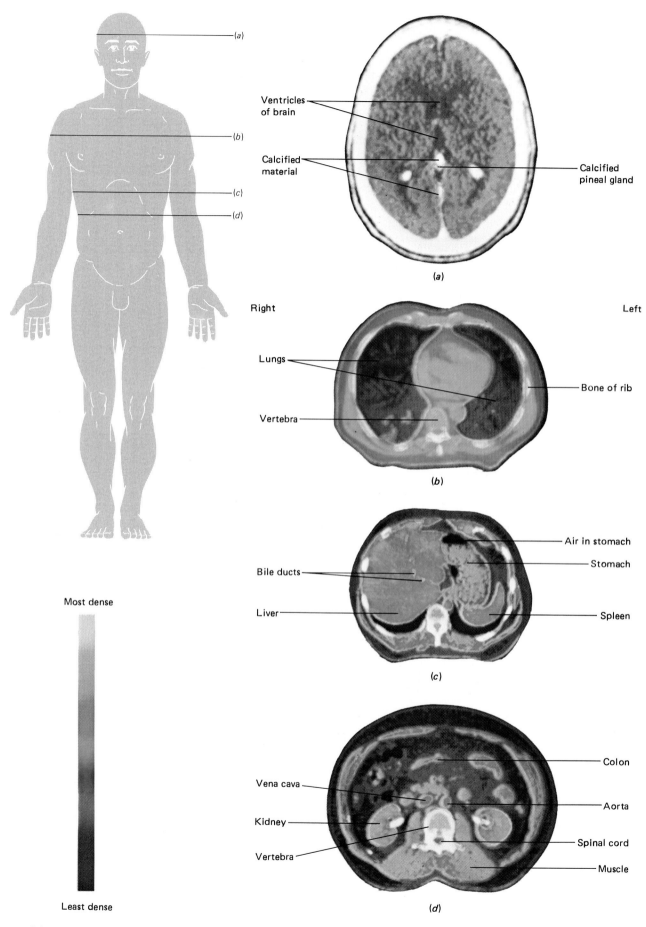

Ventricles of brain

Calcified material

Calcified pineal gland

(a)

Right   Left

Lungs

Bone of rib

Vertebra

(b)

Air in stomach

Bile ducts

Stomach

Liver

Spleen

(c)

Most dense

Colon

Vena cava

Aorta

Kidney

Spinal cord

Vertebra

Muscle

Least dense

(d)

FIGURE **1–14** *See legend on opposite page*

SUMMARY

I. Anatomy is the science of body structure; physiology is the study of function, or how the body works.

II. We can identify several levels of organization within the human body.

A. The simplest level of organization is the chemical level consisting of atoms and molecules.

B. Atoms and molecules associate to form cellular organelles and cells.

C. Cells associate to form tissues such as muscle or bone tissue.

D. Tissues may be organized to form organs such as the brain or heart.

E. Certain tissues and organs may function together to make up a body system.

F. The body systems work together to make up the human organism.

III. The body can be divided into ten different body systems that operate to maintain life.

A. The integumentary system provides a protective covering for the body and helps to regulate body temperature.

B. The skeletal and muscular systems work together as a mechanical system to permit effective movement.

C. The nervous and endocrine systems regulate the activities of the body.

D. The digestive system breaks down food so that nutrients can be absorbed into the blood.

E. The respiratory system delivers oxygen to the blood and removes carbon dioxide from the body.

F. The circulatory system transports nutrients and oxygen to all body cells and carries wastes from the cells to the excretory organs. The cardiovascular and lymphatic systems are part of the circulatory system.

G. Waste disposal and regulation of blood composition are the functions of the urinary system.

H. The reproductive system of the male produces and delivers sperm; the reproductive system of the female produces ova and incubates the developing offspring. Both systems release hormones that establish and maintain sexuality.

IV. Homeostasis is the body's automatic tendency to maintain a constant internal environment, or steady state. In general, homeostasis is maintained by negative feedback mechanisms.

V. Anatomical directional terms are applied to the body when it is in the anatomical position. In this position the body is standing erect, eyes looking forward, arms at the sides, and palms and toes directed forward. The principal directional terms are:

Term	Orientation
Superior (cephalic)	Upward; toward the head
Inferior	Downward; toward the feet
Anterior (ventral)	Belly surface; toward the front of the body
Posterior (dorsal)	Back surface; toward the back of the body
Medial	Toward the midline
Lateral	Toward the side
Proximal	Toward the midline or point of attachment to the trunk
Distal	Away from the midline or point of attachment to the trunk
Superficial	Toward the body surface
Deep	Within the body

FIGURE 1–14 A series of CT scans through various regions of the body. The level of the scan is indicated on the figure of the body. The color spectrum bar indicates the gradient of structure density as represented by color. The most dense structures, such as bone, appear white in the CT scans. The least dense structures appear orange. (CT scans courtesy of Professor Jon H. Ehringer.)

VI. The body or its organs may be cut along planes to produce different types of sections.
   A. A sagittal section divides the body into right and left parts.
   B. A transverse (or cross) section divides the body into superior and inferior parts.
   C. A frontal (or coronal) section divides the body into anterior and posterior parts.
VII. The body may be divided into axial and appendicular regions.
   A. The axial portion consists of head, neck, and trunk.
   B. The appendicular portion consists of the limbs.
   C. Terms such as abdominal, pectoral, and lumbar are used to refer to specific body regions or structures.
VIII. Two principal body cavities are the dorsal cavity and the ventral cavity.
   A. The dorsal cavity includes the cranial cavity and the vertebral canal.
   B. The ventral cavity is principally subdivided into the thoracic and abdominopelvic cavities.

POST TEST

1. The science of body structure is _____ ; the study of body function is _____ .

2. The chemical processes that take place in the body are collectively referred to as its _____ .

3. The breaking-down part of metabolism is called _____ .

4. The automatic tendency of the body to maintain a constant internal environment is called _____ .

5. Atoms combine chemically to form _____ .

6. The basic building blocks of the body are _____ .

7. Various types of tissues may be organized to form _____ .

8. Chemical messengers released by endocrine glands are called _____ .

Match
Select the most appropriate match in Column B for each item in Column A.

Column A
9. The body's principal regulatory system
10. Includes the skin
11. Functions to support and protect the body
12. Transportation system
13. Maintains adequate blood oxygen content
14. Its organs are the ductless glands that release hormones

Column B
a. endocrine system
b. integumentary system
c. circulatory system
d. nervous system
e. respiratory system
f. skeletal system

Match

15. Heart in relation to lung
16. Wrist in relation to elbow
17. Knee in relation to ankle
18. Skin in relation to muscle

a. superficial
b. medial
c. lateral
d. deep

19. Stomach in relation to backbone   e. proximal
                                             f. distal
                                             g. anterior
                                             h. posterior

20. A cut that divides the body into right and left parts is a
    _____ section.

21. A cut at right angles to the body axis is a _____ section.

22. The head, neck, and trunk make up the _____ portion of the
    body, while the limbs make up the _____ portion.

23. The internal organs within the body cavities are referred to as
    _____ .

Match
Select the most appropriate match in Column B for each item in Column A.

Column A   *Column B*
24. Head   a. cervical
25. Skull   b. cephalic
26. Skin   c. cranial
27. Chest   d. cutaneous
28. Neck   e. pectoral
29. Armpit   f. axillary

30. Thoracic and abdominopelvic cavities are separated by the
    _____ .

31. Label the diagram on the following page.

REVIEW QUESTIONS

1. Describe the position of each of the following using anatomic terms: (a) navel;
   (b) ear; (c) great toe; (d) elbow; (e) backbone.

2. Define homeostasis and give an example. Tell how your example is regulated by
   negative feedback mechanisms.

3. List in sequence the levels of organization within the human organism, from
   atom to organism.

4. What are the functions of each body system?

5. Define anatomical position.

6. Identify the body cavities given in this chapter and identify an organ or structure found in each.

7. Define each of the following: (a) cephalic; (b) cervical; (c) cranial; (d) abdominal; (e) sagittal; (f) proximal; (g) distal; (h) bilateral symmetry.

POST TEST ANSWERS

1. anatomy; physiology   4. homeostasis
2. metabolism   5. molecules
3. catabolism   6. cells

7. organs
8. hormones
9. d
10. b
11. f
12. c
13. e
14. a
15. b
16. f
17. e
18. a
19. g

20. (mid)sagittal
21. transverse (or cross)
22. axial; appendicular
23. viscera
24. b
25. c
26. d
27. e
28. a
29. f
30. diaphragm
31. see Figure 1–10

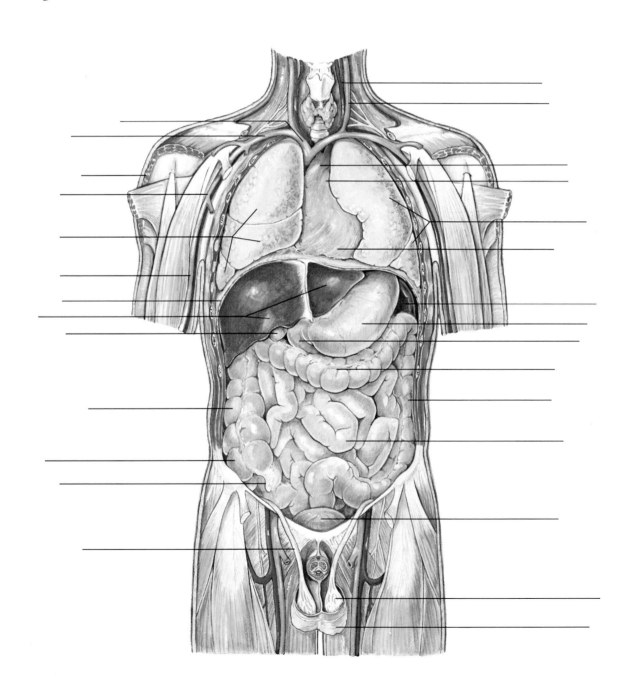

Two

CELLS AND TISSUES

CHAPTER OUTLINE

I. The cell contains organelles that perform specific functions
II. Materials move through the plasma membrane by both passive and active processes
III. Cells divide, forming genetically identical cells
IV. Tissues are the fabric of the body
    A. Epithelial tissue protects the body
    B. Connective tissue joins body structures
    C. Muscle tissue is specialized to contract
    D. Nervous tissue controls muscles and glands
V. Membranes cover or line body surfaces

LEARNING OBJECTIVES

After you have studied this chapter, you should be able to:
1. Describe the general characteristics of cells.
2. Describe, locate, and list the functions of the principal organelles and label them on a diagram.
3. Explain how materials pass through cell membranes, distinguishing among passive and active processes.
4. Predict whether cells will swell or shrink under various osmotic conditions.
5. Describe the stages of a cell's life cycle, and summarize the significance of mitosis with respect to maintaining a constant chromosome number.
6. Define the term tissue and give the functions of the principal types of tissue.
7. Compare epithelial tissue with connective tissue.
8. Compare the three types of muscle tissue.
9. Compare connective tissue membranes with epithelial membranes and contrast the types of epithelial membranes.

In Chapter 1, we learned that cells are the living building blocks of the body and that cells associate to form tissues. Each of us began life as a single cell, the fertilized egg. That cell gave rise to the millions of cells that make up the complex tissues, organs, and systems of the body. In this chapter we examine more closely the structure and function of cells and tissues.

THE CELL CONTAINS ORGANELLES THAT PERFORM SPECIFIC FUNCTIONS

The cell is an amazingly complex structure. It has a control center, internal transportation system, power plants, factories for making needed materials, and packaging plants. Despite their complexity, most cells are so small that they can be studied only under a microscope.

The microscope is one of the biologist's most important tools for studying the internal structure of cells. Most cell structures were first identified with an ordinary light microscope that uses visible light as the source of illumination. (This is the kind of microscope used by students in most college laboratories.) During the last three or four decades, the development of the electron microscope has enabled researchers to study the fine detail (ultrastructure) of cells and their parts. Whereas the ordinary light microscope may magnify a structure about a thousand times, the electron microscope can magnify it 250,000 times or more.

The size and shape of a cell are related to the specific functions it must perform (Fig. 2–1). For instance, sperm cells are tiny cells with long, whiplike tails. The tail is used to move toward the ovum, or egg. The ovum is one of the largest cells in the human body, but even it is only about as large as a period on

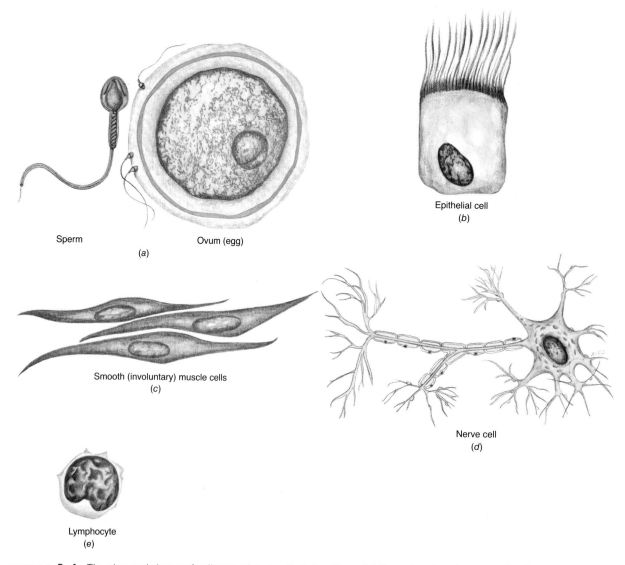

Sperm   Ovum (egg)

(a)

Epithelial cell
(b)

Smooth (involuntary) muscle cells
(c)

Nerve cell
(d)

Lymphocyte
(e)

FIGURE 2–1 The size and shape of cells are related to their functions. (a) Ovum (egg) and sperm cells. Ova are among the largest cells in the body. Sperm cells are among the smallest. Note the long tail (called a flagellum) used by the sperm cell in locomotion. (b) Epithelial cell. Epithelial cells join to form tissues that cover body surfaces and line body cavities. (c) Smooth muscle cells join to form the involuntary muscle tissues of the internal organs. For example, smooth muscle in the wall of the digestive tract moves food through the intestine. (d) A nerve cell (neuron) is specialized to transmit messages from one part of the body to another. (e) Lymphocyte, a type of white blood cell. This cell can move through the tissues of the body and destroy invading bacteria.

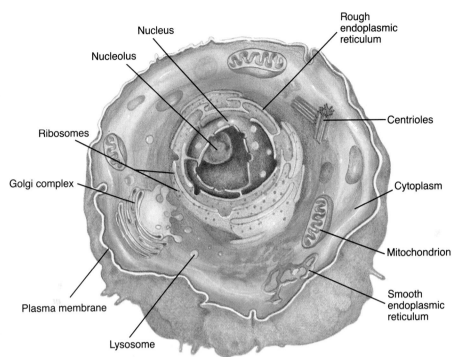

Nucleus

Nucleolus

Rough endoplasmic reticulum

Ribosomes

Centrioles

Golgi complex

Cytoplasm

Mitochondrion

Plasma membrane

Smooth endoplasmic reticulum

Lysosome

FIGURE 2–2 The structure of a cell. An artist's conception of a "typical" cell.

this page. Epithelial cells, which cover body surfaces, look like tiny building blocks. Muscle cells are elongated and specialized for contraction. Nerve cells have long extensions that permit them to transmit messages over long distances within the body. The lymphocyte, a type of white blood cell, has the ability to change its shape as it flows along through the tissues of the body, destroying invading bacteria.

The jellylike material of the cell is called **cytoplasm** (**sy′**-toe-plazm). Dissolved within the cytoplasm are a great variety of substances needed by the cell. For example, amino acids found in the cytoplasm are used to manufacture larger molecules such as proteins.

Scattered throughout the cell are specialized organelles (little organs) that perform jobs within the cell (Fig. 2–2). Many of the organelles within the cell are enclosed by membranes that partition the cytoplasm into different compartments.

Every cell is surrounded by a thin membrane, the **plasma membrane,** or simply **cell membrane.** The plasma membrane protects the cell and regulates the passage of materials into and out of the cell. The plasma membrane also communicates with other cells and organs. For example, certain proteins that project from the surface of the plasma membrane act as receptors (receivers), which receive chemical messages from endocrine glands or other types of cells.

The **endoplasmic reticulum** (ER) (en″-doe-

plaz′-mik reh-**tik′**-yoo-lum) is a system of membranes that extends throughout the cytoplasm of many cells. The ER is somewhat like a complex tunnel system through which materials can be transported from one part of the cell to another. Two types of ER can be distinguished, smooth and rough. Rough ER has a granular appearance that results from the presence of organelles called **ribosomes** (**rye′**-bow-sowms) along its outer walls. Ribosomes function as factories where proteins are manufactured.

Looking somewhat like stacks of pancakes, the **Golgi** (**goal′**-jee) **complex** is composed of layers of platelike membranes. This organelle functions as a protein processing and packaging plant. An important function of the Golgi complex is to produce **lysosomes** (**lye′**-sow-sowms). These little sacs contain powerful digestive enzymes that destroy bacteria or other foreign matter. When a cell dies, lysosomes release their enzymes into the cytoplasm, where they break down the cell itself. This "self-destruct" system accounts for the rapid deterioration of many cells when an organism dies. Some forms of tissue damage and the aging process itself may be related to leaky lysosomes.

Cells contain tiny power plants called **mitochondria** (my″-tow-**kon′**-dree-uh). Inside the mitochondria fuel molecules are broken down and energy is released. This process is called cellular respiration.

Cilia (**sil′**-ee-ah), tiny hairlike organelles projecting from the surfaces of many types of cells, help to move materials outside the cell. For example, the cells lining the respiratory passages are equipped with cilia, which continuously beat a layer of mucus away from the lungs. The mucus traps particles of dirt that are inhaled. Each human sperm cell is equipped with a whiplike tail, or **flagellum** (flah-**jel**′-um), that is used in locomotion.

The **nucleus,** a large, rounded organelle, is the control center of the cell. In a cell that is not in the process of dividing, the nucleus contains loosely coiled material called chromatin (**krow**′-muh-tin). When a cell prepares to divide, the chromatin becomes more tightly coiled and condenses to form rod-shaped bodies, the **chromosomes** (**krow**′-muh-sowms). Each chromosome contains several hundred genes arranged in a specific linear order; the genes are composed of the chemical DNA. We can think of the chromosomes as a chemical cookbook for the cell, while each gene is a recipe for making a specific protein. The nucleolus (little nucleus) is a specialized region within the nucleus. The nucleolus is a factory where ribosomes are assembled.

MATERIALS MOVE THROUGH THE PLASMA MEMBRANE BY BOTH PASSIVE AND ACTIVE PROCESSES

The plasma membrane is *selectively permeable.* This means that it can allow certain materials to enter or leave the cell while preventing the passage of other materials. Some materials move through cell membranes passively by physical processes such as diffusion, osmosis, and filtration. These processes do not require the cell to expend energy. Other materials are moved actively by processes such as active

transport and phagocytosis. Such active physiological processes require the cell to expend energy.

1. **Diffusion** is the net movement of molecules or ions from a region of higher concentration to a region of lower concentration brought about by the energy of the molecules. Molecules tend to move down a concentration gradient, that is, from where they are more concentrated to where they are less concentrated (Fig. 2–3). Diffusion depends upon the random movement of individual molecules. The molecules are propelled by collision with other molecules or with the side of the container. Eventually the molecules are evenly distributed. Gases and many nutrients move in and out of cells by diffusion.

2. **Osmosis** (oz-**mow**′-sis) is the diffusion of water molecules through a selectively permeable membrane from a region where water molecules are more concentrated to a region where they are less concentrated. The dissolved ions and molecules (solute) in the more concentrated solution "pull" the water molecules across the membrane. This pulling force is known as **osmotic pressure.**

When living cells are placed in a solution that has a solute concentration equal (isotonic) to that of the cells, the water molecule concentration is also equal, and therefore water molecules move in and out of the cells at the same rate. The net movement of the water molecules is zero (Fig. 2–4).

When cells are placed in a solution with a solute concentration (hypertonic) greater than that of the cell, water leaves the cells, causing them to dehydrate, shrink, and perhaps die. When cells are placed in a solution of lesser concentration (hypotonic) compared with that of the cell, the cell exerts an osmotic pressure on the solution. Water moves into the cells, causing them to swell and perhaps burst.

3. **Filtration** is the passage of materials through membranes by mechanical pressure. For example,

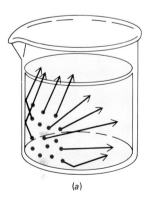 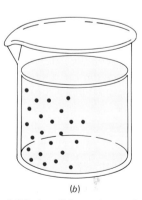 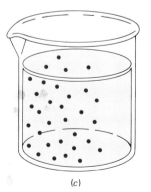 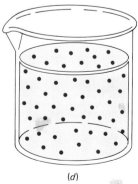

(a) (b) (c) (d)

FIGURE 2–3 *The process of diffusion. When a lump of sugar is dropped into a beaker of water, its molecules dissolve (a) and begin to diffuse (b and c). Eventually, the sugar molecules are evenly distributed throughout the water (d).*

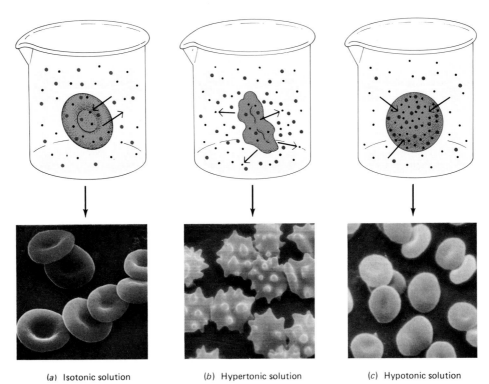

(a) Isotonic solution   (b) Hypertonic solution   (c) Hypotonic solution

FIGURE 2–4 Osmosis and the living cell. *(a)* A cell is placed in an isotonic solution, one that has the same concentration of solutes (dissolved materials) as the cell. The net movement of water molecules is zero. *(b)* A cell is placed in a hypertonic solution—one with a greater solute concentration than the cell. The solution exerts an osmotic pressure on the cell. This results in a net movement of water molecules out of the cell, causing the cell to dehydrate, shrink, and perhaps die. *(c)* A cell is placed in a hypotonic solution—a solution with a lower solute concentration than the cell. The cell contents exert an osmotic pressure on the solution, drawing water molecules inward. The net diffusion of water molecules into the cell causes the cell to swell and perhaps even to burst. *(Micrographs of human red blood cells courtesy of Dr. R.F. Baker, University of Southern California Medical School.)*

blood pressure forces some of the liquid part of the blood (plasma) through the capillary wall by filtration. This is how tissue fluid is formed.

4. **Active transport** requires cellular energy. In this process the cell moves materials from a region of lower to a region of higher concentration. Working "uphill" against a concentration gradient requires energy. The cell uses the energy of ATP to drive active transport.

5. **Phagocytosis** (fag″-oh-sigh-**tow′**-sis) means "cell eating." In phagocytosis, the cell ingests large, solid particles such as food or bacteria (Fig. 2–5). A small part of the plasma membrane surrounds the particle to be ingested, forming a small sac (vesicle or vacuole), like a tiny plastic sandwich bag, around it. This tiny vesicle then pinches off from the plasma membrane and floats around in the cytoplasm. White blood cells ingest invading bacteria in this way. Then, lysosomes fuse with the vesicle containing the bacteria. The lysosomes pour their powerful digestive enzymes on the bacteria, destroying them.

CELLS DIVIDE, FORMING GENETICALLY IDENTICAL CELLS

Certain types of cells in the body divide almost continuously. For example, as many as ten million blood cells are produced in the body every second. Other cells never divide at all after birth. The highly specialized muscle and nerve cells are ordinarily unable to replace themselves. As they wear out or are destroyed by disease, we are left with fewer and fewer.

Before a cell divides to form two cells, the chromosomes are precisely duplicated and the cell undergoes **mitosis** (my-**tow′**-sis). In mitosis a complete set of chromosomes is distributed to each end of the parent cell. After the parent cell divides, each new cell contains the identical number and types of chromosomes present in the parent cell. When a fertilized egg divides, each of the new cells receives a com-

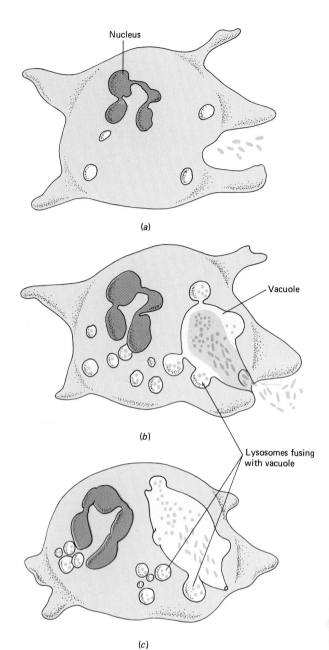

Nucleus

(a)

Vacuole

(b)

Lysosomes fusing
with vacuole

(c)

FIGURE **2–5** Phagocytosis. (a) The cell ingests large solid particles such as bacteria. Folds of the plasma membrane surround the particle to be ingested, forming a small vacuole around it. (b) This vacuole then pinches off inside the cell. (c) Lysosomes may fuse with the vacuole and pour digestive enzymes onto the ingested bacteria.

plete copy of all its genetic information. After hundreds of divisions, every cell in the body (with the exception of the sex cells) contains a complete set of the original chromosomes contributed by the sperm and egg. (The sex cells undergo a special process called meiosis, which halves their number of chromosomes; see Chap. 18.)

The life cycle of the cell may be divided into five phases: interphase, prophase, metaphase, anaphase, and telophase (Fig. 2–6). The cell spends most of its life in **interphase** (meaning between phases), the period between mitoses. During interphase the cell actively makes new materials and grows. Before mitosis actually begins, the chromosomes are duplicated.

During **prophase** (**pro′**-faze), the first stage of mitosis, the chromatin coils tightly, forming structures that are visible as dark, X-shaped bodies under the light microscope. These are the chromosomes. At this time each chromosome is doubled. During prophase, the nuclear membrane dissolves. Two pairs of organelles, the **centrioles,** function during mitosis. Each pair of centrioles migrates toward an opposite

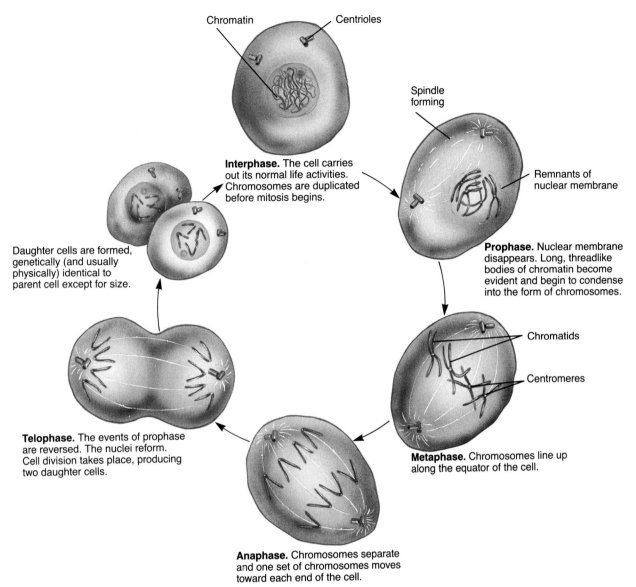

Chromatin   Centrioles

Spindle
forming

Interphase. The cell carries
out its normal life activities.
Chromosomes are duplicated
before mitosis begins.

Remnants of
nuclear membrane

Prophase. Nuclear membrane
disappears. Long, threadlike
bodies of chromatin become
evident and begin to condense
into the form of chromosomes.

Daughter cells are formed,
genetically (and usually
physically) identical to
parent cell except for size.

Chromatids

Centromeres

Telophase. The events of prophase
are reversed. The nuclei reform.
Cell division takes place, producing
two daughter cells.

Metaphase. Chromosomes line up
along the equator of the cell.

Anaphase. Chromosomes separate
and one set of chromosomes moves
toward each end of the cell.

FIGURE 2–6 *The cell cycle. Individual steps in the cycle are explained in labels within the figure. The generalized cells shown here have a chromosome number of four.*

end of the cell. Tiny threads of protein (called microtubules) in the cytoplasm form a spindle-shaped structure that extends throughout the cell.

During **metaphase,** the second phase of mitosis, threads of the spindle attach to the chromosomes. The chromosomes are then positioned along the equator of the cell. Each chromosome is now completely coiled so it appears quite thick. In fact, chromosomes can be seen so clearly in metaphase that they can be photographed and studied to determine whether any are abnormal.

During **anaphase** (**an′**-ah-faze), the doubled chromosomes separate and start to move away from one another. The protein threads of the spindle begin

to pull one set of chromosomes to one end of the spindle and the other set to the opposite end. With the arrival of a complete set of chromosomes at each end of the cell, **telophase** begins. Each chromosome now begins to uncoil and disperse. The spindle disappears and a nuclear membrane forms around each set of chromosomes.

During telophase the cell divides, forming two cells. The cell begins to constrict around its center and continues to constrict until it has completely divided to form two cells. Each new cell now enters interphase, thus beginning a new cell life.

The significance of mitosis is that all the genetic information contained within the chromosomes is

Simple squamous epithelium

Nuclei

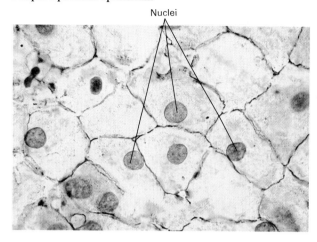

Stratified squamous epithelium

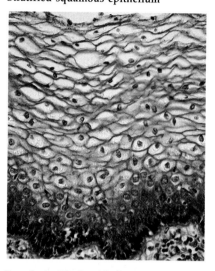

Simple cuboidal epithelium

Nuclei of cuboidal epithelial cells

Lumen of tubule

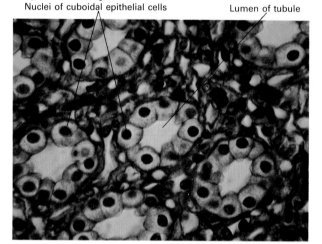

Pseudostratified epithelium

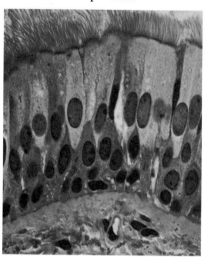

Simple columnar epithelium

Goblet cell

Nuclei of columnar cells

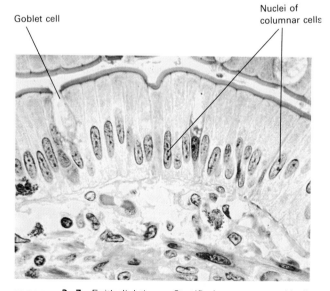

FIGURE **2–7** *Epithelial tissue. Stratified squamous epithelium makes up the outer layer of the skin.*

precisely duplicated and distributed to each new cell. No genetic information is lost and no new information is added. Each of the two new cells has the potential to function exactly like the parent cell.

TISSUES ARE THE FABRIC OF THE BODY

As defined in Chapter 1, a **tissue** is a group of closely associated cells that work together to carry out a specific function or group of functions. The cells of a tissue produce nonliving materials, called **intercellular substance,** that lie between the cells. If the body were composed only of cells, it would appear somewhat like a blob of jelly. The intercellular substances give the body strength and help maintain its shape.

Four principal types of tissue make up the body:
1. **Epithelial tissue (epithelium)** (ep″-ih-theel′-ee-um) protects the body by covering all of its free surfaces and lining its cavities. Some epithelial tissue is specialized to form glands.
2. **Connective tissue** supports and protects the organs of the body; it connects and holds parts of the body together.
3. **Muscle tissue** is specialized for moving the body and its parts.
4. **Nervous tissue** receives and transmits messages so that the various parts of the body can communicate with one another.

EPITHELIAL TISSUE PROTECTS THE BODY

Epithelial tissue has many functions. Its main job is *protection.* This tissue covers the body and lines all the body cavities. It forms a protective shield for the underlying tissues. In some epithelial tissues, certain cells are specialized to *secrete* substances. For example, goblet cells in the lining of the intestine secrete mucus, a slippery, protective substance. When large amounts of specialized secretions are needed, epithelium forms special structures called glands. In some parts of the body epithelial tissue is specialized to *absorb* certain materials. For example, epithelium lining the digestive tract absorbs molecules of digested food.

Epithelial cells lining the kidney tubules *excrete* certain materials. In the respiratory passageways, epithelium *transports* mucus containing trapped particles. Such epithelial cells are equipped with cilia that beat a thin sheet of mucus containing trapped dirt

particles away from the lungs. The taste buds in the mouth and olfactory (smelling) structures in the nose consist of epithelium specialized to receive *sensory* information.

Epithelial tissue consists of cells that fit tightly together. Very little intercellular substance is present. Epithelial tissue may be **simple,** that is, composed of one layer of cells, or **stratified,** composed of two or more layers (Fig. 2–7). Simple epithelium is usually present in areas where materials must diffuse through the tissue or where substances are secreted, excreted, or absorbed. Stratified epithelial tissue is located in regions where protection is the main function.

Many epithelial tissues are subjected to continuous wear and tear. As outer cells are shed they must be replaced by new ones from below. Some epithelial tissues have a rapid rate of mitosis so that new cells are continuously produced to take the place of those lost.

A gland consists of one or more epithelial cells that produce and discharge a particular product. Two main types of glands are endocrine and exocrine glands. **Endocrine glands** do not have ducts (tubes) through which the secretion is discharged. They release their products, called hormones, into the surrounding tissue fluid. The hormone usually diffuses into the blood, which transports it to its destination. The adrenal glands are examples of endocrine glands.

Exocrine glands, in contrast, have ducts, also made of epithelial cells, which conduct the secretion to some body surface. For example, sweat passes from sweat glands through ducts to the surface of the skin, and salivary gland ducts conduct saliva to the mouth. Exocrine glands may be unicellular (composed of one cell), such as goblet cells (Fig. 2–8), but most are multicellular (composed of many cells).

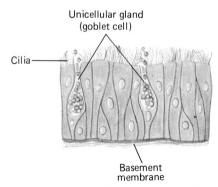

FIGURE 2–8 A goblet cell is a unicellular gland that secretes mucus. Goblet cells are found in the epithelial lining of the intestine.

CONNECTIVE TISSUE JOINS BODY STRUCTURES

The main function of **connective tissue** is to *join together* the other tissues of the body. Connective tissues also *support* the body and its structures and *protect* underlying organs. Almost every organ in the body has a supporting framework of connective tissue.

Some of the main types of connective tissue are (1) connective tissue proper, (2) adipose (fat) tissue, (3) cartilage, (4) bone, and (5) blood, lymph, and tissues that produce blood cells. Cartilage and bone will be discussed in Chapter 4, blood in Chapter 10, and lymph in Chapter 12.

Unlike the closely fitting cells of epithelial tissues, the cells of connective tissue are usually separated by large amounts of intercellular substance (Fig. 2–9). The intercellular substance usually consists of threadlike, microscopic fibers scattered throughout a thick gel, or matrix.

Three types of connective tissue fibers are col-

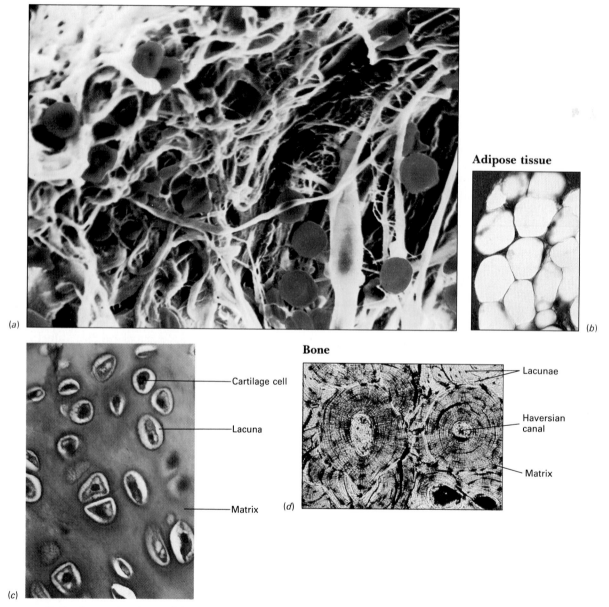

Adipose tissue

Cartilage cell

Lacuna

Matrix

Bone

Lacunae

Haversian canal

Matrix

FIGURE 2–9 Connective tissue. *(a)* Scanning electron micrograph of connective tissue (magnified approximately ×440). Collagen fibers appear as an irregular mass of yellow strands. Red blood cells are visible between the fibers. Connective tissue provides support for other tissues. *(b)* Adipose (fat) tissue. *(c)* Cartilage. The cartilage cells are separated by a tough matrix. *(d)* Bone. Bone cells are arranged in concentric circles. They are separated by a hard matrix.

lagen fibers, reticular fibers, and elastic fibers. **Collagen fibers** are the most numerous. Collagen fibers contain the protein **collagen,** the most abundant protein in the body. Collagen is a very tough substance, and collagen fibers give great strength to body structures.

Reticular fibers are very fine, branched fibers. They form a network that supports many tissues and organs. Elastic fibers stretch easily and are an important component of structures that must stretch. For example, elastic fibers in the walls of the air sacs in the lungs permit these tiny sacs to stretch as they fill with air and then snap back to force air out of the lungs during expiration.

Connective tissue proper joins body structures. It is found as a thin filling between body parts and serves as a reservoir for water and salts. Together with adipose tissue, connective tissue proper forms the tissue layer (subcutaneous tissue) that attaches the skin to the tissues and organs beneath.

Adipose (fat) tissue stores fat and releases it when the body needs energy for cellular work. Adipose tissue helps to shape the body and provides insulation.

MUSCLE TISSUE IS SPECIALIZED TO CONTRACT

Muscle tissue is composed of cells specialized to contract. When muscle cells contract they become shorter and thicker. As they shorten they move body parts attached to them. Because they are long and narrow, muscle cells are referred to as fibers. Muscle fibers are usually arranged in bundles or layers surrounded by connective tissue. Three types of muscle tissue are skeletal muscle, cardiac muscle, and smooth muscle (Table 2–1).

When we think of muscles, we normally think of the voluntary muscles that enable us to walk, run, or move the body in some other way. Such movements are the job of the **skeletal muscles,** which are attached to the bones. Skeletal muscle fibers have a striped, or striated, appearance. These fibers contract when they are stimulated by nerves.

Cardiac muscle, found in the walls of the heart, is considered involuntary because we do not generally decide to contract it. **Smooth muscle** occurs in the walls of the digestive tract, uterus, blood vessels, and other internal organs. Its fibers are not striated and its control is involuntary.

NERVOUS TISSUE CONTROLS MUSCLES AND GLANDS

Nervous tissue consists of **neurons,** cells specialized for transmitting nerve impulses and glial cells, cells that support and nourish the neurons. Typically, a neuron has a large **cell body** that contains the nucleus and from which two types of extensions project. **Dendrites** are specialized for receiving impulses, whereas the single **axon** conducts information away from the cell body (Fig. 2–10).

TABLE 2–1

The types of muscle tissues

	SKELETAL	SMOOTH	CARDIAC
Location	Attached to skeleton	Walls of stomach, intestines, etc.	Walls of heart
Type of control	Voluntary	Involuntary	Involuntary
Striations	Present	Absent	Present
Number of nuclei per fiber	Many	One	One or two
Speed of contraction	Most rapid	Slowest	Intermediate
Ability to remain contracted	Least	Greatest	Intermediate

(a) Skeletal muscle fibers   (b) Smooth muscle fibers   (c) Cardiac muscle fibers

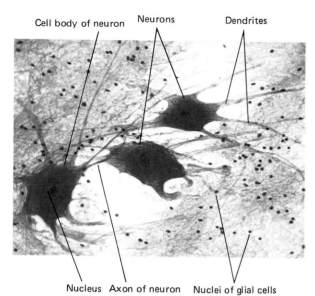

Cell body of neuron   Neurons   Dendrites

Nucleus   Axon of neuron   Nuclei of glial cells

FIGURE 2–10 *Nervous tissue consists of neurons and glial cells (approximately ×500).*

MEMBRANES COVER OR LINE BODY SURFACES

Membranes are sheets of tissue that cover or line body surfaces. **Connective tissue membranes** consist of connective tissue. The membranes that cover bone and cartilage are examples. The synovial membrane is a connective tissue membrane that lines the joint cavities. **Epithelial membranes** consist of epithelial tissue and a layer of underlying connective tissue. The main types of epithelial membranes are mucous membranes, serous membranes, and the skin, which is a cutaneous membrane.

A **mucous membrane,** or **mucosa,** lines body cavities that open to the outside of the body. The epithelial layer secretes mucus, which lubricates the tissue and prevents drying. Mucous membranes line the digestive, respiratory, urinary, and reproductive tracts.

A **serous membrane,** or **serosa,** lines a body cavity that does not open to the outside of the body. The cavity contains fluid secreted by the serous membrane. A serous membrane consists of a thin layer of loose connective tissue covered by a layer of simple epithelium. A serous membrane folds, forming a double-walled sheet of tissue. The portion of the membrane attached to the wall of the cavity is the **parietal membrane,** whereas the part of the membrane that covers the organs inside the cavity is the **visceral membrane.** Thus, the serous membrane lining the thoracic cavity is the parietal pleura, while the portion of that membrane covering the lungs is the visceral pleura. Similarly, the serous membrane lining the abdominal cavity is the parietal peritoneum; the portion of the membrane that covers the abdominal and some pelvic organs is the visceral peritoneum.

SUMMARY

I. Cells are the building blocks of the body.
II. Most cells are bounded by a plasma membrane and have a nucleus and other types of organelles dispersed within the cytoplasm.
   A. The plasma membrane protects the cell and regulates the passage of materials into and out of the cell.
   B. The endoplasmic reticulum (ER) is a system of internal membranes that play a role in the transport of materials within the cell.
   C. The rough ER is studded along its outer walls with ribosomes, granular organelles that manufacture proteins.
   D. The Golgi complex processes and packages proteins and produces lysosomes.
   E. Lysosomes function in intracellular digestion.
   F. Mitochondria, the power plants of the cell, are the sites of most of the reactions of cellular respiration, which yield energy for the cell.
   G. The nucleus, the control center of the cell, contains the chromosomes.
III. Materials move through the plasma membrane passively by physical processes such as diffusion, osmosis, and filtration, or they can be actively transported by physiological processes such as active transport and phagocytosis.
   A. Passive processes do not require the cell to expend energy.
   B. Active processes require energy input by the cell.
   C. Diffusion is the movement of molecules or ions from one region to another because of their

random molecular motion. The net movement of molecules in diffusion is from a region of greater concentration to a region of lower concentration.

    D. Osmosis is a kind of diffusion in which molecules of water diffuse through a selectively permeable membrane.

    E. In filtration, substances are forced through a membrane.

    F. In active transport, cells expend energy to transport materials across membranes from a region of lower to a region of higher concentration.

    G. In phagocytosis, the cell ingests large, solid particles by enclosing them in a vesicle pinched off from the plasma membrane.

IV. The stages in the life cycle of a cell include interphase, prophase, metaphase, anaphase, and telophase. A cell reproduces itself by undergoing mitosis and then dividing to form two new cells.

V. A tissue is a group of closely associated cells that work together to perform a specific function or group of functions. Four main types of tissue are epithelial, connective, muscle, and nervous tissue.

    A. Epithelial tissue covers the body surfaces and lines its cavities; some epithelial tissue is specialized to form glands.

    B. Connective tissue joins other tissues of the body, supports the body, and protects underlying organs. Some main types of connective tissue are ordinary connective tissue, adipose tissue, cartilage, bone, and blood, lymph, and tissues that produce blood cells.

    C. Muscle tissue is specialized to contract; three types are skeletal, cardiac, and smooth.

    D. Nervous tissue is specialized to transmit information.

VI. Membranes cover or line body surfaces.

    A. Connective tissue membranes include the membranes that cover bone and cartilage and synovial membranes that line joint cavities.

    B. The main types of epithelial membranes are mucous membranes, serous membranes, and the skin.

POST TEST

Match
Select the most appropriate match in Column B for each item in Column A.
The same answer may be used as many times as appropriate or not at all.

Column A

1. Regulates passage of materials into the cell
2. Network of internal membranes that extends throughout cytoplasm
3. Site of energy capture from fuel molecules
4. Membranous sacs containing digestive enzymes
5. Chromosomes located here
6. Propels sperm
7. Packages secretions
8. Granules that manufacture protein

Column B

a. ribosomes
b. endoplasmic reticulum (ER)
c. mitochondria
d. plasma membrane
e. nucleus
f. lysosomes
g. Golgi complex
h. flagellum

9. If a cell is placed in a very salty (hypertonic) solution the net passage of water molecules will be from _____ to _____ .

10. A cell engulfs a bacterium; this is an example of _____ .

11. Active transport requires the expenditure of _____ by the cell.

12. A complete set of chromosomes is distributed to each end of the cell during the phase of mitosis known as _____ .

13. Tiny hairlike structures that project from the surface of some cells and function in movement of materials outside the cell are called _____ .

Match

Select the most appropriate match in Column B for each item in Column A.

Column A
14. Covers body surfaces
15. Specialized to contract
16. Contains collagen fibers
17. Supports and protects
18. Contains neurons and glial cells

Column B
a. muscle tissue
b. nervous tissue
c. connective tissue
d. epithelial tissue

19. Endocrine glands do not have _____ .

20. Bone and cartilage are examples of _____ tissue.

21. Label the diagram.

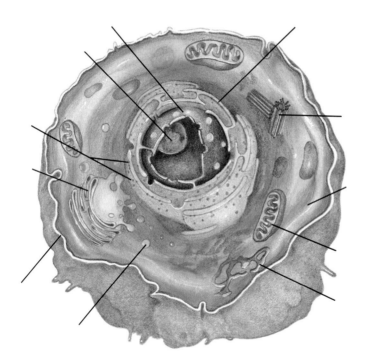

REVIEW QUESTIONS

1. What are the functions of the plasma membrane?
2. What is the function of mitochrondria?
3. Draw a diagram of a cell and label at least eight organelles. Give the function of each organelle you labeled.
4. Explain why the nucleus is considered the control center of the cell.
5. Compare diffusion with active transport.

6. If red blood cells are accidentally placed in a hypotonic solution (one containing less solute than the cells), what happens to them? What would happen if red blood cells were placed in a hypertonic solution (one containing more solute than the cell)? An isotonic solution?

7. Why is mitosis important?

8. What are some of the differences between epithelial and connective tissue?

9. The heart (like most organs) contains epithelial, connective, muscle, and nervous tissue. What function might each of these tissues perform in the heart?

10. What are the functions of epithelial tissue?

11. Where would you expect to find connective tissue membranes? Epithelial membranes? What are two types of epithelial membranes?

POST TEST ANSWERS

1. d
2. b
3. c
4. f
5. e
6. h
7. g
8. a
9. inside the cell; the solution outside the cell
10. phagocytosis
11. energy

12. anaphase
13. cilia
14. d
15. a
16. c
17. c
18. b
19. ducts
20. connective tissue
21. see Figure 2–2

Three

THE SKIN

CHAPTER OUTLINE

    I. The skin functions as a protective barrier
   II. The skin consists of epidermis and dermis
      A. The epidermis continuously replaces itself
      B. The dermis provides strength and elasticity
      C. The subcutaneous layer attaches the skin to underlying tissues
  III. Sweat glands and sebaceous glands are found in the skin
  IV. Hair and nails are appendages of the skin
   V. Melanin helps determine skin color

LEARNING OBJECTIVES

After you have studied this chapter, you should be able to:
1. List six functions of the skin and explain how each is important in homeostasis.
2. Compare the structure and function of the epidermis with that of the dermis.
3. Describe the subcutaneous layer.
4. Describe the functions of sweat glands and sebaceous glands.
5. Give the function of hair and nails and describe the structure of a hair.
6. Explain the function of melanin.

The skin is the body's tough, outer protective covering. Together with its glands, hair, and nails, the skin makes up the **integumentary system** (in-teg″u-**men**′-tar-y). This is the body system with which you are most familiar because it is at least partly exposed to view. Perhaps for this reason we give the skin a lot of attention. We scrub it, cream it, and coat it with makeup; we cut, shave, and curl its hair; and we manicure its nails.

The skin is also important in communication. You may shake hands, stroke, kiss, squeeze, or slap it. Involuntary changes in the skin reflect emotional states. For example, you may blush with embarrassment, blanch with fear or rage, redden with exertion, or sweat excessively when anxious. In addition, the appearance, coloration, temperature, and feel of the skin are important indicators of general health and of many disease states.

THE SKIN FUNCTIONS AS A PROTECTIVE BARRIER

The skin is the outer boundary of the body—the part in direct contact with the external environment. The 20 or so square feet of skin that cover the body must resist continuous wear and tear, drying, and exposure to cold, heat, and toxic substances. The skin is frequently cut, bruised, or scraped and must be able to heal such wounds. The skin is important in maintaining the balanced internal environment. The skin:

1. Protects the body against injury and against disease organisms. The skin is the body's first line of defense against harmful bacteria and other agents of disease.

2. Receives information about the outside world. Located within the skin are sensory receptors that detect touch, pressure, heat, cold, and pain.

3. Prevents drying out. The cells of the body are bathed in an internal sea, a carefully regulated, dilute salt solution essential to life. We humans move about in the relatively dry environment of air. The skin prevents loss of fluid so that the cells do not dry out.

4. Helps maintain body temperature. Capillary (tiny blood vessels) networks and sweat glands in the skin are an important part of the body's temperature-regulating system.

5. Has sweat glands that excrete excess water and some wastes from the body.

6. Contains a compound that is converted to vi-

tamin D when the skin is exposed to the ultraviolet rays of the sun.

THE SKIN CONSISTS OF THE EPIDERMIS AND DERMIS

Skin consists of two main layers: an outer **epidermis** (ep″-ih-**der′**-mus) and an inner **dermis** (**der′**-mus). Beneath the skin is an underlying **subcutaneous layer** (sub-koo-**tay′**-nee-us) (Fig. 3–1).

THE EPIDERMIS CONTINUOUSLY REPLACES ITSELF

Over most parts of the body the epidermis is only about as thick as a page of this book, yet it consists of several sublayers. The epidermis consists of stratified epithelial tissue. The outer cells of the epidermis continuously wear off. They are immediately replaced by new cells. New epidermal cells are con-

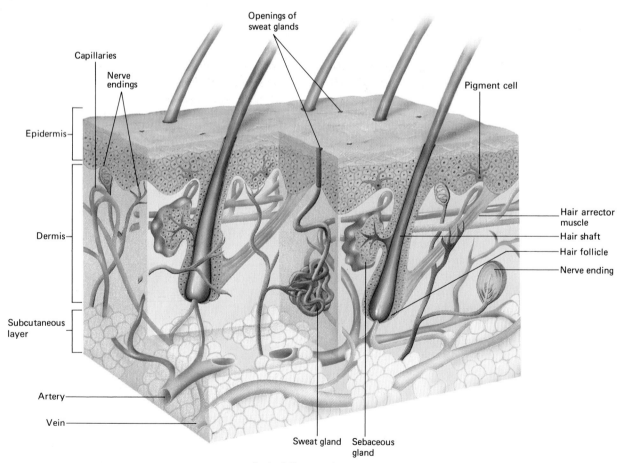

FIGURE 3–1 Microscopic structure of skin.

stantly produced in the deepest sublayer of the epidermis. These cells mature as they are pushed toward the outer surface by newer cells beneath. As they move through the outer sublayer of epidermis, the cells die. **Keratin** (**ker′**a-tin), a tough waterproofing protein, fills most of each cell. The cells at the surface of the skin resemble dead scales. They are closely packed together and serve as a waterproof protective covering for the body.

THE DERMIS PROVIDES STRENGTH AND ELASTICITY

The dermis is the thick layer of skin beneath the epidermis (Fig. 3–1). Dermis consists of dense connective tissue composed mainly of collagen fibers. Collagen is largely responsible for the mechanical strength of the skin. It also permits the skin to stretch and then return to its normal form again. Blood vessels and nerves, which are generally absent in the epidermis, are found throughout the dermis. Specialized skin structures such as hair follicles and glands are found in the dermis. They develop from cells of the epidermis that push down into the dermis.

The upper portion of the dermis has many small, fingerlike elevations that project into the epidermal tissue. Extensive networks of capillaries in these elevations deliver oxygen and nutrients to the cells of the epidermis and also function in temperature regulation. The patterns of ridges and grooves visible on the skin of the soles and palms (including the fingertips) reflect the arrangement of the dermal elevations beneath. Unique to each individual, these patterns provide the fingerprints so useful to law-enforcement officials. They also serve as friction ridges that help us hold onto the objects we grasp.

THE SUBCUTANEOUS LAYER ATTACHES THE SKIN TO UNDERLYING TISSUES

The subcutaneous layer beneath the dermis is also known as the **superficial fascia** (**fash′**-ee-ah). This layer consists of loose connective tissue, usually containing a lot of adipose (fat) tissue. The subcutaneous layer attaches the skin to the muscles and other tissues beneath. This thick fatty layer helps protect underlying organs from mechanical shock. It also insulates the body, thus conserving heat. Fat stored within the adipose tissue can be mobilized and used as an energy source when adequate food is not available. Distribution of fat in the subcutaneous layer is largely responsible for characteristic male and female body shapes.

SWEAT GLANDS AND SEBACEOUS GLANDS ARE FOUND IN THE SKIN

Each **sweat gland** is a tiny coiled tube in the dermis or subcutaneous tissue, with a duct that extends up through the skin and opens onto the surface (Fig. 3–1). About 3 million sweat glands (also called sudoriferous glands) in the skin help maintain body temperature. Muscle movement and metabolic activity generate heat and so raise body temperature. Because heat is required for evaporation, the body becomes cooler as sweat evaporates from the skin.

Sweat glands excrete excess water, salts, and small amounts of nitrogen wastes. About 1 quart of water is excreted in sweat each day. Normally, perspiration is not noticed. Only when it is produced more quickly than it can evaporate does it accumulate on the skin and cause annoyance. This is most apt to happen on a humid day when the air already contains a great deal of water vapor. When profuse sweating occurs, proportionately more salt is lost in the sweat. This is why people engaged in strenuous physical exercise must replace salts lost in sweat.

Certain sweat glands found in association with hairs are concentrated in a few specific areas of the body such as the armpits and genital areas. These glands discharge into hair follicles. Their secretion is thick, sticky, and initially odorless. However, certain bacteria that inhabit the skin surface begin to decompose this secretion, causing it to become odorous. Deodorants kill these bacteria and replace the odor with a more perfumed scent; antiperspirants reduce moisture and so inhibit the growth of bacteria. Emotional stress or sexual stimulation promotes secretion of these glands.

Sebaceous glands (see-**bay′**-shus), also known as oil glands, are generally attached to hair follicles. They are connected to each hair follicle by little ducts through which they release their secretion. These glands are most numerous on the face and scalp. Sebaceous glands secrete an oily substance called **sebum** (**see′**-bum) that oils the hair, lubricates the surface of the skin, and helps prevent water loss. Sebum inhibits the growth of certain bacteria and may also have antifungal action.

During childhood, sebaceous glands are relatively inactive. At puberty they are activated by increased secretion of male hormone in both males and females. This stepped-up activity can lead to acne, a condition very common during adolescence.

Sometimes sebum accumulates in the duct of the sebaceous gland and hair follicle and blocks it, forming a blackhead (comedo). In a blackhead, sebum and dead cells containing the dark pigment melanin block the duct. The black color is due to the melanin rather than to dirt. Sometimes the duct of a sebaceous gland ruptures, allowing sebum to spill into the dermis. The skin may become inflamed and a pimple may form.

HAIR AND NAILS ARE APPENDAGES OF THE SKIN

Hair serves a protective function. It is found on all skin surfaces except the palms and the soles. The part of the hair that we see is the **shaft;** the portion below the skin surface is the **root.** The root, together with its epithelial and connective tissue coverings, is called the **hair follicle** (Fig. 3–2). At the bottom of the follicle is a little mound of connective tissue containing capillaries that deliver nutrients to the cells of the follicle. Each hair consists of cells that multiply, manufacture keratin as they move outward, and then die. The shaft of the hair consists of dead cells and their products. That is why hair can be cut without any sensation of pain. As long as the follicle remains intact, new hair will continue to grow. If the follicle is destroyed, as by electrolysis, no new hair can form.

Tiny bundles of smooth muscle are associated with hair follicles. These arrector pili muscles contract in response to cold or fear, making the hairs stand up straight. Skin around the hair shaft is pulled up into "gooseflesh."

Nails help protect the ends of the fingers and toes. They develop from horny epidermal cells and consist mainly of a closely compressed, tough keratin. Nails appear pink because of underlying capillaries. The actively growing area is the white crescent (lunula) at the base of the nail.

MELANIN HELPS DETERMINE SKIN COLOR

Scattered throughout the lowest layer of the epidermis are cells that produce pigment granules. These granules are composed of a type of protein called **melanin** (mel′-uh-nin) that gives color to hair as well as skin. Skin color is inherited. In dark-skinned individuals the pigment cells are more active and produce more melanin. Asians have the yellowish pigment carotene in their skin as well as melanin. The pinkish hue of light skin is due to the color of blood in the vessels of the dermis. An albino is a per-

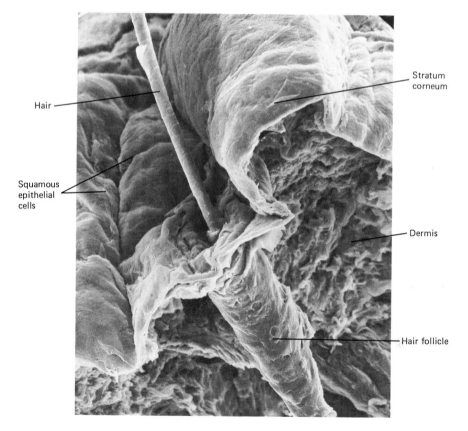

FIGURE **3–2** Scanning electron micrograph of human skin showing hair follicle (approximately ×250). *(Courtesy of Dr. Karen A. Holbrook.)*

Hair

Squamous epithelial cells

Stratum corneum

Dermis

Hair follicle

son of any race who has inherited the inability to produce pigment.

Melanin is an important protective screen against the sun because it absorbs harmful ultraviolet rays. Exposure to the sun stimulates an increase in the amount of melanin produced and causes the skin to become darker. This suntan is a protective response.

The tan so prized by sun worshippers is actually

a sign that the skin has been exposed to too much ultraviolet radiation. When the melanin is not able to absorb all the ultraviolet rays the skin becomes inflamed, or sunburned. Excessive exposure to sun over a period of years, especially in fair-skinned individuals, eventually results in wrinkling of the skin and sometimes in skin cancer. Because dark-skinned people have more melanin they suffer less sunburn, wrinkling, and skin cancer.

SUMMARY

I. The integumentary system consists of the skin and its hair, nails, and glands.
II. The skin:
 A. Protects the body against injury and disease organisms.
 B. Receives information about the outside world.
 C. Prevents drying out.
 D. Helps maintain constant body temperature.
 E. Helps excrete water and some wastes.
 F. Produces vitamin D.
III. As a cell moves outward through the layers of the epidermis it produces keratin, then dies, becoming scalelike, and finally is sloughed off the skin surface.
IV. The dermis consists of connective tissue containing large amounts of collagen. It gives strength to the skin and holds the blood vessels that nourish the epidermal cells.
V. The subcutaneous layer consists of connective tissue, including fat. This tissue cushions underlying structures against mechanical injury, connects skin with tissues beneath, and stores energy in the form of fat.
VI. Sweat glands excrete a dilute salt water that evaporates, cooling the body.
VII. Sebaceous glands secrete an oily substance that lubricates the surface of the skin and helps prevent water loss.
VIII. Hair and nails both serve a protective function.
IX. Pigment cells in epidermis produce melanin that gives color to skin and hair. Melanin absorbs ultraviolet rays from the skin, preventing damage to dermis and blood vessels.

POST TEST

1. The skin with its glands, hair, nails, and other structures makes up the _Integumentary_ system.
2. The two main layers of the skin are the outer _Epidermis_ and the inner _Dermis_.
3. The tough waterproofing protein of the epidermis is _Keratin_.
4. The _Superficial Fascia_ layer beneath the dermis consists of loose connective tissue.
5. _Sebaceous_ glands are attached to each hair follicle by ducts; they secrete an oily substance called _Sebum_.
6. Sweat consists mainly of _Water_ with some _Salt_, and small amounts of nitrogen wastes.
7. The root of a hair together with its coverings is called a _hair follicle_.
8. Nails consist mainly of tough, compressed _____.

9. Pigment granules in the skin produce the dark pigment _____ .

10. Melanin protects against the sun by absorbing _____ rays.

11. Label the diagram.

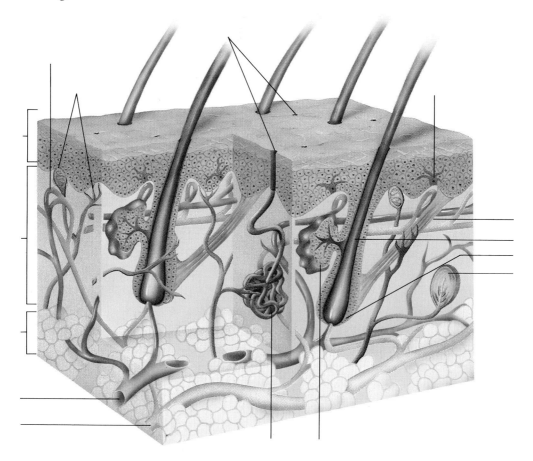

REVIEW QUESTIONS

1. In what ways does the skin help preserve homeostasis?

2. Compare the structure of the epidermis with that of the dermis.

3. Which cells of the epidermis actively divide? Which are dead?

4. What are the functions of the dermis? The subcutaneous layer?

5. What is the function of the sebaceous glands? What happens when they malfunction?

6. Why is melanin important?

POST TEST ANSWERS

1. integumentary
2. epidermis; dermis
3. keratin
4. subcutaneous
5. Sebaceous; sebum
6. water; salts

7. follicle
8. keratin
9. melanin
10. ultraviolet
11. see Figure 3–1

Four

THE SKELETAL SYSTEM

CHAPTER OUTLINE

I. Functions of the skeletal system include support and protection
II. A typical long bone consists of a shaft with flared ends
III. Two types of bone tissue are compact and cancellous bone
IV. Bone develops by replacing existing connective tissue
V. The skeleton may be divided into the axial and the appendicular skeleton
VI. The skull is the bony framework of the head
VII. The vertebral column supports the body
VIII. The thoracic cage protects the organs of the chest
IX. The pectoral girdle attaches the upper limbs to the axial skeleton
X. The upper limb consists of 30 bones
XI. The pelvic girdle supports the lower limbs
XII. The lower limb consists of 30 bones
XIII. Joints are junctions between bones
    A. Joints can be classified according to the degree of movement they permit
    B. A diarthrosis is surrounded by a joint capsule

LEARNING OBJECTIVES

After you have studied this chapter, you should be able to:
1. List five functions of the skeletal system.
2. Label a diagram of a long bone, and describe the microscopic structure of a bone.
3. Contrast endochondral with intramembranous bone development, and describe the role of osteoblasts and osteoclasts in bone production.
4. List and describe the bones of the axial skeleton and identify each on a diagram or skeleton.
5. List and describe the bones of the appendicular skeleton and identify each on a diagram or skeleton.
6. Compare the main types of joints, and describe the structure and functions of a diarthrosis.

The skeleton found in science laboratories consists of dry, dead bones. In the living body, the skeletal system consists of bone, cartilage, and other connective tissues that are alive—their cells must have nutrients and oxygen, they consume energy in their metabolism, they produce waste products, some of their metabolism is regulated by hormones, and they function closely with the muscular system.

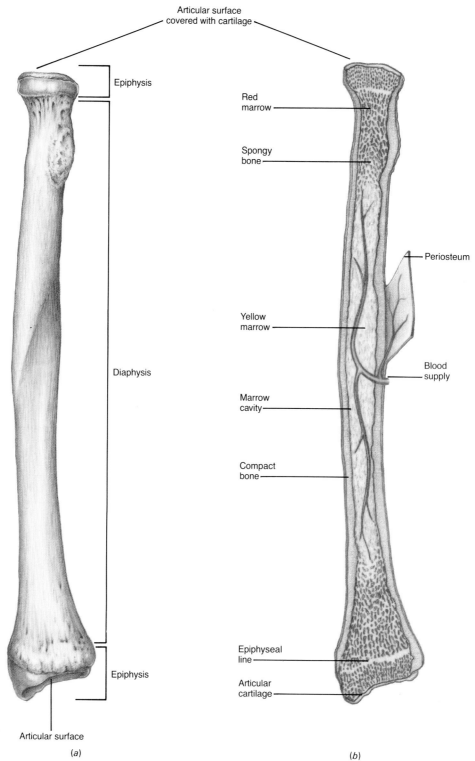

Articular surface
covered with cartilage

Epiphysis

Red
marrow

Spongy
bone

Diaphysis

Periosteum

Yellow
marrow

Blood
supply

Marrow
cavity

Compact
bone

Epiphysis

Epiphyseal
line

Articular
cartilage

Articular surface

(a)

(b)

FIGURE **4–1**   Anatomy of a bone. *(a)* The structure of a typical long bone. *(b)* Internal structure of a long bone.

FUNCTIONS OF THE SKELETAL SYSTEM INCLUDE SUPPORT AND PROTECTION

The skeletal system serves several important functions:

1. It *supports* the body by serving as a bony framework for the other tissues and organs.

2. It *protects* delicate vital organs. For example, the bones of the skull surround and protect the brain; the sternum (breastbone) and ribs protect the heart and lungs. For their weight, bones are nearly as strong as steel.

3. Bones serve as levers that *transmit muscular forces.* Muscles are attached to bones by bands of connective tissue called **tendons.** When muscles contract they pull on bones, and in this way they move parts of the body. Bones are held together at joints by bands of connective tissue called **ligaments.** Most joints are movable. The interaction of bones and muscles also makes breathing possible.

4. The marrow within some bones *produces blood cells.*

5. Bones serve as banks for the *storage and release of minerals* such as calcium and phosphorus. When the concentration of calcium in the blood increases above normal, calcium is deposited in the bones. When the concentration of calcium decreases, calcium is withdrawn from the bones and enters the blood.

A TYPICAL LONG BONE CONSISTS OF A SHAFT WITH FLARED ENDS

The main shaft of a long bone is known as its **diaphysis** (die-**af′**-i-sis) (Fig. 4–1). The expanded ends of the bone are called **epiphyses** (e-**pif′**-i-sees). In children, a disc of cartilage, the metaphysis, is found between the epiphyses and the diaphysis. The **metaphyses** (meh-**taf′**-ih-sees) are growth centers that disappear at maturity, becoming vague epiphyseal lines.

Within the long bone is a central marrow cavity filled with a fatty connective tissue known as yellow bone marrow. The marrow cavity is lined with a thin layer of cells, the **endosteum** (end-**oss′**-tee-um).

Each bone is covered by a layer of specialized connective tissue, the **periosteum** (per″-ee-**os′**-tee-um). The inner layer of the periosteum contains cells that produce bone. At its joint surfaces the outer layer of a bone consists of a thin layer of hyaline cartilage, the **articular cartilage.**

TWO TYPES OF BONE TISSUE ARE COMPACT AND CANCELLOUS BONE

Two types of bone tissue are compact bone and spongy bone. **Compact bone,** which is very dense and hard, is found near the surfaces of the bone, where great strength is needed. Compact bone consists of interlocking, spindle-shaped units called **osteons** (**os′**-tee-ons), or haversian systems (Fig. 4–2). Within an osteon, **osteocytes** (**os′**-tee-o-sites″), the mature bone cells, are found in small cavities called **lacunae** (la-**koo′**-nee). The lacunae are arranged in concentric circles around central **haversian canals.** Blood vessels that nourish the bone tissue pass through the haversian canals. Threadlike extensions of the cytoplasm of the osteocytes extend through narrow channels (called canaliculi). These cellular extensions connect the osteocytes.

Spongy bone is found within the epiphyses and makes up the inner part of the wall of the diaphysis. Spongy bone consists of a network of thin strands of bone. The spaces within the spongy bone are filled with **bone marrow.** The **red marrow,** found in certain bones, produces blood cells. **Yellow marrow** consists mainly of fat cells.

BONE DEVELOPS BY REPLACING EXISTING CONNECTIVE TISSUE

Bone formation is called **ossification** (os″-ih-fih-**kay′**-shun). During fetal development bones form in two ways. The long bones develop from cartilage models, a process called **endochondral** (en″-doe-**kon′**-dral) **bone development.** The flat bones of the skull, the irregular vertebrae, and some other bones develop from a noncartilage connective tissue scaffold. This is known as **intramembranous** (in″-trah-**mem′**-brah-nus) **bone development.**

Osteoblasts are cells that produce bone. They secrete the protein collagen that forms the strong, elastic fibers of bone. A complex calcium phosphate called apatite is present in the tissue fluid. This compound automatically crystallizes around the collagen fibers, forming the hard matrix of bone. As the matrix

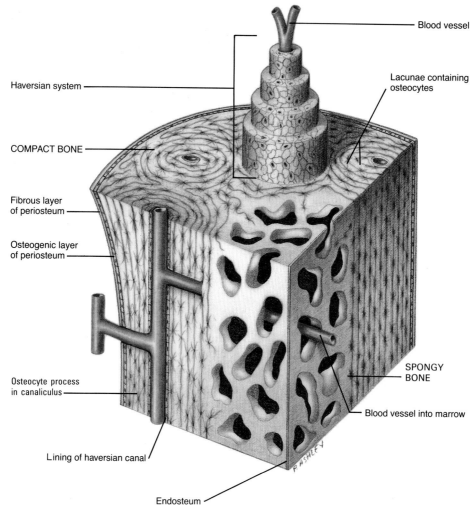

Blood vessel

Lacunae containing osteocytes

Haversian system

COMPACT BONE

Fibrous layer of periosteum

Osteogenic layer of periosteum

SPONGY BONE

Osteocyte process in canaliculus

Blood vessel into marrow

Lining of haversian canal

Endosteum

FIGURE 4–2 A three-dimensional diagram showing the microscopic structure of bone. A cross section and longitudinal section of compact bone are shown.

forms around the osteoblasts they become isolated within small spaces called lacunae. When osteoblasts become embedded in the bone matrix, they are referred to as osteocytes.

Bones are modeled during growth and remodeled continuously throughout life in response to physical stresses on the body. As muscles develop in response to physical activity, the bones to which they are attached thicken and become stronger. As bones grow, bone tissue must be removed from the interior, especially from the walls of the marrow cavity. This process keeps bones from getting too heavy.

Osteoclasts (**os'**-tee-oh-klasts″) are the cells that break down bone, a process referred to as bone resorption. Osteoclasts are very large cells that move about secreting enzymes that digest bone. Osteoclasts and osteoblasts work side by side to shape bones and to form the precise grain needed in the

finished bone. Some important types of bone markings are described in Table 4–1.

THE SKELETON MAY BE DIVIDED INTO THE AXIAL SKELETON AND THE APPENDICULAR SKELETON

The human skeleton (Figs. 4–3 and 4–4) may be divided into two groups of bones:

1. The axial (**ak'**-se-al) skeleton consists of the skull, vertebral column, ribs, and sternum.

2. The appendicular (ap-en-**dik'**-u-lar) skeleton consists of the upper and lower limbs (arms and legs), the shoulder girdle, and the pelvic girdle (with the exception of the sacrum).

TABLE 4–1

Bone markings

PROCESS: ANY PROMINENT BONY PROJECTION

Processes That Help Form Joints

Condyle (**kon'**-dil)	Rounded projection
Head	Rounded projection supported by narrow neck (constricted region); usually the upper or proximal extremity of a bone; often bears the ball of ball-and-socket joint
Facet	Smooth, flat surface; found on vertebrae for articulation with ribs

Processes That Are Sites of Attachment for Tendons and Ligaments

Crest	Projecting line or ridge, often on long border of bone
Epicondyle	Bony bulge adjacent to condyle
Spine	Sharp projection; sometimes a long, strongly raised ridge
Trochanter (tro-**kan'**-ter)	Pulley-like process found only on femur
Tubercle (**too'**-ber-kul)	Small, rounded process
Tuberosity	Large, rounded, often roughened process

DEPRESSIONS AND OPENINGS

Fissure (**fish'**-ur)	Narrow cleft or groove between adjacent bones through which blood vessels and nerves pass
Foramen (foe-**ray'**-men)	Natural opening or passage into or through bony structure, often round; term means "hole"
Fossa	Trench or shallow depression on surface of bone; term means "basin-like depression"
Sulcus	Elongated groove through which blood vessel or nerve may pass
Meatus (me-**a'**-tus)	Opening into some passageway in body, not necessarily bony; usually lengthy and tunnel-like
Sinus	Air-filled cavity (paranasal sinuses are connected to nasal cavity)

THE SKULL IS THE BONY FRAMEWORK OF THE HEAD

The **skull,** the bony framework of the head, is divided into the cranial and the facial bones. The **cranium** consists of eight cranial bones that enclose the brain. Fourteen bones make up the facial portion of the skull. Also within the head are six very small bones in the middle ears. The bones of the head are described in Table 4–2 and are illustrated in Figures 4–5 through 4–8.

Most of the bones of the skull are joined by immovable joints called **sutures.** The **sagittal suture** is the joint between the two parietal bones. The coronal suture joins the parietal bones to the frontal bone.

The lambdoidal suture is the joint between the parietal bones and the occipital bone.

At birth, ossification at the skull joints is not complete. Many of these bones are loosely joined by fibrous connective tissue or cartilage. Six such joints, called **fontanelles** (fon-tah-**nells'**), occur at the angles of the parietal bone.

The largest is the anterior fontanelle at the junction of the sagittal, coronal, and frontal sutures. The fontanelles, popularly referred to as soft spots, permit the baby's head to be compressed slightly as it passes through the bony pelvis during birth. They also allow the infant's brain to grow during the latter weeks of prenatal development and permit growth of the skull bones.

Sinuses are air spaces lined with mucous mem-
Text continued on page 61

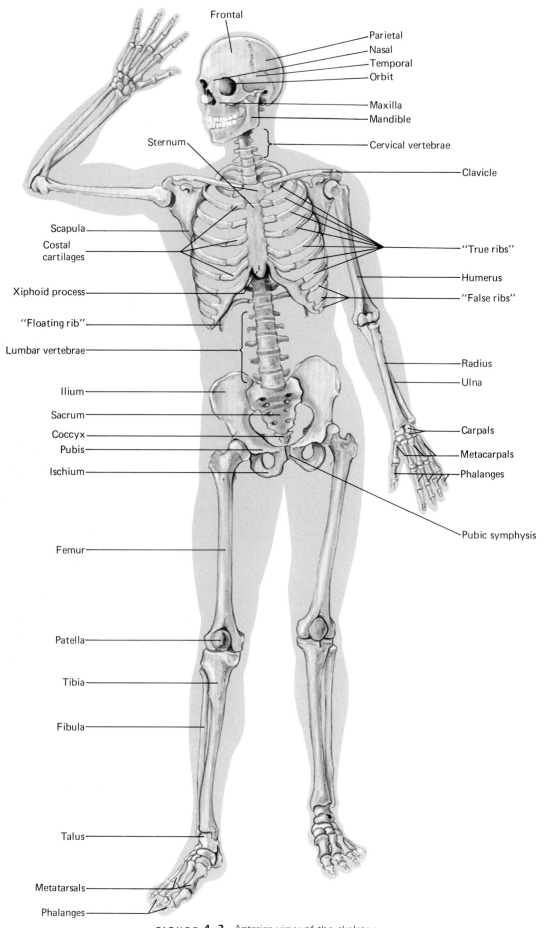

Frontal

Parietal
Nasal
Temporal
Orbit

Maxilla
Mandible

Cervical vertebrae

Clavicle

Sternum

Scapula

Costal
cartilages

"True ribs"

Humerus

Xiphoid process

"False ribs"

"Floating rib"

Lumbar vertebrae

Radius
Ulna

Ilium

Sacrum

Coccyx

Carpals

Pubis

Metacarpals

Ischium

Phalanges

Pubic symphysis

Femur

Patella

Tibia

Fibula

Talus

Metatarsals

Phalanges

52

FIGURE 4–3 Anterior view of the skeleton.

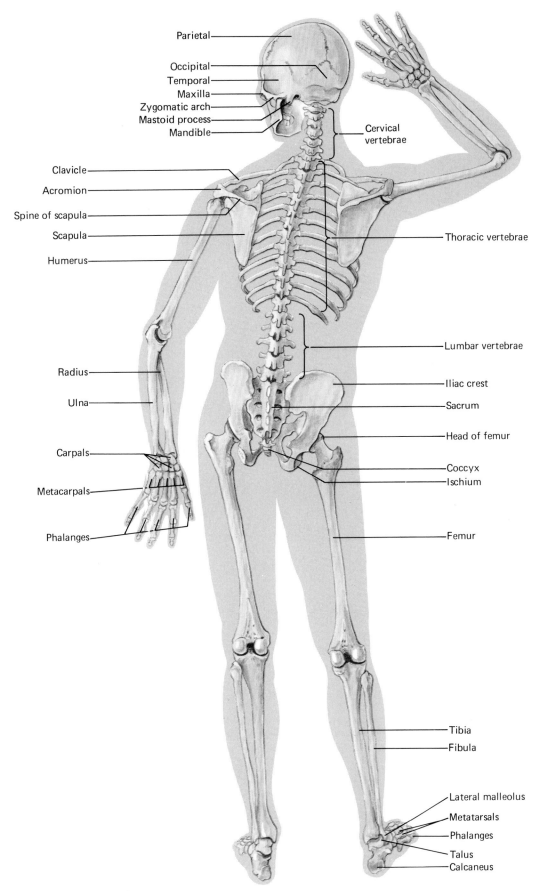

Parietal
Occipital
Temporal
Maxilla
Zygomatic arch
Mastoid process
Mandible
Cervical vertebrae
Clavicle
Acromion
Spine of scapula
Scapula
Humerus
Thoracic vertebrae
Lumbar vertebrae
Radius
Ulna
Iliac crest
Sacrum
Head of femur
Carpals
Coccyx
Ischium
Metacarpals
Phalanges
Femur
Tibia
Fibula
Lateral malleolus
Metatarsals
Phalanges
Talus
Calcaneus

FIGURE 4–4 Posterior view of the skeleton.

TABLE 4–2

Bones that make up the skeleton

NAME OF BONE (Number)	FUNCTION	DESCRIPTION
Cranial Bones		
Frontal (1)	Forms forehead and front part of cranium floor; forms part of roof over eyes and nasal cavity	Large, curved bone **Frontal sinuses:** air-filled cavities lined with mucous membrane **Supraorbital ridge:** just below eyebrows
Parietal (2) (pah-**rye**'-eh-tal)	Form much of walls and roof of cranium	Curved, flattened bones that meet at midline of cranium just behind frontal bone
Temporal (2)	Helps form floor and lateral wall of cranial cavity; contains ear canal, middle ear bones, and sensory portions of ear; bears temporomandibular joint (see mandible below)	Pointed **styloid process** serves as point of attachment for certain neck muscles; **mastoid process** contains air sinuses that may become infected when a middle ear infection spreads; **zygomatic process** helps form cheek
Occipital (1)	Forms most of floor and posterior part of skull; articulates with neck	Contains **foramen magnum** through which spinal cord passes; **occipital condyles** articulate with first vertebra of spinal column
Sphenoid (1) (**sfee**'-noyd)	Forms floor of cranium; helps form eye orbits	Shaped like butterfly **Sella turcica** (**sell**'-ah-**tur**'-si-kah): saddle-shaped depression on superior surface holds pituitary gland; also called Turkish saddle **Sphenoid sinus:** air-filled spaces lined with mucous membrane
Ethmoid (1) (**eth**'-moyd)	Forms roof of nasal cavity and part of medial walls of eye orbits	Has irregular shape **Crista galli:** beak-shaped process to which an extension (falx cerebri) of outermost membrane surrounding brain attaches **Cribriform plate:** area of ethmoid perforated by tiny holes through which fibers of olfactory nerves pass from nose to brain **Superior and middle turbinates (conchae):** projections that form ledges along lateral walls of nasal cavity **Ethmoid sinuses:** air spaces lined with mucous membrane
Facial Bones		
Mandible (1) (**man**'-dih-bal)	Lower jawbone; joins with temporal bone on each side forming **temporomandibular joints** (only freely movable joints in the skull); used in many mouth movements, especially chewing	U-shaped bone; its body (horizontal part) forms chin; its rami (vertical parts) have condyles (heads) that articulate with temporal bones **Alveolar process:** bony ridge in which lower teeth are rooted
Maxilla (2) (mak-**sil**'-ah)	Fuse to form upper jaw bone; form lateral walls of nose, floor of orbits, anterior part of hard palate (roof of mouth)	Very irregular shape; all facial bones except mandible touch maxilla **Palatine processes:** form anterior part of hard palate **Alveolar process:** bony ridge in which upper teeth are rooted **Maxillary sinuses:** largest sinuses; drain into nasal passages and throat

TABLE 4–2 *Continued*

Bones that make up the skeleton

NAME OF BONE (Number)	FUNCTION	DESCRIPTION
Facial Bones		
Palatine (2)	Forms posterior part of hard palate	Irregular shape; cleft palate occurs when these bones (or palatine processes) do not fuse
Malar (zygomatic) (2)	Cheekbones; form walls and floors of orbits	Curved, irregular shape
Nasal (2)	Form upper part of bridge of nose	Small, thin, triangular shape
Lacrimal (2) (**lak**'-rih-mal)	Help form medial wall of orbit; contain a groove through which tears pass into nasal cavity	About size and shape of a fingernail
Vomer (1) (**voe**'-mer)	Forms inferior, back part of nasal septum	Trapezoid-shaped
Inferior turbinate (2)	Forms ledge along lateral walls of nose; increases surface area of nasal cavity	Scroll-shaped
Ear Bones		
A chain of 3 tiny bones, or ossicles, in each middle ear cavity.		
Malleus (2)	Transmits vibration from eardrum	Attached to eardrum; shaped somewhat like hammer
Incus (2)	Transmits vibration in middle ear	Shaped somewhat like anvil
Stapes (2)	Transmits vibration to oval window	Shaped like stirrup
Hyoid (1)	Important during swallowing	U-shaped, located in neck between mandible and larynx; does not articulate directly with any other bone
Vertebral Column		
Cervical vertebrae(7)		
Atlas (C1)	First cervical vertebra; forms joints with occipital condyles that allow head to nod "yes"	Has no centrum; no neural spine
Axis (C2)	Second cervical vertebra; its odontoid process serves as pivot for rotation of atlas and skull; permits you to shake your head "no"	**Odontoid process** (dens) projects upward from centrum
Inferior cervical vertebrae	**Spines** serve as points of attachment for neck and back muscles	Can be identified by its **transverse foramina** through which vertebral arteries and veins pass
Thoracic vertebrae (12)	Ribs attach to these vertebrae; part of thoracic cage	Have facets for articulation with ribs
Lumbar vertebrae (5)	Make up part of vertebral column in small of back; support most of body weight; responsible for much of flexibility of trunk; many of back muscles attach to them	Large, heavy vertebrae
Sacrum (1) (**say**'-krum)	Part of pelvic girdle	5 separate vertebrae in child; fuse to form a single bone in adult
Coccyx (1) (**kok**'-six)	Several pelvic and hip muscles originate on coccyx	3–5 separate vertebrae in child; fuse in adult

Table continued on following page

TABLE 4–2 *Continued*

Bones that make up the skeleton

NAME OF BONE (Number)	FUNCTION	DESCRIPTION
Thoracic Cage		
Ribs (24)	Protect organs of thoracic cavity; form part of thoracic cage	Long, curved bones **True ribs** Upper 7 pairs; attach directly to sternum by way of costal cartilages **False ribs** Pairs 8, 9, and 10; attach to sternum by way of common bar of cartilage that joins costal cartilage of seventh ribs **Floating ribs** Pairs 11 and 12; not connected to sternum
Sternum (1)	Breastbone; protects heart and anchors anterior ends of ribs; produces red blood cells in its marrow cavity	Consists of 3 parts: thick, superior **manubrium;** long **body;** inferior **xiphoid process** composed of cartilage (xiphoid process important landmark for CPR)
Pectoral Girdle		
Scapula (2) (**skap'**-u-lah)	Shoulder blade	Somewhat flat, triangular bone **Spine:** sharp ridge that runs diagonally across posterior surface of shoulder blade **Acromion process:** helps hold head of humerus in place **Glenoid fossa:** socket that receives head of humerus
Clavicle (2) (**klav'**-ih-kle)	Collarbone; connects scapula with sternum; helps form shoulder joint	Small, curved bone
Upper Limb		
Humerus (2) (**hu'**-mer-us)	Upper arm bone; forms joint with scapula above and with the radius and ulna at the elbow	Longest, largest bone of upper limb **Head:** fits into glenoid process of scapula
Radius (2)	Bone on thumb side of lower arm	Curved with lengthwise ridge
Ulna (2)	Medial bone of forearm; main forearm bone in elbow joint	**Styloid process:** sharp projection at distal end
Carpal bones (16) (**kar'**-pal)	Wrist bones	Irregular bones at proximal end of hand
Metacarpal bones (10)	Form palm of hand	Heads of metacarpals are knuckles
Phalanges (28) (fah-**lan'**-jeez)	Bones of fingers; 3 in each finger, 2 in each thumb	
Pelvic Girdle		
Coxal (innominate) (2)	Hipbone; supports weight of upper body	Formed by fusion of 3 bones: ilium, ischium, and pubis **Acetabulum:** hip socket; receives head of femur

TABLE 4–2 Continued

Bones that make up the skeleton

NAME OF BONE (Number)	FUNCTION	DESCRIPTION
Pelvic Girdle		
Ilium (**il**'-ee-um)	Large flaring part of coxal bone; connects posteriorly with sacrum at sacroiliac joint	**Iliac crest:** upper edge of ilium (feels somewhat like a shelf) **Anterior superior spine:** projection at anterior end of iliac crest
Ischium (**iss**'-kee-um)	Lower, posterior portion of coxal bone	**Ischial tuberosity:** large, rough area on which body rests when sitting erect **Ischial spine:** superior to tuberosity; narrows pelvic outlet through which baby passes during delivery
Pubis (**pu**'-bis)	Most anterior part of coxal bone	**Obturator foramen:** largest foramen in body; formed by pubis and ischium **Pubic symphysis:** joint between pubic bones; made of fibrocartilage **Pelvic brim (inlet):** opening within flaring parts of ilia that leads into true pelvis **True (lesser) pelvis:** space inferior to pelvic brim; bounded by muscle and bone; pelvic organs located here; superior opening is **pelvic inlet;** inferior opening is **pelvic outlet** (true pelvis must be large enough in female to permit passage of infant's head during childbirth)
Lower Limb		
Femur (2) (**fee**'-mer)	Thigh bone; largest bone in body	Slightly curved bone **Head:** Ball-like end; fits into acetabulum **Condyles:** rounded projections at distal end; articulate with tibia **Greater trochanter:** prominent projection from upper part of shaft; large muscles (including gluteus maximus) attach here **Lesser trochanter:** smaller projection located inferiorly and medially to greater trochanter
Patella (2) (pah-**tell**'-ah)	Kneecap	Largest sesamoid bone (one that occurs in a tendon or other soft tissue and does not articulate with any other bone) in body
Tibia (2) (**tib**'-ee-ah)	Larger and more medial of the two shank bones	**Medial and lateral condyles:** articulate with condyles of femur, forming knee joint **Medial malleolus:** medial, rounded process at distal end
Fibula (2) (**fib**'-u-lah)	Smaller bone of shank; foot muscles attach to it	Slender bone **Lateral malleolus:** lateral, rounded process at distal end. The medial and lateral malleoli are popularly referred to as the anklebones
Tarsals (14)	Ankle and proximal foot bones; 4 (3 cuneiforms and cuboid) articulate with long bones (metatarsals) of foot; the largest tarsal is the calcaneus (kal-**kay**'-nee-us), or heelbone	2 longitudinal and 1 transverse arch are formed by arrangement of tarsals and metatarsals; these bones are held in arched position by tendons and ligaments; arches permit bones and their ligaments to act as shock absorbers

Table continued on following page

TABLE **4–2** _Continued_		
Bones that make up the skeleton		
NAME OF BONE [Number]	FUNCTION	DESCRIPTION
Lower Limb		
Metatarsals [10]	Form middle part of foot	
Phalanges [28]	Toe bones; 3 in each toe; 2 in each great toe	

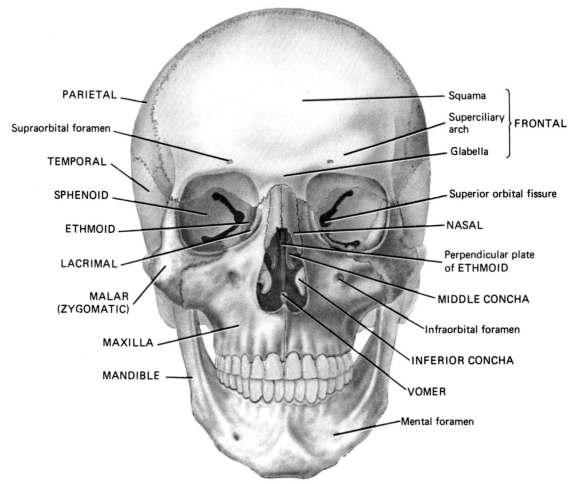

FIGURE **4–5** Anterior view of the skull.

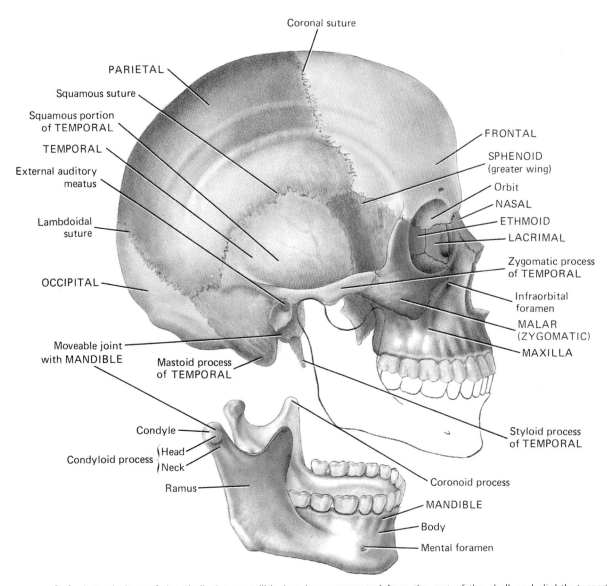

FIGURE **4–6** Lateral view of the skull; the mandible has been separated from the rest of the skull and slightly turned.

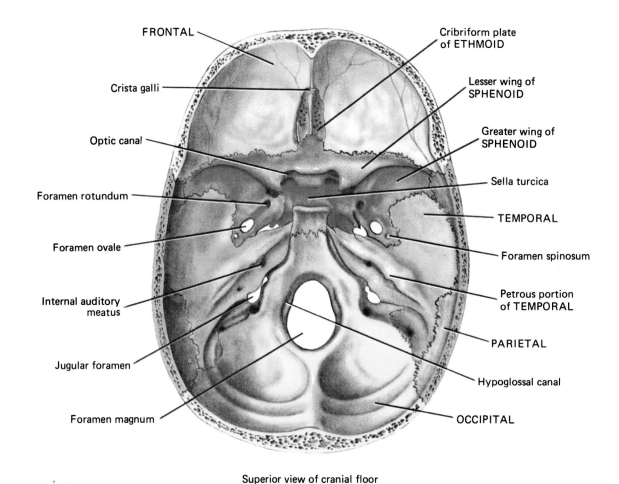

FRONTAL

Crista galli

Optic canal

Foramen rotundum

Foramen ovale

Internal auditory
meatus

Jugular foramen

Foramen magnum

Cribriform plate
of ETHMOID

Lesser wing of
SPHENOID

Greater wing of
SPHENOID

Sella turcica

TEMPORAL

Foramen spinosum

Petrous portion
of TEMPORAL

PARIETAL

Hypoglossal canal

OCCIPITAL

Superior view of cranial floor

FIGURE **4–7** The top of the skull has been removed to expose the superior surface of the cranial floor. Portions of the superior views of the ethmoid and sphenoid bones can be seen in the floor of the cranial cavity.

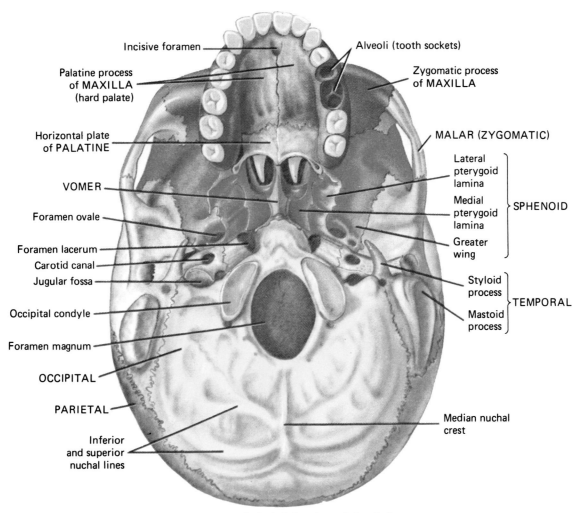

Incisive foramen

Palatine process
of MAXILLA
(hard palate)

Horizontal plate
of PALATINE

VOMER

Foramen ovale

Foramen lacerum
Carotid canal
Jugular fossa

Occipital condyle

Foramen magnum

OCCIPITAL

PARIETAL

Inferior
and superior
nuchal lines

Alveoli (tooth sockets)

Zygomatic process
of MAXILLA

MALAR (ZYGOMATIC)

Lateral
pterygoid
lamina

Medial
pterygoid
lamina

Greater
wing

SPHENOID

Styloid
process

Mastoid
process

TEMPORAL

Median nuchal
crest

FIGURE 4–8 Inferior view of the skull.

brane found in some of the cranial bones. Four pairs of sinuses, the paranasal sinuses, (located in the frontal, maxillary, sphenoid, and ethmoid bones) are continuous with the nose and throat. Sometimes the mucous membranes of the sinuses become swollen and inflamed, the condition we know as sinusitis.

THE VERTEBRAL COLUMN SUPPORTS THE BODY

The **vertebral column,** or spine, supports the body and bears its weight. It consists of 24 vertebrae and 2 fused bones, the **sacrum** (**say′**-krum) and **coccyx** (**kok′**-six) (Fig. 4–9). The regions of the vertebral column are the **cervical** (neck), composed of 7 vertebrae; the **thoracic** (chest), which consists of 12

vertebrae; the **lumbar** (back), composed of 5 vertebrae; the **sacral** (pelvic), which consists of 5 fused vertebrae; and the **coccygeal,** also consisting of fused vertebrae.

The vertebral column is S-shaped because of four curves that develop before birth and during childhood. These curves provide strength and flexibility for the vertebral column.

Vertebrae articulate with each other by means of synovial joints and by means of **intervertebral discs** composed of cartilage. The intervertebral discs are tiny pads that act as shock absorbers. Occasionally an intervertebral disc herniates (ruptures) and puts pressure on the root of a spinal nerve. This condition, popularly known as a slipped disc, can be extremely painful.

A "typical" vertebra has certain structural features (Fig. 4–10):

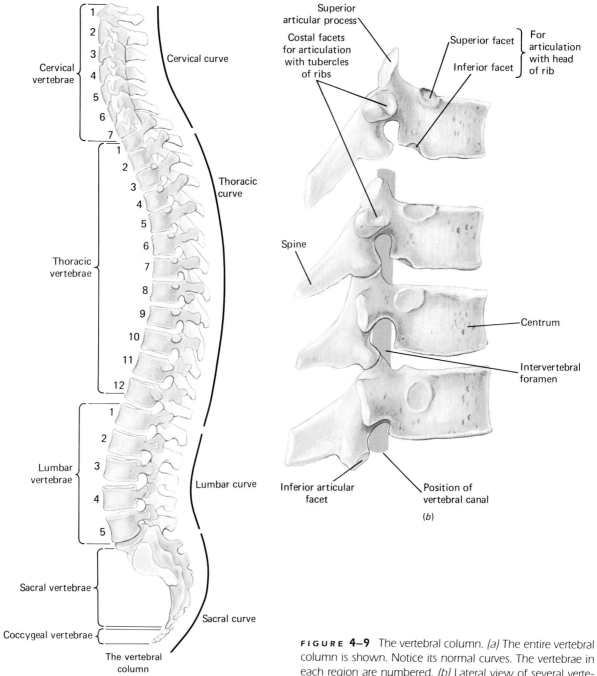

FIGURE 4–9 The vertebral column. *(a)* The entire vertebral column is shown. Notice its normal curves. The vertebrae in each region are numbered. *(b)* Lateral view of several vertebrae, showing how they articulate.

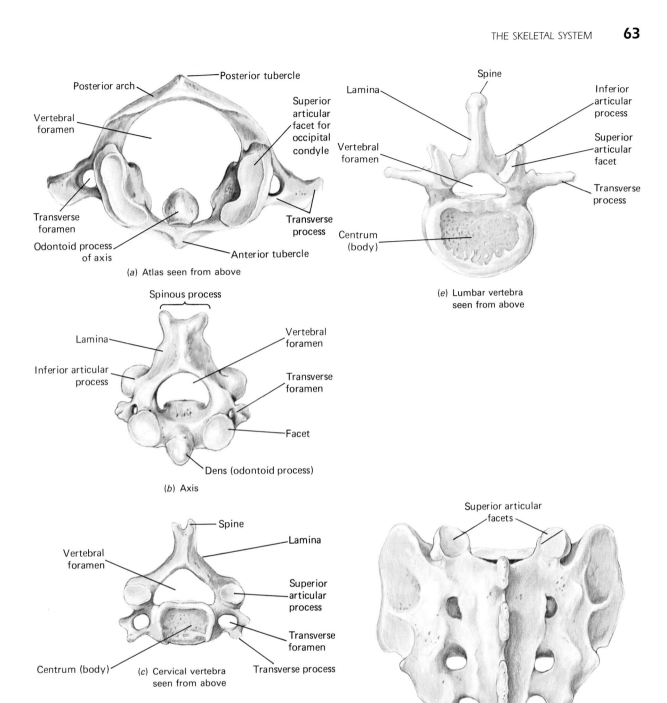

(a) Atlas seen from above

Posterior arch — Posterior tubercle — Superior articular facet for occipital condyle — Vertebral foramen — Transverse foramen — Odontoid process of axis — Anterior tubercle — Transverse process

(b) Axis

Spinous process — Lamina — Inferior articular process — Vertebral foramen — Transverse foramen — Facet — Dens (odontoid process)

(c) Cervical vertebra seen from above

Spine — Lamina — Vertebral foramen — Superior articular process — Transverse foramen — Transverse process — Centrum (body)

(e) Lumbar vertebra seen from above

Spine — Lamina — Inferior articular process — Superior articular facet — Vertebral foramen — Transverse process — Centrum (body)

(f) Sacrum and coccyx

Superior articular facets — Coccyx

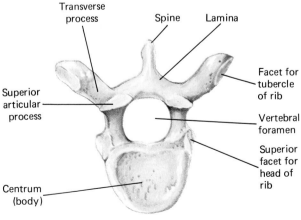

(d) Thoracic vertebra

Transverse process — Spine — Lamina — Superior articular process — Facet for tubercle of rib — Vertebral foramen — Superior facet for head of rib — Centrum (body)

FIGURE 4–10 The vertebrae. *(a)* The first cervical vertebra, the atlas, seen from above. *(b)* The second cervical vertebra, the axis. *(c)* A typical lower cervical vertebra seen from above. *(d)* A thoracic vertebra. *(e)* A lumbar vertebra. *(f)* The sacrum and coccyx.

Structural feature	Definition
Centrum (or body)	The bony central part of the vertebra that bears most of the body weight
Lamina	Arch
Vertebral foramen	Passageway through which the spinal cord passes
Spinous process	Posterior projection from the lamina; back muscles attach to this process
Transverse processes	Lateral projections from the centrum; provided with articular surfaces for joining with other vertebrae and ribs
Superior and inferior articular processes	Projections lateral to the vertebral foramen; where vertebra forms joints with adjacent vertebrae

THE THORACIC CAGE PROTECTS THE ORGANS OF THE CHEST

The **thoracic cage,** or rib cage, protects the internal organs of the chest including the heart and lungs. The thoracic cage provides support for the bones of the pectoral girdle and upper limbs and is also important in breathing. The thoracic cage is a bony cage formed by the sternum (breastbone), the thoracic vertebrae, and 12 pairs of ribs.

THE PECTORAL GIRDLE ATTACHES THE UPPER LIMBS TO THE AXIAL SKELETON

The **pectoral girdle,** or shoulder girdle, attaches the upper limbs to the axial skeleton. Each pectoral girdle consists of a scapula (shoulderblade)

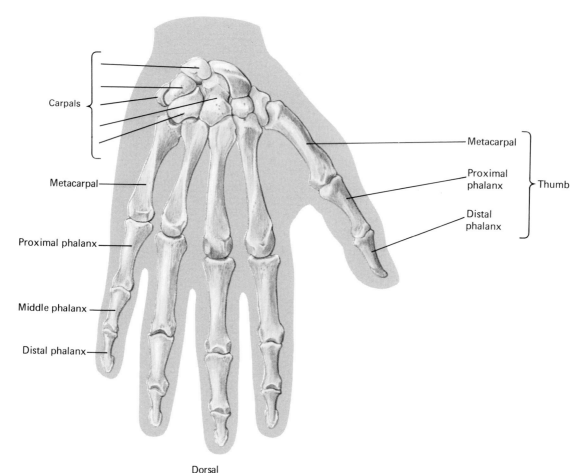

Carpals

Metacarpal

Proximal phalanx

Middle phalanx

Distal phalanx

Metacarpal

Proximal phalanx

Distal phalanx

Thumb

Dorsal

FIGURE **4–11** *The skeleton of the hand.*

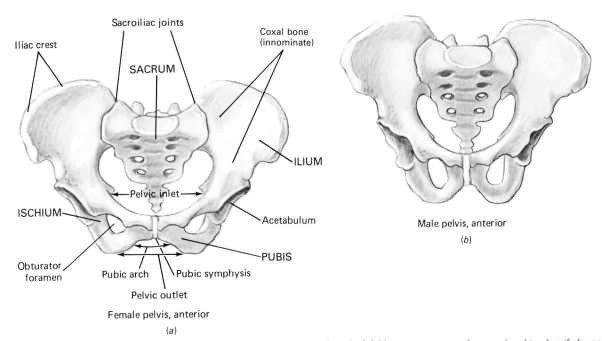

Iliac crest

Sacroiliac joints

SACRUM

Coxal bone
(innominate)

ILIUM

← Pelvic inlet →

ISCHIUM

Acetabulum

Obturator
foramen

PUBIS

Pubic arch

Pubic symphysis

Pelvic outlet

Female pelvis, anterior
(a)

Male pelvis, anterior
(b)

FIGURE 4–12 Generally, the male pelvis (b) is narrower than the female (a). However, some pelves are hard to classify by sex. In this illustration extreme examples are shown. In the adult, the ilium, ischium, and pubis are fused with one another and should be considered regions of the coxal bone rather than separate bones.

and a clavicle (collarbone). The pectoral girdles articulate with the sternum but not with the vertebral column.

THE UPPER LIMB CONSISTS OF 30 BONES

Each upper limb consists of 30 bones—the **humerus** (**hu′**-mer-us) in the upper arm, **ulna** (**ul′**-nuh) and **radius** (**ray′**-dee-us) in the forearm, **carpal** (**kar′**-pal) **bones** in the wrist, **metacarpals** in the palm of the hand, and **phalanges** (fay-**lan′**-jeez) in the fingers (Fig. 4–11).

THE PELVIC GIRDLE SUPPORTS THE LOWER LIMBS

The **pelvic girdle** is a broad basin of bone that encloses the pelvic cavity. The pelvic girdle supports the lower limbs and is the site of attachment of major muscles of the trunk and lower limbs. It supports the weight of the upper body and protects the organs that lie within the pelvic cavity—the reproductive organs, urinary bladder, and part of the large intestine. The hip bones are called **coxal bones** (also called os coxae or innominate bones). The coxal

bones, together with the sacrum and coccyx, form the pelvic girdle (Fig. 4–12).

Each coxal bone is formed from the fusion of three bones during development. The largest of the three, the **ilium,** lies on top of the other two bones. The most posterior bone is the **ischium** (**is′**-kee-um). The anterior bone is the **pubis.** In the adult, they are not separate bones, but are parts of the coxal bone. The joint where the coxal bones come together anteriorly is called the **pubic symphysis** (**sim′**-fih-sis).

The female pelvis is adapted for holding a developing baby and permitting its passage to the outside world at birth. Accordingly, it is broader and shallower than the male pelvis (Fig. 4–12). The pelvic inlet in the female is larger and more circular. The ischial spines of the female are shorter so there is a greater relative distance between them. The female pelvis also has a greater angle between the pubic bones.

THE LOWER LIMB CONSISTS OF 30 BONES

The lower limb consists of 30 bones—the **femur** (**fee′**-mer) in the upper leg, or thigh; the **patella** (pah-**tel′**-uh), or kneecap; the **tibia** (**tib′**-ee-ah)

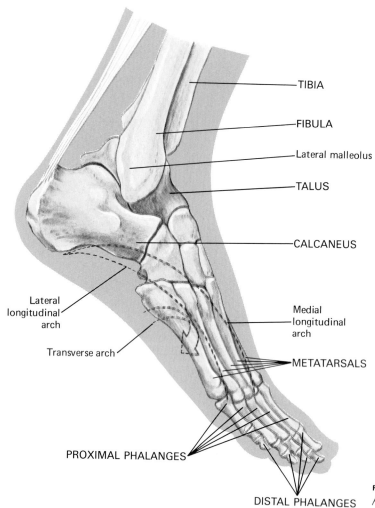

TIBIA

FIBULA

Lateral malleolus

TALUS

CALCANEUS

Lateral
longitudinal
arch

Medial
longitudinal
arch

Transverse arch

METATARSALS

PROXIMAL PHALANGES

DISTAL PHALANGES

Lateral

FIGURE 4–13 The bones of the right foot. As indicated in the figure, these bones form several arches.

and **fibula** (fib′-u-lah) in the lower leg, or shin; the **tarsal bones** in the back part of the foot and heel; the **metatarsals** in the main part of the foot; and the **phalanges** in the toes (Fig. 4–13).

JOINTS ARE JUNCTIONS BETWEEN BONES

A **joint,** or **articulation,** is the point of contact between two bones. Joints hold bones together and many of them permit flexibility and movement.

JOINTS CAN BE CLASSIFIED ACCORDING TO THE DEGREE OF MOVEMENT THEY PERMIT

Joints can be classified into three main groups according to the degree of movement they permit:

1. **Synarthroses** (sin″-ar-**throw**′-sees) do not permit movement. They connect bones by means of fibrous connective tissue. The sutures that join skull bones together are synarthroses (Fig. 4–14(a)).

2. **Amphiarthroses** (am″-fee-ar-**throw**′-sees) permit slight movement. In this type of joint, bones are joined by cartilage. The pubic symphysis of the pelvis and the intervertebral joints of the vertebral column are examples of amphiarthroses (Fig. 4–14(b)).

3. **Diarthroses** (die″-ar-**throw**′-sees), or **synovial joints,** are referred to as freely movable joints, but their flexibility varies. Most of the body's joints are diarthroses.

The six types of synovial joints are: gliding, condyloid, saddle, pivot, hinge, and ball-and-socket. These are described in Table 4–3 and are shown in Figure 4–14(c) and (d). Some of the types of movement at the joints are described and illustrated in Table 4–4.

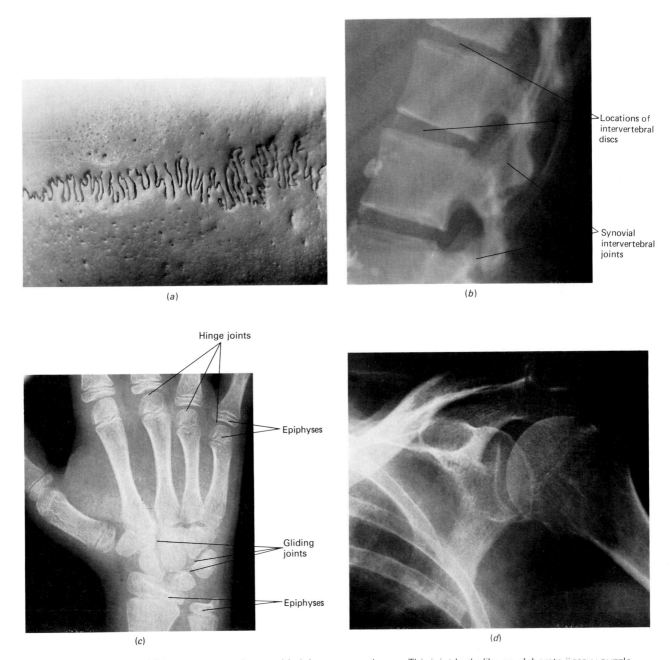

Locations of intervertebral discs

Synovial intervertebral joints

Hinge joints

Epiphyses

Gliding joints

Epiphyses

(a)   (b)   (c)   (d)

FIGURE **4–14** Joints. (a) Skull sutures are immovable joints, or synarthroses. This joint looks like an elaborate jigsaw puzzle. (b) Intervertebral joints are amphiarthroses, or slightly movable joints. (c) Synovial joints. Gliding joints between the wrist bones and hinge joints between the phalanges are synovial joints. (d) The shoulder joint, also a synovial joint, is a ball-and-socket joint. It is one of the most freely movable joints and also the loosest joint in the body. The shoulder joint is held together partly by the steady contraction of the surrounding muscles.

TABLE 4–3

Some types of synovial joints

TYPE	EXAMPLE	SHAPE OF JOINT SURFACE	RANGE OF MOVEMENT
Gliding	Carpal joints of wrist; tarsal joints of ankle	Flat or slightly curved	One bone glides over another without circular movement
Saddle	Carpometacarpal joint of thumb	Saddle-shaped	Permits wide range of movement
Pivot	Atlantoaxial joint of first 2 cervical vertebrae; radioulnar joint of elbow	Small projection of one bone pivots in ring-shaped socket of another bone	Rotation
Hinge	Elbow; knee	Convex surface of one bone fits into concave surface of another bone	Motion in one plane only; permits only flexion and extension
Ball-and-socket	Shoulder; hip joint	Ball-shaped end of one bone fits into cup-shaped socket of another bone	Permits widest range of movement, including rotation

TABLE 4–4

Types of body movements

MOVEMENT	DESCRIPTION	ILLUSTRATION
Flexion (**flek**'-shun)	Bending of joint; usually a movement that reduces angle of joint and brings two bones closer together (when you crouch, your knees are flexed; when you touch your shoulder, your elbow is flexed)	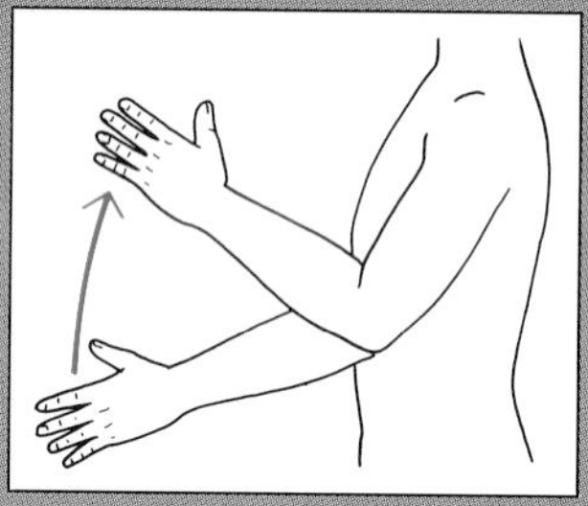
Extension	Opposite of flexion; increases angle of joint, increasing distance between two bones; examples of extension include straightening the knee or the elbow	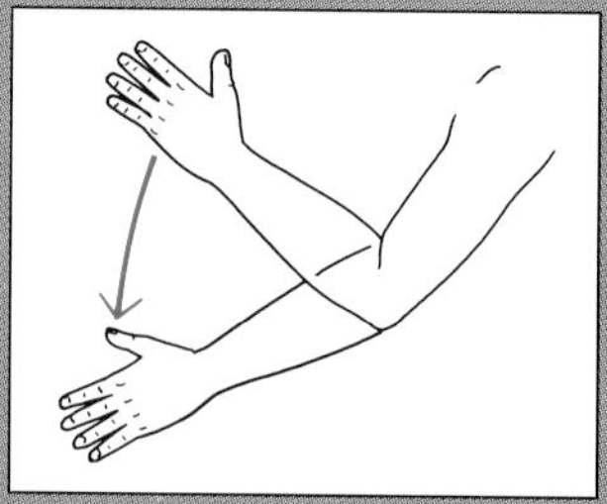
Abduction (ab-**duk**'-shun)	Movement of bone or limb away from midline, or median plane of body; abduction in hands and feet is movement of digit away from central axis of limb (one abducts fingers by spreading them apart)	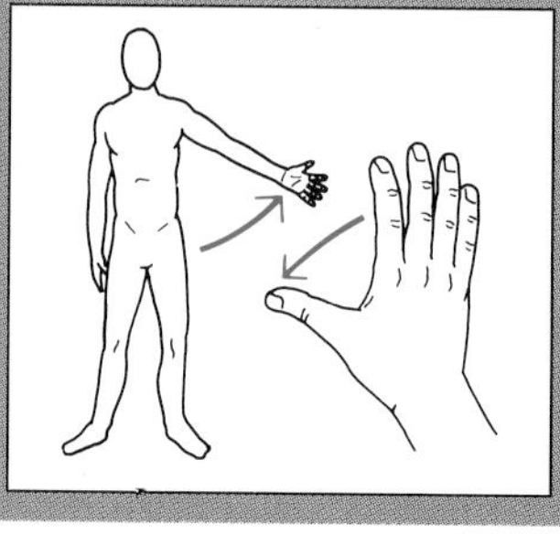

TABLE 4–4 *Continued*

Types of body movements

MOVEMENT	DESCRIPTION	ILLUSTRATION
Adduction	Movement of bone or limb toward the midline of body or, for extremities, movement toward axis of limb; opposite of abduction	
Circumduction (ser"-kum-**duk**'-shun)	Combination of movements that makes body part describe a circle; characteristic of ball-and-socket joints such as shoulder	
Rotation	Pivoting of body part around its axis, as in shaking the head "no"; no rotation of any body part is complete (i.e., 360 degrees)	
Pronation	Movement of forearm that in extended position brings palm of hand from upward-facing to downward-facing position; applies only to arm; this action moves distal end of radius across ulna	
Supination	Opposite of pronation; when forearm is in extended position, this movement brings palm of hand upward	
Inversion	Ankle movement that turns sole of foot medially; applies only to foot	Medial side

Table continued on following page

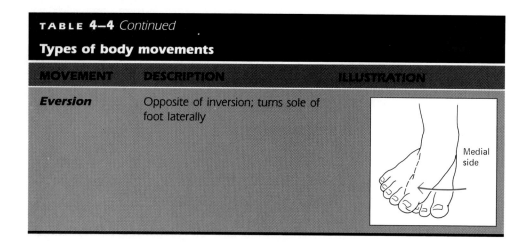

TABLE **4–4** Continued		
Types of body movements		
MOVEMENT	DESCRIPTION	ILLUSTRATION
Eversion	Opposite of inversion; turns sole of foot laterally	Medial side

A DIARTHROSIS IS SURROUNDED BY A JOINT CAPSULE

The ends of the bones forming a diarthrodial joint are covered with hyaline cartilage that lacks any sort of covering membrane. This articular cartilage also lacks nerves and blood vessels. The joint is surrounded by a connective tissue capsule, the **joint capsule,** made of tough fibrous connective tissue (Fig. 4–15). This tissue is continuous with the periosteum of the bones, but does not cover the articular cartilage. The joint capsule is generally reinforced with ligaments, bands of fibrous connective tissue

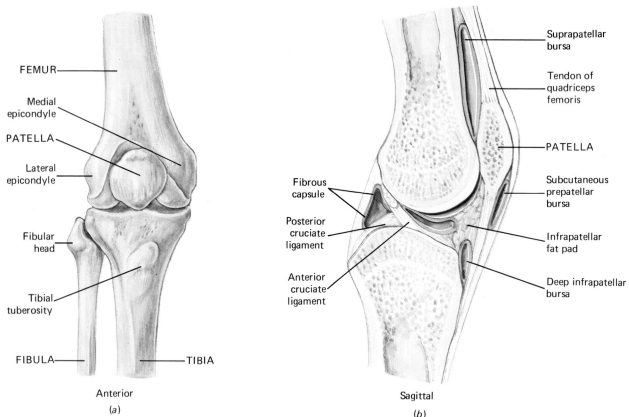

FIGURE **4–15** The knee joint is a complex synovial joint. *(a)* Anterior view of the knee joint. *(b)* Sagittal section of the knee joint.

that connect the bones and also limit movement at the joint. The joint capsule is lined with a membrane that secretes a lubricating **synovial fluid.**

Fluid-filled sacs called **bursae** are located be-tween bone and tendons and between bone and some other tissues. Bursae cushion the movement of bone over other tissues. Inflammation of a bursa is a painful condition known as bursitis.

SUMMARY

I. The skeletal system supports and protects the body, transmits muscular forces, produces blood cells, and stores calcium and phosphorus.
II. A long bone consists of a diaphysis (shaft) with flared ends called epiphyses. It has a central marrow cavity and is covered by a periosteum.
III. Compact bone consists of osteons; spongy bone consists of thin strands of bone. The spaces within spongy bone are filled with bone marrow.
IV. Endochondral bones develop from a cartilage model; intramembranous bones develop from a noncartilage connective tissue model.
V. Osteoblasts are cells that produce bone; osteoclasts break down bone.
VI. The axial skeleton consists of the skull, vertebral column, ribs, and sternum.
  A. The skull is formed by the cranial and facial bones. The cranial bones include the frontal, oc-cipital, ethmoid, sphenoid, and the paired parietal and temporal bones. The facial bones in-clude the maxilla, mandible, vomer, and the paired malars, palatines, nasals, lacrimals, and in-ferior turbinates.
  B. The vertebral column consists of 7 cervical vertebrae, 12 thoracic vertebrae, 5 lumbar verte-brae, the sacrum, and the coccyx.
    1. The first cervical vertebra is the atlas; the second is the axis.
    2. A typical vertebra consists of a centrum, lamina, vertebral foramen, transverse processes, and superior and inferior articular processes.
  C. The thoracic cage is formed by the sternum, thoracic vertebrae, and 12 pairs of ribs.
VII. The appendicular skeleton consists of the upper and lower limbs, the pectoral girdle, and the pelvic girdle.
  A. The pectoral girdle attaches the upper limbs to the axial skeleton; it consists of the scapulae and clavicles.
  B. Each upper limb consists of the humerus, ulna, radius, 8 carpal bones, 5 metacarpals, and 14 phalanges.
  C. The pelvic girdle consists of the coxal bones together with the sacrum and coccyx.
    1. Each coxal bone consists of three fused bones: an ilium, ischium, and pubis.
    2. The female pelvis is broader and shallower than the male pelvis; the pelvic inlet is larger and more circular.
  D. Each lower limb consists of a femur, tibia, fibula, 7 tarsal bones, 5 metatarsals, and 14 phalan-ges.
VIII. An articulation, or joint, is the junction between two or more bones.
  A. Synarthroses are immovable joints such as sutures in the skull.
  B. Amphiarthroses are slightly movable joints such as the pubic symphysis.
  C. Diarthroses, also called synovial joints, are movable joints. The body has several types of diarthroses. The ball-and-socket joint permits the greatest freedom of movement.
  D. In diarthroses, the articulating bone surfaces are covered with hyaline cartilage and are en-closed in a joint capsule. Ligaments are bands of fibrous connective tissue that bind bones together at joints.

POST TEST

1. The _____ within some bones produces blood cells.
2. Bone is covered by a connective tissue membrane, the _____

3. The main shaft of a long bone is its _____ .

4. Compact bone consists of spindle-shaped units called _____ .

5. Osteocytes are found in small cavities called _____ .

6. Osteoclasts are cells that _____ .

7. The skull and ribs are part of the _____ skeleton.

8. The skull consists of the _____ and _____ bones.

9. _____ are air spaces found in some of the cranial bones.

10. The vertebral foramen is a passageway for the _____ _____ .

11. The scapula is part of the _____ _____ .

12. The ribs are attached to the _____ vertebrae.

13. The bony central body of a vertebra is its _____ .

14. An example of an immovable joint is a cranial _____ .

15. _____ fluid is found in diarthroses.

16. The bending of a joint is known as _____ ; movement of a limb away from the midline of the body is _____ .

17. A joint, like the elbow joint, that moves in one plane only is a _____ joint.

Match
Select the most appropriate match in Column B for each item in Column A.

Column A	*Column B*
18. Lower jaw bone	a. atlas
19. Breastbone	b. mandible
20. Longest bone in body	c. calcaneus
21. Articulates with occipital condyles	d. sternum
22. Heelbone	e. femur
23. Contains sella turcica	f. humerus
24. Forms posterior part of hard palate	g. palatine
25. Label the diagrams.	h. sphenoid

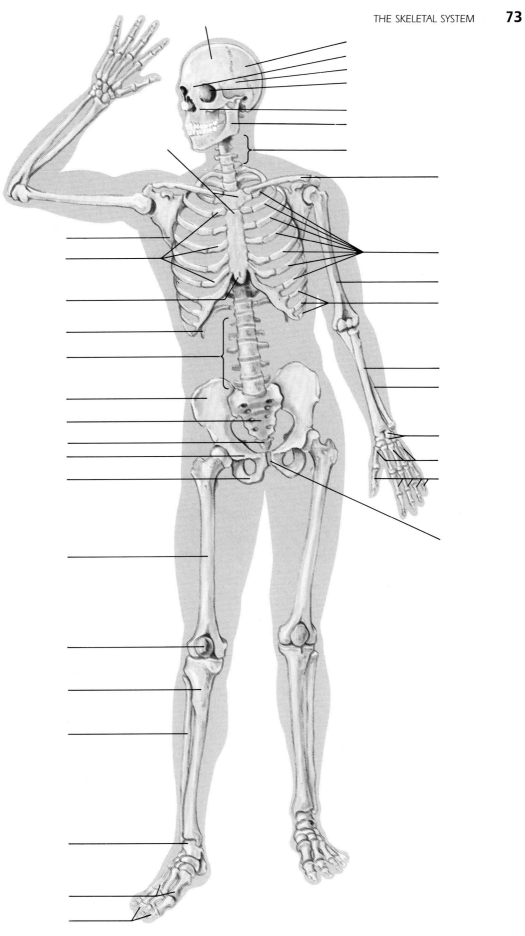

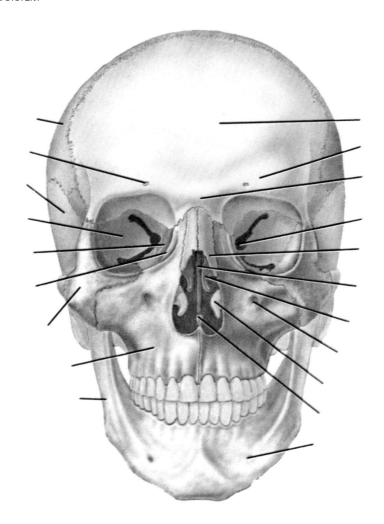

REVIEW QUESTIONS

1. What are the functions of the skeletal system? How does the skeletal system help maintain homeostasis?

2. Compare spongy bone with compact bone.

3. How does the development of a skull bone differ from the development of a long bone such as the femur?

4. How do osteoblasts and osteoclasts function together in bone remodeling?

5. Describe the structure of the vertebral column. What are the advantages of a curved vertebral column rather than a straight one?

6. Where is the vertebral foramen? Why is it important?

7. Locate the following and give their functions: (a) sella turcica; (b) cribriform plate; (c) occipital condyles; (d) temporomandibular joint.

8. Locate each of the following: (a) metacarpals; (b) malar; (c) palatine; (d) axis.

9. How do false ribs differ from true ribs? How many pairs of ribs are there in a male? In a female?

10. Contrast the three main types of joints. What are ligaments? What are bursae?

11. What are the functions of: (a) condyles; (b) foramina; (c) facets?

POST TEST ANSWERS

1. marrow
2. periosteum
3. diaphysis
4. osteons
5. lacunae
6. break down bone
7. axial
8. cranial; facial
9. Sinuses
10. spinal cord
11. pectoral girdle
12. thoracic
13. centrum
14. suture
15. Synovial
16. flexion; abduction
17. hinge
18. b
19. d
20. e
21. a
22. c
23. h
24. g
25. see Figures 4–3 and 4–5

Five

THE MUSCULAR SYSTEM

CHAPTER OUTLINE

    I. Each skeletal muscle is an organ
    II. Muscle fibers are specialized for contraction
    III. Muscle contraction occurs when actin and myosin filaments slide past each other
    IV. ATP provides energy for muscle contraction
    V. Muscle tone is a state of partial contraction
    VI. Two types of contraction are isotonic and isometric
    VII. Muscles work antagonistically to one another
    VIII. We can study muscles in functional groups

LEARNING OBJECTIVES

After you have studied this chapter, you should be able to:
1. Describe the structure of a skeletal muscle.
2. Relate the structure of a muscle fiber to its function.
3. Trace the sequence of events that occur during muscle contraction.
4. Identify ATP as the source of energy for muscle contraction and identify the source of energy for making ATP.
5. Define muscle tone and explain why muscle tone is important.
6. Distinguish between isotonic and isometric contraction.
7. Explain how muscles work antagonistically to one another.
8. Locate and give the actions of the principal muscles as indicated in Table 5–1.

Walking, talking, chewing food, circulating blood—all body movements depend upon the action of muscles. The three types of muscles—skeletal, smooth, and cardiac—were compared in Chapter 2 (Table 2–3). In this chapter we will focus on skeletal muscle, the voluntary muscles attached to bones. About 600 skeletal muscles working together permit us to carry on our daily activities and to move effectively through our world.

EACH SKELETAL MUSCLE IS AN ORGAN

A skeletal muscle is an organ composed of hundreds of muscle cells, or **fibers.** The muscle has a nerve supply and a system of blood vessels that supply it with nutrients and oxygen and carry away its wastes. Each muscle is surrounded by a covering of connective tissue called the **epimysium** (ep″-ih-**mis′**-ee-um) (Fig. 5–1). The muscle fibers are arranged in bundles known as **fascicles** (**fas′**-ih-kuls). Each fascicle is wrapped by connective tissue, the **perimysium** (per″-ih-**mis′**-ee-um). Finally, individual muscle fibers are surrounded by a connective tissue covering, the **endomysium** (end″-o-**mis′**-ee-um).

The epimysium, perimysium, and endomysium are continuous with one another. Extensions of epimysium form tough cords of connective tissue, the **tendons,** that anchor muscles to bones.

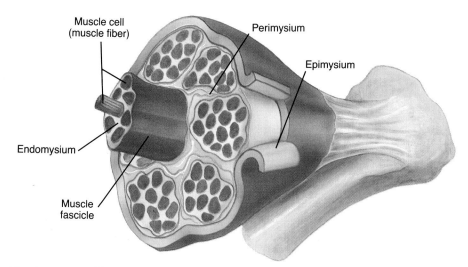

FIGURE 5–1 *Muscle structure. The muscle consists of bundles of muscle fibers called fascicles. Each fascicle is wrapped in connective tissue, the perimysium. Individual muscle fibers are surrounded by endomysium.*

MUSCLE FIBERS ARE SPECIALIZED FOR CONTRACTION

Each muscle fiber is a spindle-shaped cell with many nuclei. The plasma membrane has many inward extensions that form a set of transverse tubules (T tubules). Each muscle fiber is almost filled with tiny protein threads, or **filaments.** Thick filaments, called **myosin** (**my′**-o-sin) **filaments,** consist mainly of the protein myosin. Thin filaments, called **actin filaments,** consist of the protein actin. Myosin and actin are contractile proteins; this means they are capable of shortening. The myosin and actin filaments are largely responsible for muscle contraction.

Myosin and actin filaments are arranged lengthwise in the muscle fibers so they overlap. Their overlapping produces a pattern of bands, or **striations;** skeletal and cardiac muscles are both striated.

MUSCLE CONTRACTION OCCURS WHEN ACTIN AND MYOSIN FILAMENTS SLIDE PAST EACH OTHER

Body movement generally occurs when muscles pull on bones. A muscle pulls on a bone by contracting, or shortening. A muscle contracts when its fibers (cells) contract. Muscle fibers contract when the actin and myosin filaments actively pull themselves past and between one another.

A **motor nerve** is a nerve that controls muscle contraction. Nerve fibers (neurons) from a motor nerve transmit impulses (messages) to muscle fibers (Fig. 5–2). Each nerve fiber controls from one to several hundred muscle fibers. The junction of a nerve and muscle fiber is called a neuromuscular junction (or motor end plate). We can summarize the process of muscle contraction as follows:

1. A motor neuron releases a compound known as **acetylcholine** (as″-eh-til-**koe′**-lin).

2. The acetylcholine diffuses across the neuromuscular junction and combines with receptors on the surface of the muscle cell. This triggers an impulse (an electric current) that spreads over the plasma membrane of the muscle cell. The electric current generated is known as an **action potential.** Excess acetylcholine is broken down by an enzyme called **cholinesterase** (ko″-lin-**es′**-ter-ase).

3. The impulse spreads through the T tubules and stimulates the release of calcium.

4. The calcium stimulates the myosin and actin filaments to slide past each other in such a way that the muscle shortens. This movement of the filaments requires energy.

ATP PROVIDES ENERGY FOR MUSCLE CONTRACTION

The immediate source of energy for muscle contraction comes from the energy storage molecule, **ATP.** Muscle cells are often called upon to perform strenuously and must be provided with large amounts of energy. Large amounts of ATP cannot be stored. After the first few seconds of strenuous activ-

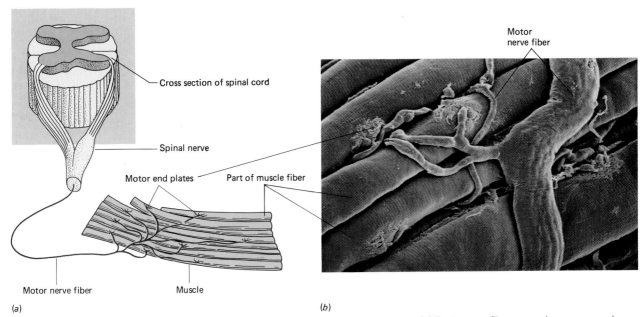

Cross section of spinal cord

Spinal nerve

Motor end plates   Part of muscle fiber

Motor nerve fiber   Muscle

Motor
nerve fiber

(a)   (b)

FIGURE 5–2   Nerve fibers from a motor nerve transmit impulses to muscle fibers. (a) Each nerve fiber controls many muscle fibers. (b) Photomicrograph of neuromuscular junctions (×100) (Ed Reschki/Peter Arnold.)

ity, ATP supplies are used up. To solve this problem, muscle cells also have an energy storage compound known as **creatine phosphate.** This compound can be stockpiled, and its stored energy is transferred to ATP as needed.

During vigorous exercise, the supply of creatine phosphate is soon used up. As ATP and creatine phosphate stores are depleted, muscle cells must replenish their supply of these high-energy compounds.

The energy for making creatine phosphate and ATP comes from fuel molecules. Glucose, a simple sugar, is stored in muscle cells in the form of a large molecule called glycogen. As needed, glycogen is degraded, yielding glucose, which is then broken down in cellular respiration. When sufficient oxygen is available, enough energy is captured from the glucose to produce needed quantities of ATP.

During strenuous exercise sufficient oxygen may not be available to meet the needs of the rapidly metabolizing muscle cells. Under these conditions muscle cells are capable of breaking down fuel anaerobically (without oxygen) for short periods of time. However, anaerobic metabolism does not yield very much ATP. The depletion of ATP results in weaker contractions, and **muscle fatigue.**

A waste product, called **lactic acid,** is produced during anaerobic metabolism of glucose. Lactic acid buildup contributes to muscle fatigue. During muscle exertion an **oxygen debt** develops. The oxygen debt is paid back during the period of rapid breathing that typically follows strenuous exercise.

MUSCLE TONE IS A STATE OF PARTIAL CONTRACTION

Even when we are not moving, our muscles are in a state of partial contraction known as **muscle tone.** Messages from nerve cells continuously stimulate muscle fibers so that some fibers are contracted at any given moment. Muscle tone is an unconscious process that helps keep muscles prepared for action. Muscle tone is also responsible for helping the muscles of the abdominal wall hold the internal organs in place and for helping our muscles keep us upright. When the motor nerve to a muscle is cut, the muscle becomes limp, or flaccid.

TWO TYPES OF CONTRACTION ARE ISOTONIC AND ISOMETRIC

When you lift a heavy object or bend your elbow, muscles shorten and thicken as they contract. Muscle tone remains the same. We usually think of muscle contraction in terms of this type of contraction, called **isotonic contraction.** However, if you push against a table or wall, no movement results. Muscle length does not appreciably change, but muscle tension may increase greatly. This type of muscle contraction is referred to as **isometric contraction** (Fig. 5–3).

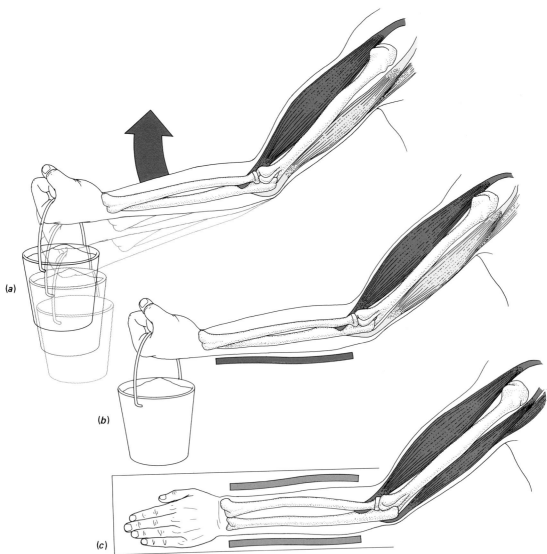

FIGURE 5–3 Isotonic and isometric exercise. *(a)* Isotonic exercise. The force of muscle contraction is greater than the opposing force of the weight. The muscle shortens, pulling the forearm toward it. *(b)* and *(c)* Two forms of isometric exercise. The force of muscle contraction is met by an equal opposing force. The muscle cannot shorten and no movement occurs. However, the tension within the muscle is great.

MUSCLES WORK ANTAGONISTICALLY TO ONE ANOTHER

Muscles can only pull; they cannot push. Skeletal muscles produce movements by pulling on tendons, which in turn pull on bones. Most muscles pass across a joint and are attached to the bones that form the joint. When the muscle contracts it draws one bone toward or away from the bone with which it articulates. The attachment of the muscle to the less movable bone is called its **origin.** The attachment of the muscle to the more movable bone is its **insertion.**

When you flex your elbow, your biceps contracts, pulling the radius (and thus, your forearm) upward so that you can touch your shoulder (Fig. 5–4). Your biceps cannot push your radius back down, however. To move your forearm down again, the triceps muscle contracts pulling on the ulna. Thus, the biceps and triceps work **antagonistically** to one another. What one does, the other can undo.

The muscle that contracts to produce a particular action is known as the **agonist,** or **prime mover.** The muscle that produces the opposite movement is the **antagonist.** When the agonist is contracting, the antagonist is relaxed. Generally, movements are accomplished by groups of muscles working together so several agonists and several antagonists may take part in any action. Note that muscles that are agonists in one movement may be antagonists in another.

Synergists and fixators are muscles that help the agonist by reducing unnecessary movement. Synergists stabilize joints so that undesirable movement does not occur. Fixators stabilize the origin of an agonist so that its force is fully directed upon the bone on which it inserts. Several common shapes of muscles are shown in Fig. 5–5.

WE CAN STUDY MUSCLES IN FUNCTIONAL GROUPS

Many of the superficial muscles are shown in Figures 5–6 and 5–7. Every muscle is important, but including them all is beyond the scope of this book. Instead, we have selected some functional groups of muscles and present them in Table 5–1 along with their actions, origins, and insertions. (Also see Figures 5–8 through 5–10.)

Text continued on page 88

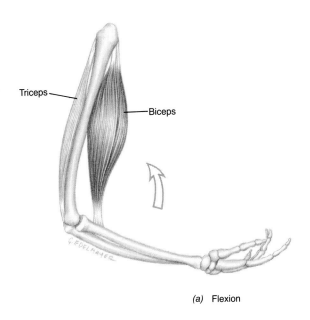

(a) Flexion

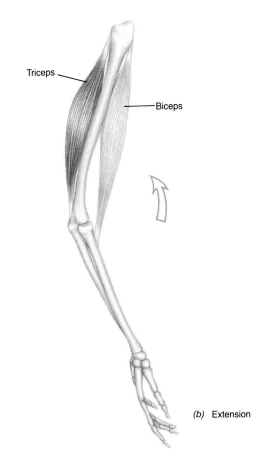

(b) Extension

FIGURE 5–4 *The antagonistic arrangement of the biceps and triceps muscles. (a) In flexion, the biceps is the agonist and the triceps the antagonist. (b) In extension, the triceps is the agonist, and the biceps is the antagonist.*

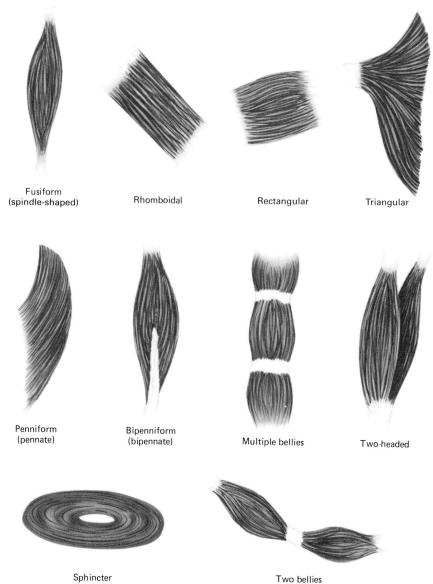

Fusiform
(spindle-shaped)

Rhomboidal

Rectangular

Triangular

Penniform
(pennate)

Bipenniform
(bipennate)

Multiple bellies

Two-headed

Sphincter

Two bellies

FIGURE 5–5 Some common muscle shapes.

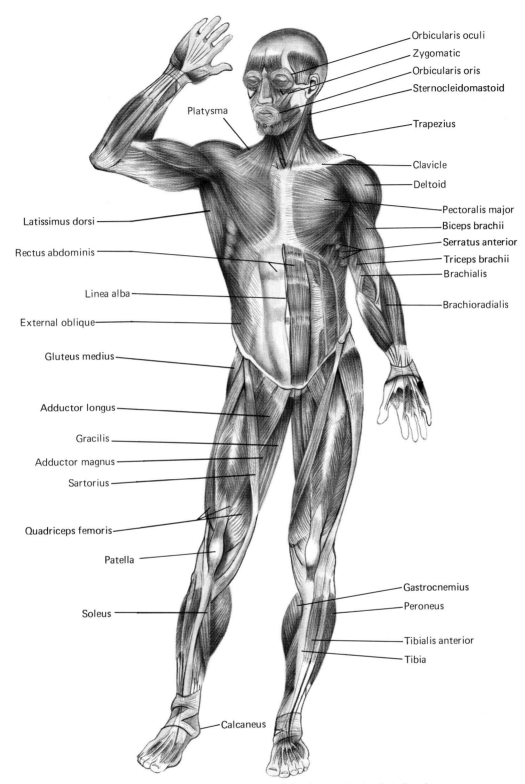

Orbicularis oculi
Zygomatic
Orbicularis oris
Sternocleidomastoid
Trapezius
Clavicle
Deltoid
Pectoralis major
Biceps brachii
Serratus anterior
Triceps brachii
Brachialis
Brachioradialis

Platysma
Latissimus dorsi
Rectus abdominis
Linea alba
External oblique
Gluteus medius
Adductor longus
Gracilis
Adductor magnus
Sartorius
Quadriceps femoris
Patella
Soleus
Calcaneus

Gastrocnemius
Peroneus
Tibialis anterior
Tibia

FIGURE 5–6 Superficial muscles of the human body. Anterior view.

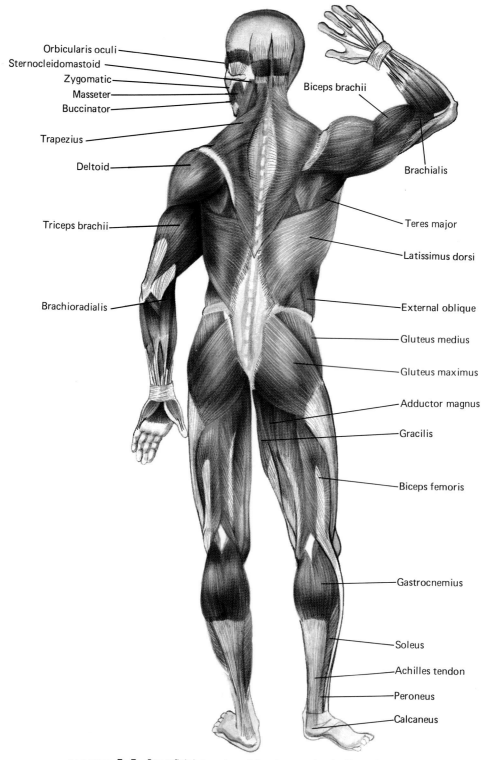

Orbicularis oculi

Sternocleidomastoid

Zygomatic

Masseter

Buccinator

Trapezius

Deltoid

Triceps brachii

Brachioradialis

Biceps brachii

Brachialis

Teres major

Latissimus dorsi

External oblique

Gluteus medius

Gluteus maximus

Adductor magnus

Gracilis

Biceps femoris

Gastrocnemius

Soleus

Achilles tendon

Peroneus

Calcaneus

FIGURE 5–7 Superficial muscles of the human body. Posterior view.

TABLE 5-1

Selected muscles—functionally grouped

MUSCLE	ACTION	ORIGIN	INSERTION
Facial Muscles			
Orbicularis oculi (or-bik"-u-**lar**'-is **ok**'-u-li)	Closes eyes; these are sphincter muscles of eyelids	Frontal bone; maxilla	Eyelids
Frontalis (fron-**tal**'-is)	Raises brows; moves entire scalp backwards	Occipital	Skin of scalp and face
Orbicularis oris	Closes lips; protrudes lips	Tissue around lips	Lips
Zygomatic (zy-go-**mat**'-ik)	Elevates upper corners of mouth	Malar (zygomatic)	Corners of mouth

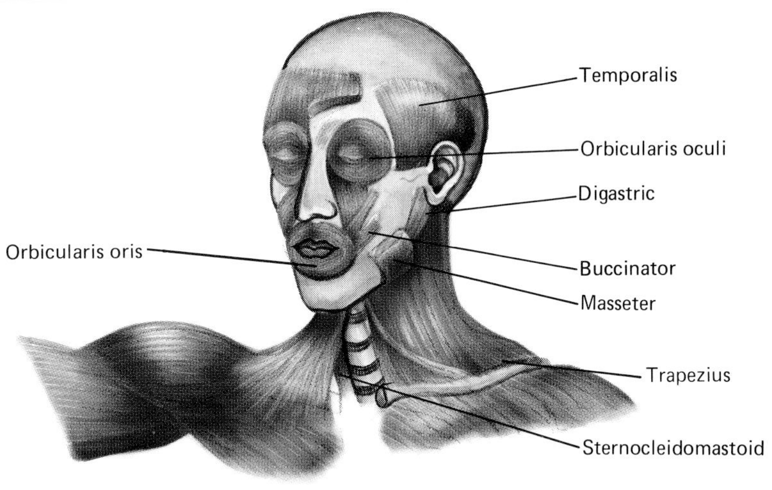

FIGURE 5-8 Some muscles of the head and anterior neck.

MUSCLE	ACTION	ORIGIN	INSERTION
Chewing Muscles			
Digastric (di-**gas**'-trik)	Opens mouth; can elevate hyoid	Mastoid process of temporal	Hyoid; mandible
Buccinator (**buk**'-sih-nay"-tor)	Flattens cheek (as in whistling)	Lateral side of mandible	Maxilla
Masseter (mas-**see**'-ter)	Raises jaw; mastication	Maxilla (zygomatic arch)	Ramus of mandible
Temporalis (tem-po-**ra**'-lis)	Raises jaw; mastication	Temporal bone	Coronoid process of mandible
Muscles of the Head and Trunk			
Sternocleidomastoid (ster-no-kly-do-**mas**'-toid) (paired)	Contraction of both muscles flexes neck; contractions of one muscle rotates head to opposite side	Sternum and clavicle	Mastoid process of occipital

Table continued on following page

TABLE 5–1

Selected muscles—functionally grouped

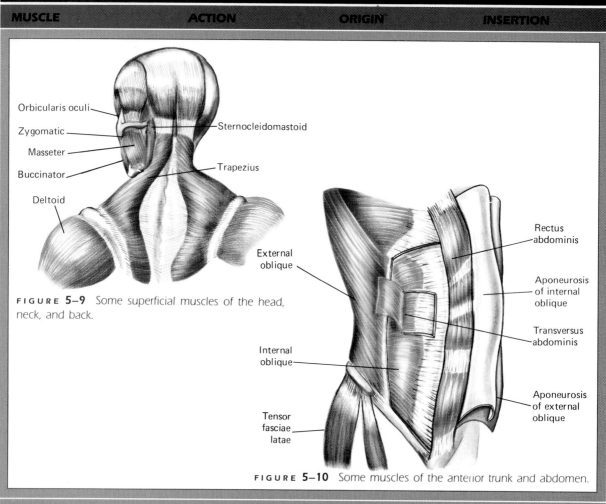

FIGURE 5–9 Some superficial muscles of the head, neck, and back.

FIGURE 5–10 Some muscles of the anterior trunk and abdomen.

Muscles of the Head and Trunk

MUSCLE	ACTION	ORIGIN	INSERTION
Trapezius (trah-**pee**'-zee-us) (paired)	Adducts scapula and rotates it; draws shoulder upward; extends, bends neck	Occipital bone and thoracic vertebrae	Scapula
External oblique	Contain the abdominal viscera; increase intraabdominal pressure (as in defecation); contraction of both compresses abdomen; contraction of one side bends vertebral column laterally	Lateral surface of lower 8 ribs	Linea alba (midline connective tissue), iliac crest
Transversus abdominis	Compresses abdominal contents	Cartilages of lower 6 ribs; iliac crest	Linea alba, pubis, xiphoid process
Rectus abdominis	Flexes trunk; compresses abdominal contents	Pubis	Xiphoid process of sternum and costal cartilages of ribs 5 to 7

TABLE 5–1 *Continued*

Selected muscles—functionally grouped

MUSCLE	ACTION	ORIGIN	INSERTION
Muscles of the Head and Trunk			
Pectoralis minor	Pulls scapula forward and downward	Ribs 2 to 5	Coracoid process of scapula
Serratus (ser-**ray**'-tus) anterior	Pulls scapula forward and downward	Upper 8 ribs	Scapula
Muscles Used in Breathing			
External intercostals	Elevate ribs	Inferior borders of ribs	Superior borders of ribs
Internal intercostals	Depress ribs	Inferior borders of ribs	Superior borders of ribs
Diaphragm	Increases volume of chest cavity	Xiphoid process, internal surfaces of lower 6 ribs, and first 3 lumbar vertebrae	Central tendon
Muscles That Move the Arm			
Pectoralis (pek-to-**ray**'-lis) major	Adducts, rotates arm medially	Clavicle, sternum	Humerus
Teres major	Adducts, rotates arm medially	Scapula	Humerus
Latissimus (lah-**tis**'-i-mus) dorsi	Adducts, rotates arm medially; lowers shoulder	Spines of thoracic vertebrae; ilium, ribs	Humerus
Deltoid	Abducts upper arm	Clavicle, scapula	Humerus
Muscles That Move the Forearm			
Biceps brachii (**bray**'-kee-i)	Flexes elbow; supinates forearm	Scapula	Radius
Brachialis	Flexes elbow	Humerus	Ulna
Brachioradialis	Flexes elbow	Humerus	Radius
Triceps brachii	Extends elbow	Scapula, humerus	Ulna
Muscles That Move the Thigh			
Iliacus	Flexes and rotates thigh	Ilium	Femur
Gluteus maximus (**gloo**'-te-us **mak**'-si-mus)	Extends and rotates thigh laterally; tilts pelvis	Sacrum, coccyx, ilium	Femur
Gluteus medius	Abducts, rotates thigh medially	Ilium	Femur
Gluteus minimus	Abducts, rotates thigh laterally	Ilium	Femur
Abductor longus and magnus	Adducts, flexes, rotates thigh	Symphysis pubis; pubis, ischium	Femur

Table continued on following page

TABLE 5–1 *Continued*

Selected muscles—functionally grouped

MUSCLE	ACTION	ORIGIN	INSERTION
Muscles That Move the Thigh			
Gracilis	Adducts thigh; flexes knee	Pubis	Tibia
Muscles That Move the Leg			
Sartorius	Flexes knee and thigh; abducts, rotates thigh laterally	Ilium	Tibia
Quadriceps femoris (**kwod**'-re-seps **fem**'-or-is)	Extends leg at knee	Ilium, femur	Tibia
Biceps femoris	Flexes knee; extends thigh	Ischium, femur	Tibia, fibula
Muscles That Move the Foot and Ankle			
Tibialis anterior (tib-ee-**a**'-lis)	Dorsiflexes foot	Tibia	Metatarsals
Peroneus (per-o-**nee**'-us)	Plantarflexes and everts foot	Fibula, tibia	Metatarsals
Gastrocnemius (gas-trok-**nee**'-me-us)	Plantarflexes foot; flexes knee	Femur	Calcaneus
Soleus (**so**'-lee-us)	Plantarflexes foot	Tibia, fibula	Calcaneus

SUMMARY

I. A skeletal muscle consists of hundreds of fibers arranged in fascicles.
  A. Each fiber is wrapped in an endomysium.
  B. The fascicle is surrounded by perimysium, and the entire muscle is covered by epimysium.
II. Each muscle fiber contains thick myosin and thin actin filaments; these filaments are largely responsible for muscle contraction.
III. Muscle contraction occurs when the actin and myosin filaments slide past one another.
  A. A muscle fiber is signaled to contract by acetylcholine released by a motor nerve.
  B. The acetylcholine generates an action potential in the muscle fiber.
  C. The action potential spreads through the T tubules and stimulates the release of calcium ions.
  D. The calcium stimulates the actin filaments and myosin filaments to slide past one another.
IV. The immediate source of energy for muscle contraction is ATP.
  A. Creatine phosphate is an energy storage compound; its energy can be transferred to ATP.
  B. Fuel molecules such as glucose provide the energy for making creatine phosphate and ATP.
  C. During vigorous exercise muscle cells can break down glucose without oxygen (that is, anaerobically); a waste product called lactic acid is produced and can cause muscle fatigue.
V. Muscle tone is the state of partial contraction that keeps muscle prepared for action.
VI. In isotonic contraction, muscles shorten and thicken as they contract; in isometric contraction, muscle length does not change much, but muscle tension may increase greatly.
VII. Muscles work antagonistically to one another. The muscle that contracts to produce a particular action is the agonist; the muscle that produces the opposite action is the antagonist.
VIII. Use Table 5–1 to review the functional groups of muscles in the body.

POST TEST

1. Muscle cells are referred to as muscle _____ .
2. The _____ is the connective tissue covering around the muscle.
3. Cords of connective tissue that connect muscles to bones are called _____ .
4. Thick filaments consist mainly of the protein _____ ; thin filaments consist of _____ .
5. A muscle is stimulated to contract by acetylcholine released by a _____ _____ .
6. The action potential stimulates the release of _____ .
7. The immediate source of energy for muscle contraction is _____ .
8. Creatine phosphate is a compound that stores _____ .
9. The state of partial contraction that exists in a muscle even when we are not moving it is called _____ _____ .
10. A muscle that opposes an agonist is called an _____ .
11. Synergists are muscles that stabilize _____ .

Match
Select the most appropriate match from Column B for each item in Column A. You may use an answer once, more than once, or not at all.

Column A
12. Used in chewing
13. Extends thigh
14. Flexes trunk
15. Extends elbow
16. Extends leg at knee
17. Plantarflexes foot
18. Abducts upper arm

Column B
a. triceps brachii
b. gluteus maximus
c. quadriceps femoris
d. masseter
e. rectus abdominis
f. deltoid
g. gastrocnemius

19. Label the diagram on the following page.

REVIEW QUESTIONS

1. We can think of each muscle as an organ. Explain why.
2. What are actin and myosin filaments? Why are they important?
3. What are the functions of: (a) acetylcholine; (b) creatine phosphate; (c) glycogen?
4. List the steps in muscle contraction.
5. What happens when the motor nerve to a muscle is cut?
6. Give an example of the antagonistic action of muscles.
7. List four abdominal muscles. What are their functions?
8. Which muscles function in breathing?
9. Identify two muscles that move the arm; identify three muscles that move the forearm.

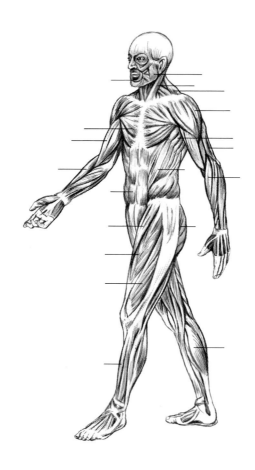

POST TEST ANSWERS

1. fibers
2. epimysium
3. tendons
4. myosin; actin
5. motor nerve
6. calcium
7. ATP
8. energy
9. muscle tone
10. antagonist

11. joints
12. d
13. b
14. e
15. a
16. c
17. g
18. f
19. see Figures 5–6 and 5–7

Six

THE CENTRAL NERVOUS SYSTEM

CHAPTER OUTLINE

   I. The nervous system consists of central nervous system and peripheral nervous system
  II. Neurons and glial cells are the cells of the nervous system
 III. Bundles of axons make up nerves
 IV. Neural function includes reception, transmission, integration, and response
  V. The human brain is the most complex mechanism known
     A. The medulla contains vital centers
     B. The pons is a bridge to other parts of the brain
     C. The midbrain contains centers for visual and auditory reflexes
     D. The diencephalon includes the thalamus and hypothalamus
     E. The cerebellum is responsible for coordination of movement
     F. The cerebrum is the largest part of the brain
        1. The cerebrum is divided into hemispheres
        2. White matter of the cerebrum consists of myelinated neurons
        3. The cerebrum has sensory, motor, and association functions
        4. Lobes of the cerebrum specialize in specific functions
 VI. The spinal cord transmits information to and from the brain
VII. The central nervous system is well protected
     A. The meninges are connective tissue coverings
     B. The cerebrospinal fluid cushions the CNS
VIII. A reflex action is a simple neural response

LEARNING OBJECTIVES

After you have studied this chapter, you should be able to:

1. List the divisions of the nervous system.
2. Draw a neuron, label its parts, and give the functions of each.
3. Distinguish between nerve and tract; ganglion and nucleus.
4. Briefly describe the four basic processes on which all neural responses depend—reception, transmission, integration, and response.
5. Label on a diagram the structures of the brain described in this chapter.
6. Describe the structure and functions of the main parts of the brain: medulla, pons, midbrain, diencephalon (thalamus and hypothalamus), cerebellum, cerebrum.
7. Name the principal areas and functions associated with the lobes of the cerebrum.
8. List two functions of the spinal cord and describe its structure.
9. Describe the structures that protect the brain and spinal cord.
10. Diagram a withdrawal reflex, identifying the essential structures and indicating the direction of impulse transmission.

The nervous system coordinates the activities of the other body systems so the body functions smoothly. The nervous system also serves as the body's link with the outside world. This system enables us to detect stimuli (changes within the body or in the outside world) and to respond to them. Together with the endocrine system, the nervous system works continuously to preserve homeostasis.

THE NERVOUS SYSTEM CONSISTS OF CENTRAL NERVOUS SYSTEM AND PERIPHERAL NERVOUS SYSTEM

The two principal divisions of the nervous system are the **central nervous system (CNS)** and the **peripheral nervous system (PNS)** (Fig. 6–1). The CNS consists of the brain and spinal cord. Serving as a control center for the entire organism, these organs integrate incoming information and determine appropriate responses.

The PNS is made up of the sense organs—the eyes, ears, taste buds, olfactory receptors, and touch receptors—and the nerves, which are the communication lines to and from the CNS. Twelve pairs of **cranial nerves** link the brain, and 31 pairs of **spinal nerves** link the spinal cord with sense organs, muscles, and other parts of the body. The nerves continually inform the CNS of changing conditions and then transmit its "decisions" to appropriate muscles and glands that make the adjustments needed to preserve homeostasis.

For convenience the PNS may be subdivided into **somatic** and **autonomic** divisions. Receptors and nerves concerned with changes in the outside environment are somatic; those that regulate the internal environment are autonomic. Both systems have **afferent nerves,** also called sensory nerves, that transmit messages from receptors to the CNS and **efferent nerves,** also called motor nerves, that transmit information back from the CNS back to the structures that must respond. The autonomic system has two kinds of efferent pathways—sympathetic and parasympathetic nerves. These will be discussed in Chapter 7.

NEURONS AND GLIAL CELLS ARE THE CELLS OF THE NERVOUS SYSTEM

Cell types unique to nervous tissue are glial cells and neurons. **Glial cells** protect and support the neu-

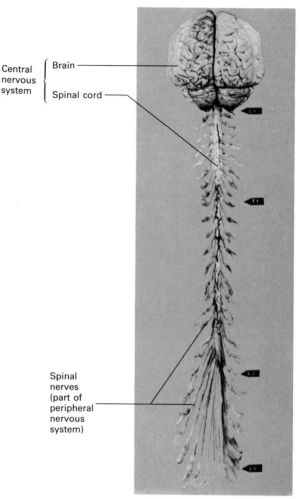

FIGURE 6–1 The brain and spinal cord with attached spinal nerve roots, photographed from the posterior aspect. The nerves that extend caudally from the lower region of the cord have been fanned out on the left. (Dissection by Dr. M.C.E. Hutchinson, Department of Anatomy, Guy's Hospital Medical School, London. From Williams, P., and Warwick, R. (eds.): Gray's Anatomy, 36th ed. Edinburgh, Churchill Livingstone, 1980.)

rons. **Neurons** are highly specialized to receive and transmit messages in the form of neural impulses. The neuron is distinguished from all other cells by its fibers, long threadlike extensions of the cytoplasm. The nucleus and most of the organelles are contained in the main part of the cell, the **cell body** (Fig. 6–2).

The two types of nerve fibers are dendrites and axons. **Dendrites** (**den'**-drites) are highly branched fibers that project from the cell body. Dendrites are specialized to *receive* neural impulses. The single **axon** (**ax'**-ahn) transmits neural messages *from* the cell body toward another neuron (or toward a muscle or gland). At its distal end the axon branches extensively. These branches have tiny enlargements called synaptic knobs. The synaptic knobs re-

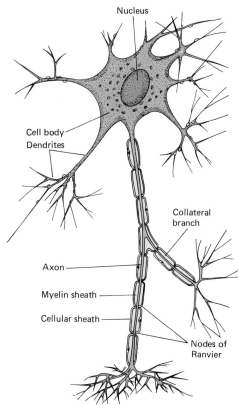

Nucleus

Cell body
Dendrites

Collateral
branch

Axon

Myelin sheath

Cellular sheath

Nodes of
Ranvier

F I G U R E **6–2** Structure of a neuron. The axon of this neuron is myelinated, and therefore the myelin sheath is shown as well as the cellular sheath. Cellular sheaths are found only around axons of peripheral neurons.

lease **neurotransmitters** (new-row-**trans′**-mit-ers), chemical substances that transmit impulses from one neuron to another.

Axons of many neurons of the PNS are covered by two sheaths—an inner **myelin** (**my′**-eh-lin) **sheath** and an outer **cellular sheath** or neurilemma. The cellular sheath is important in the repair of injured neurons. Myelin, a white, fatty substance, is an excellent electrical insulator that speeds the conduction of nerve impulses. Myelin is responsible for the white color of the white matter of the brain and spinal cord and of myelinated peripheral nerves. In the disease multiple sclerosis, patches of myelin deteriorate at irregular intervals along neurons in the CNS. The myelin is replaced by glial cells that form a hard matrix around the neurons. Such neurons are not able to conduct impulses effectively, and neural function is impaired.

BUNDLES OF AXONS MAKE UP NERVES

A **nerve** is a large bundle of axons wrapped in connective tissue. We can compare a nerve to a telephone cable. The axons are like the individual wires,

and the myelin, cellular, and connective tissue sheaths are like the insulation. The cell bodies attached to the axons of a nerve are often grouped together in a mass known as a **ganglion.** Many ganglia are located just outside the spinal cord.

Within the CNS, bundles of axons are known as **tracts** or **pathways** instead of nerves. Masses of cell bodies are referred to as **nuclei** rather than ganglia.

NEURAL FUNCTION INCLUDES RECEPTION, TRANSMISSION, INTEGRATION AND RESPONSE

Imagine that you are driving down the street and the traffic light on the corner ahead turns red. Automatically you step on the brake and bring your vehicle to a smooth stop. Each day you make hundreds of such responses. The following processes are involved in even very simple responses.

1. **Reception.** First, you must receive the information that the traffic light has turned red. This process is called reception. In this example the information that the light is red is received by visual receptors in the eyes.

2. **Transmission.** The information must be delivered by afferent (sensory) neurons to the CNS, the process of transmission. The transmission of a neural impulse is an electrical process that depends on changes in the distribution of certain ions.

3. **Integration.** In the CNS the information provided by the sensory neurons is interpreted as a "red light" and an appropriate response is determined. This process is known as integration.

4. **Transmission.** Appropriate efferent (motor) neurons transmit the message to the muscles.

5. **Actual response.** The message directs the muscles to contract, lifting the foot from the gas pedal and pressing down on the brake. This is the actual response.

Neural messages travel over sequences of neurons. Neurons are arranged so that the axon of one neuron forms junctions with the dendrites of other neurons. A junction between two neurons is called a **synapse** (**sin′**-aps). At a synapse neurons are separated by a tiny gap known as the synaptic cleft. Neurotransmitters conduct the "message" across the synaptic cleft.

THE HUMAN BRAIN IS THE MOST COMPLEX MECHANISM KNOWN

The most advanced computer does not even come close to matching the complexity of the human brain. The brain is a soft, wrinkled mass of tissue. Each of its 25 billion neurons is connected to as many as 1000 others. No wonder that scientists have barely begun to unravel the tangled neural circuits that govern human physiology and behavior.

What we do know is that at any moment millions of neural messages are flashing through the brain. They bring information to the brain about the state of the body and transmit "decisions" back to the organs maintaining an appropriate heart rate, blood pressure, respiration rate, temperature, muscle tone, and blood chemistry. At the same time the brain receives and responds to hundreds of messages from the outer environment—a ringing telephone, the aroma of a steak dinner, the sounds of traffic, the printed words on this page.

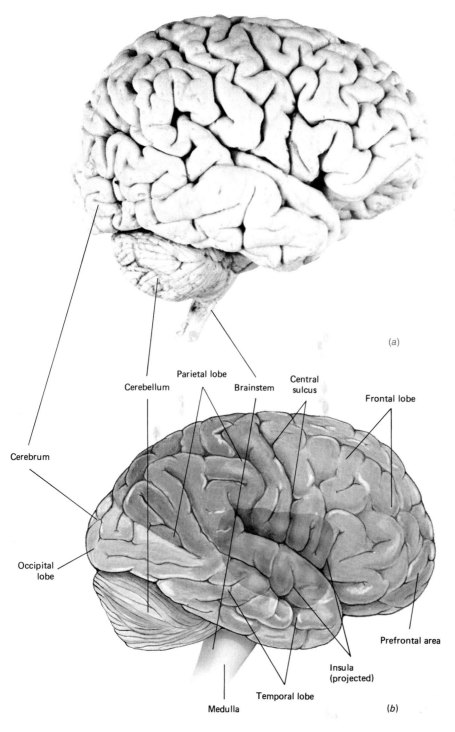

FIGURE **6–3** *Structure of the human brain. (a) Photograph of the human brain, lateral view. Note that the cerebrum covers the diencephalon and part of the brain stem. (b) Lateral view of the human brain showing the lobes of the cerebrum. Part of the brain has been made transparent so that the underlying central lobe can be located. (a) From Williams, P., and Warwick, R. (eds.): Gray's Anatomy, 36th ed. Edinburgh, Churchill, Livingstone, 1980.)*

(a)

Cerebellum

Parietal lobe

Brainstem

Central sulcus

Frontal lobe

Cerebrum

Occipital lobe

Prefrontal area

Insula (projected)

Temporal lobe

Medulla

(b)

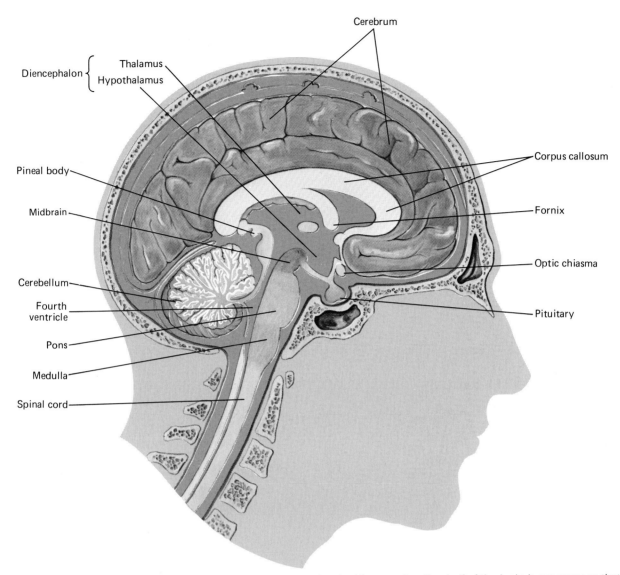

FIGURE **6–4** A midsagittal section through the brain. Note that in this type of section half of the brain is cut away so that structures normally covered by the cerebrum are exposed.

Brain cells require a continuous supply of oxygen and glucose. The brain is so dependent on its blood supply that when it is deprived of it, consciousness may be lost very quickly, and irreversible damage may occur within a few minutes. In fact, the most common cause of brain damage is a stroke, or cerebrovascular accident (CVA). In a CVA a portion of the brain is deprived of its blood supply (often because a blood vessel has been blocked by a blood clot).

The main divisions of the brain are the medulla, pons, midbrain, diencephalon (which includes the thalamus and hypothalamus), cerebellum, and cerebrum (Figs. 6–3 through 6–7 and Table 6–1). The medulla, pons, and midbrain make up the **brain stem,** the elongated portion of the brain that looks like a stalk for the cerebrum. The brain is a hollow organ. Its fluid-filled spaces are called **ventricles** (see Fig. 6–5).

THE MEDULLA CONTAINS VITAL CENTERS

More formally known as the **medulla oblongata** (meh-**dul′**-ah ob″-long-**gah′**-tuh), the medulla is the most posterior portion of the brain stem. It is continuous with the spinal cord (see Fig. 6–4). Its cavity, the **fourth ventricle,** is continuous with the central canal of the spinal cord. The medulla consists of white matter and gray matter. The white matter consists mainly of nerve tracts passing between the

TABLE 6–1
Divisions of the brain

	DESCRIPTION	FUNCTIONS
Medulla	Most inferior portion of the brain stem; continuous with spinal cord; its white matter consists of nerve tracts passing between the spinal cord and various parts of the brain; its gray matter consists of neuclei; contains nuclei of cranial nerves IX through XII*; its cavity is the fourth ventricle	Contains vital centers (within its reticular formation) that regulate heartbeat, respiration, and blood pressure; contains reflex centers that control swallowing, coughing, sneezing, and vomiting; relays messages to the other parts of the brain
Pons	Consists mainly of nerve tracts passing between the medulla and other parts of the brain; forms a bulge on the anterior surface of the brain stem; contains respiratory centers and nuclei of cranial nerves V through VIII	Connects various parts of the brain; helps regulate respiration
Midbrain	Just superior to the pons; cavity is the cerebral aqueduct; within midbrain are nuclei of cranial nerves III and IV	Regulates visual and auditory reflexes
Diencephalon		
Thalamus	Contains many important nuclei	Main relay center between spinal cord and cerebrum; incoming messages are sorted and partially interpreted here before being relayed to the appropriate centers in the cerebrum
Hypothalamus	Forms ventral floor of third ventricle; contains many nuclei; optic chiasma mark the crossing of the optic nerves; connected to the pituitary gland	Contains centers for control of body temperature, appetite, and water balance; regulates pituitary gland and links nervous and endocrine systems; helps control autonomic system; involved in some emotional and sexual responses
Cerebellum	Second largest part of the brain; superior to the fourth ventricle; consists of two hemispheres	Responsible for smooth, coordinated movement; maintains posture and muscle tone; helps maintain equilibrium
Cerebrum	Largest, most prominent part of the brain; longitudinal fissure divides the cerebrum into right and left hemispheres, each containing a lateral ventricle; each hemisphere is divided into six lobes; frontal, parietal, occipital, temporal, limbic, and central	Center of intellect, memory, language, and consciousness; receives and interprets sensory information from all sense organs; controls motor functions
Cerebral cortex	Convoluted, outer layer of gray matter covering the cerebrum; functionally divided into:	
	(1) Sensory areas	Receive incoming sensory information from eyes, ears, touch, and pressure receptors, and other sense organs; sensory association areas interpret incoming sensory information
	(2) Motor areas	Control voluntary movement and certain types of involuntary movement
	(3) Association areas	Responsible for thought, learning, language, judgment, and personality; store memories; connect sensory and motor areas
White matter	Consists of fibers that connect the two hemispheres and fibers that are part of ascending and descending tracts; basal ganglia are located within the white matter	Links various areas of the brain

*Cranial nerves are discussed in more detail in Table 7-1.

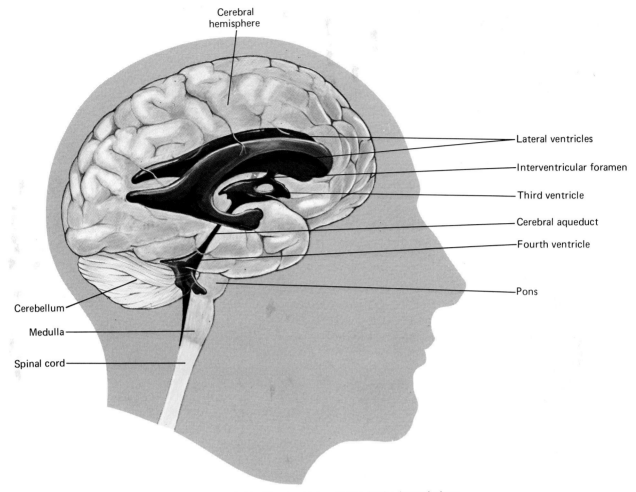

Cerebral hemisphere

Lateral ventricles

Interventricular foramen

Third ventricle

Cerebral aqueduct

Fourth ventricle

Pons

Cerebellum

Medulla

Spinal cord

FIGURE 6–5 The ventricles of the brain. Lateral view.

spinal cord and the various portions of the brain. Because of its position, all nerve tracts carrying messages from the spinal cord to the brain must pass through the medulla. Similarly, all the motor tracts transmitting messages back from the decision-making parts of the brain pass through the medulla. The gray matter of the medulla consists mainly of various nuclei (groups of cell bodies).

Within the medulla, most of the motor fibers cross. This is why the right side of the brain controls the movement of the left side of the body and vice versa.

A vast complex of gray and white matter known as the **reticular formation** extends from the spinal cord through the medulla and upward through the brain stem and thalamus. The reticular formation is important in keeping the cerebrum conscious and alert. Within the reticular formation of the medulla are several vital reflex centers.

The medulla contains discrete nuclei that serve as vital centers. The following are among the vital centers.

1. **Cardiac centers** that control heart rate.
2. **Vasomotor centers** that help regulate blood pressure by controlling the diameter of the blood vessels.
3. **Respiratory centers** that initiate and regulate breathing. Centers for other reflex actions such as vomiting, sneezing, coughing, and swallowing are also found within the medulla.

Four cranial nerves, designated cranial nerves IX through XII, originate within the medulla, and their nuclei are located there.

THE PONS IS A BRIDGE TO OTHER PARTS OF THE BRAIN

The **pons** forms a bulge on the anterior (ventral) surface of the brain stem. The pons is just superior to the medulla with which it is continuous; its posterior surface is hidden by the cerebellum. The word pons means bridge, and indeed the pons serves as a link connecting various parts of the brain. In fact, the pons consists mainly of nerve fibers passing between the medulla and other parts of the brain. The pons contains centers that help regulate respiration. Centers for the reflexes mediated by cranial nerves V through VII are also located within the pons.

THE MIDBRAIN CONTAINS CENTERS FOR VISUAL AND AUDITORY REFLEXES

The midbrain is the shortest portion of the brain stem. It extends from the pons to the diencephalon. Its cavity, the cerebral aqueduct, connects the third and fourth ventricles.

Anteriorly (ventrally), the midbrain consists of large bundles of neurons connecting the cerebrum with lower portions of the brain and with the spinal cord. The nuclei of cranial nerves III and IV are found in the midbrain. The roof of the midbrain consists of four rounded bodies that serve as reflex centers for visual and auditory (ear) reflexes. For example, constriction of the pupil in response to light is controlled by this area of the midbrain.

THE DIENCEPHALON INCLUDES THE THALAMUS AND THE HYPOTHALAMUS

The **diencephalon** (die″-en-**seph**′-ah-lon) is the part of the brain between the cerebrum and the midbrain. Its cavity is the third ventricle (see Fig. 6–5). Among its important structures are the thalamus and hypothalamus.

The **thalamus** (**thal**′-ah-mus) consists of two oval masses, one located on each side of the third ventricle. The thalamus is a major relay center. Nuclei in the thalamus serve as relay stations for all sensory information (except smell) to the cerebrum. Afferent neurons coming from the sense organs synapse within these nuclei. Neural messages arriving from these afferent neurons are sent on into the cerebrum. Many motors neurons carrying messages from the cerebrum also synapse within nuclei of the thalamus.

The thalamus also interprets many types of sensory information. We become vaguely aware of sensory input when impulses reach the thalamus. If sensory areas of the cerebrum are destroyed, an individual can still be conscious of pain, temperature, touch, and pressure.

The **hypothalamus** (hy″-poe-**thal**′-ah-mus) lies below the thalamus. Many nuclei are located within the hypothalamus. Afferent and efferent neurons connect these centers with all other parts of the central nervous system. The optic chiasma (crossing) is located in the floor of the hypothalamus. This prominent X-shaped structure is formed by the crossing of part of each optic nerve. A stalk of tissue connects the pituitary gland to the hypothalamus.

A small but mighty part of the brain, the hypothalamus helps regulate an impressive number of mechanisms essential to maintaining homeostasis. Here are some of its functions:

1. The hypothalamus is the most important relay station between the cerebral cortex and the lower autonomic centers. It is sometimes called the control center of the autonomic system. For example, stimulation of certain areas in the hypothalamus results in a decrease in heart rate. In this role the hypothalamus serves as an important link between "mind" (cerebrum) and "body" (physiological mechanisms).

2. The hypothalamus is the link between the nervous and endocrine systems. It produces several releasing hormones that regulate the secretion of hormones from the anterior lobe of the pituitary gland. In addition, the hypothalamus manufactures two hormones—antidiuretic hormone (ADH) and oxytocin. (Oxytocin stimulates contraction of the uterus during childbirth and release of milk from the breast.) ADH and oxytocin are stored in the posterior lobe of the pituitary gland and are released from the pituitary gland when needed.

3. The hypothalamus helps maintain fluid balance. ADH produced by its cells regulates the volume of water excreted by the kidneys. In addition, a thirst center in the hypothalamus lets us know when we need fluids.

4. Body temperature is regulated by the hypothalamus.

5. The appetite and satiety (fullness) centers within the hypothalamus regulate food intake.

6. The hypothalamus influences sexual behavior and the affective (emotional) aspects of sensory input. Centers there help us decide whether something is pleasant or painful.

THE CEREBELLUM IS RESPONSIBLE FOR COORDINATION OF MOVEMENT

The second largest part of the brain, the **cerebellum,** consists of two lateral masses called hemispheres and a connecting portion. The outer layer of the cerebellum, called the cerebellar cortex, consists of gray matter; beneath it, the cerebellum is composed mainly of white matter.

The cerebellum is responsible for coordination of movements. We can identify three main functions:

1. The cerebellum helps make movements smooth instead of jerky and steady rather than trembling. When the cerebellum is damaged, movements essential in running, walking, writing, talking, and many other activities become uncoordinated.

2. The cerebellum helps maintain muscle tone and thus posture.

3. Impulses from the vestibular apparatus (organ of balance) in the inner ear are continuously delivered to the cerebellum (see Figs. 6–3 and 6–4), which uses that information to help maintain equilibrium.

THE CEREBRUM IS THE LARGEST PART OF THE BRAIN

The **cerebrum** (seh-**ree'**-brum) is the largest and most prominent part of the human brain. It controls motor activities, interprets sensation, and serves as the center of intellect, memory, language, and consciousness.

The Cerebrum Is Divided into Hemispheres

The thin outer layer of the cerebrum consists of gray matter and is called the **cerebral cortex.** Beneath it lies white matter. Within the white matter lie the **basal ganglia,** paired nuclei that play an important role in movement. The two cavities within the cerebrum are the **lateral ventricles.**

In the embryo the cerebrum grows rapidly, enlarging out of proportion to the rest of the brain. It grows backward over the brain stem and also folds upon itself, forming **convolutions.** The convolutions are separated by shallow grooves, called **sulci** (**sul'**-si) and by deep grooves called **fissures.**

The cerebrum is partially divided into right and left halves, the **right** and **left cerebral hemispheres,** by a deep groove called the **longitudinal fissure** (see Fig. 6–6). The cerebrum is separated from the cerebellum by the **transverse fissure.**

FIGURE **6–6** Superior view of the cerebrum.

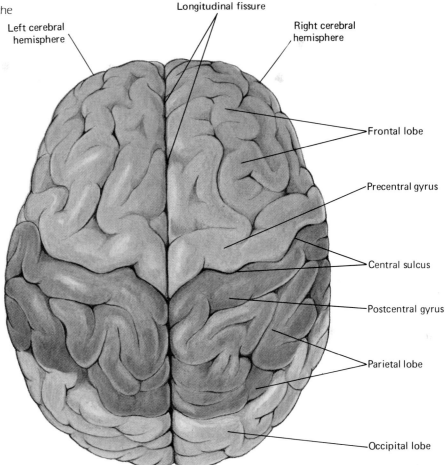

Longitudinal fissure

Left cerebral hemisphere

Right cerebral hemisphere

Frontal lobe

Precentral gyrus

Central sulcus

Postcentral gyrus

Parietal lobe

Occipital lobe

White Matter of the Cerebrum Consists of Myelinated Neurons

The white matter of the cerebrum is composed of myelinated neurons. These neurons transmit impulses between neurons in the cerebrum and connect the cerebrum with other parts of the nervous system. A large band of white matter, the **corpus callosum,** connects the right and left hemispheres. The **fornix** connects the cortex with the thalamus.

The Cerebrum Has Sensory, Motor, and Association Functions

The cerebrum is responsible for the human qualities that we cherish—ability to reason, communicate by language, create poetry and art, and invent machines such as computers and artificial hearts.

For convenience we can divide the functions performed by the cerebrum into three categories:

1. **Sensory functions.** The cerebrum receives information from the sense receptors and then interprets these messages so that we "know" what we are seeing, hearing, tasting, smelling, or feeling. These functions are carried out by areas of the cerebrum known as **sensory areas.**

2. **Motor functions.** The **motor areas** of the cerebrum are responsible for all voluntary movement and for some involuntary movement.

3. **Association functions.** Association is a term used to describe all of the intellectual activities of the cerebral cortex. These include learning and reasoning, memory storage and recall, language abilities, and even consciousness. **Association areas** also link sensory with motor areas.

Lobes of the Cerebrum Specialize in Specific Functions

Fissures and sulci divide each cerebral hemisphere into six lobes: frontal, parietal, occipital, temporal (named after the bones that protect them), central (insula), and limbic. The first five of these lobes are shown in Figures 6–3 and 6–6. Each frontal lobe is separated from a parietal lobe by a **central sulcus.** Each lobe has certain functions.

1. **Frontal lobe.** The anterior portion of each frontal lobe is an association area known as the prefrontal area. Just anterior to the central fissure lies the **precentral gyrus** of the frontal lobe. Because voluntary movements of skeletal muscles are controlled from this area, it is known as the **motor cortex.** One part of the frontal lobe (Broca's speech area) is concerned with directing the formation of words.

2. **Parietal lobe.** The parietal lobe has a primary sensory area, the **postcentral gyrus,** which receives information from the sensory receptors in the skin and joints. Important sensory association areas in the parietal lobe receive and integrate information about visual, auditory, and taste sensations from other areas of the cortex and thalamus. Through this integration process, persons become aware of themselves in relation to their environment. They are able to interpret characteristics of objects that they feel with their hands and to comprehend spoken and written language.

3. **Occipital lobe.** The occipital lobe receives information from the thalamus about what we see and integrates the information in order to formulate an appropriate response. The area that receives the visual information is known as the **primary visual area;** the portion that integrates the information is the **visual association area.**

4. **Temporal lobe.** The temporal lobe is concerned with reception and integration of auditory messages. Part of the temporal lobe is concerned with emotion, personality, and behavior.

5. **Limbic lobe.** The limbic lobe is the ring of cortex and associated structures that surrounds the ventricles of the cerebrum. This lobe is thought to be a link between emotional and cognitive (thought) processes.

6. **Central lobe.** Hidden from surface view, the central lobe is located deep within the cerebrum. The central lobe is thought to be involved in both autonomic and somatic activities.

Investigators have drawn maps of the brain, indicating which area is most responsible for each function. Brodmann's classification, one of the most widely used, is shown in Figure 6–7.

THE SPINAL CORD TRANSMITS INFORMATION TO AND FROM THE BRAIN

The spinal cord has two main functions: (1) it controls many reflex activities of the body; and (2) it transmits information back and forth from the nerves of the PNS to the brain.

The spinal cord is a slightly flattened hollow cylinder that extends downward from the brain. It extends caudally to the level of the second lumbar vertebra. The spinal cord occupies the vertebral canal of the vertebral column.

Several grooves, called fissures, divide the spinal

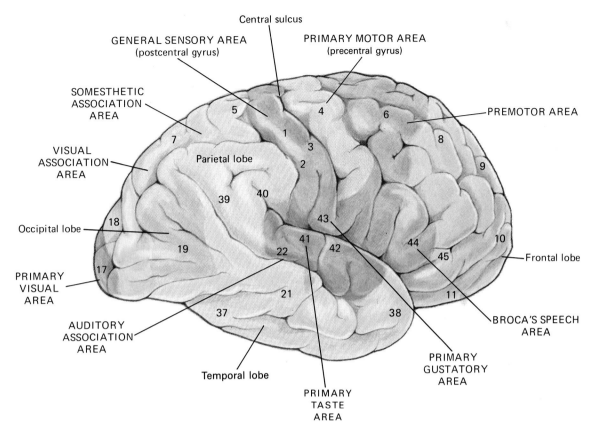

FIGURE 6–7 Map of the lateral surface of the cerebral cortex showing some of the functional areas. Areas 4, 6, and 8 are motor areas; areas 1, 2, 3, 17, 41, 42, and 43 are primary sensory areas; and areas 9, 10, 11, 18, 19, 22, 38, 39, and 40 are association areas.

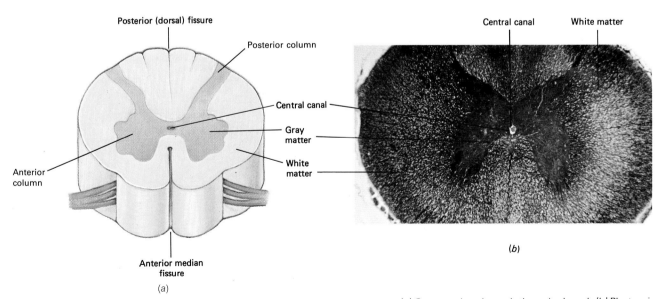

FIGURE 6–8 The spinal cord consists of gray matter and white matter. *(a)* Cross section through the spinal cord. *(b)* Photomicrograph of a cross section through the spinal cord (approximately ×25).

cord into regions. The deepest groove, the anterior median fissure, lies in the midanterior line. Opposite this, on the posterior (dorsal) surface, is the more shallow posterior (dorsal) fissure. When we examine a cross section through the spinal cord, we can see a small central canal surrounded by an area of gray matter. The gray matter is shaped somewhat like the letter H (Fig. 6–8). Outside the gray matter the cord is composed of white matter.

The gray matter of the spinal cord is subdivided into columns. The anterior (ventral) portions of the letter H are the anterior columns; the posterior (dorsal) regions are the posterior columns. The white matter consists of myelinated axons arranged in bundles, called tracts or pathways. **Ascending tracts** transmit sensory information up the spinal cord to the brain. **Descending tracts** transmit impulses (the "decisions") from the brain back down the spinal cord to efferent nerves.

THE CENTRAL NERVOUS SYSTEM IS WELL PROTECTED

The soft, fragile brain and spinal cord are the most carefully protected organs in the body. Both are encased in bone, covered by three layers of connective tissue, and bathed in a cushioning fluid.

THE MENINGES ARE CONNECTIVE TISSUE COVERINGS

The three connective tissue layers covering the brain and spinal cord are the **meninges** (meh-**nin'**-jeez). The outermost of the meninges is the **dura mater** (**do'**-rah **may'**-ter), a tough, double-layered membrane (Fig. 6–9). Inside the skull, the two layers of the dura mater are separated in some regions by large blood vessels called sinuses. These vessels receive blood leaving the brain and deliver it to the jugular veins in the neck. The dura mater forms four partitions (septa) that subdivide the cranium into compartments. The largest of these partitions (the falx cerebri) dips down between the cerebral hemispheres.

The second of the meninges is the **arachnoid** (ah-**rak'**-noyd), a thin, delicate membrane. Thread-like fibers of the arachnoid extend like the threads of a web to the innermost meningeal layer, the **pia mater** (**pee'**-ah **may'**-ter). The pia mater is a very thin membrane that adheres closely to the brain and spinal cord, following each curve or indentation of tissue. It has many blood vessels.

Meningitis, an inflammation of the meninges, is usually due to infection by bacteria or viruses. Viral meningitis is usually a self-limited disease from which the patient recovers fully. However, some viruses that cause meningitis can spread, causing inflamma-

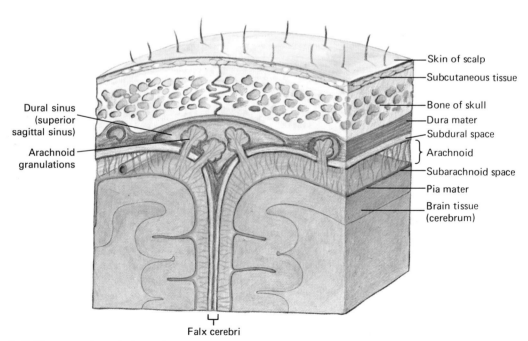

Dural sinus (superior sagittal sinus)

Arachnoid granulations

Skin of scalp
Subcutaneous tissue
Bone of skull
Dura mater
Subdural space
Arachnoid
Subarachnoid space
Pia mater
Brain tissue (cerebrum)

Falx cerebri

FIGURE 6–9 *The protective coverings of the brain. Note the large blood sinus shown between two layers of the dura mater. Blood leaving the brain flows into such sinuses and then circulates to the larger jugular veins in the neck. The falx cerebri, the partition between the cerebral hemispheres, is shown in this illustration.*

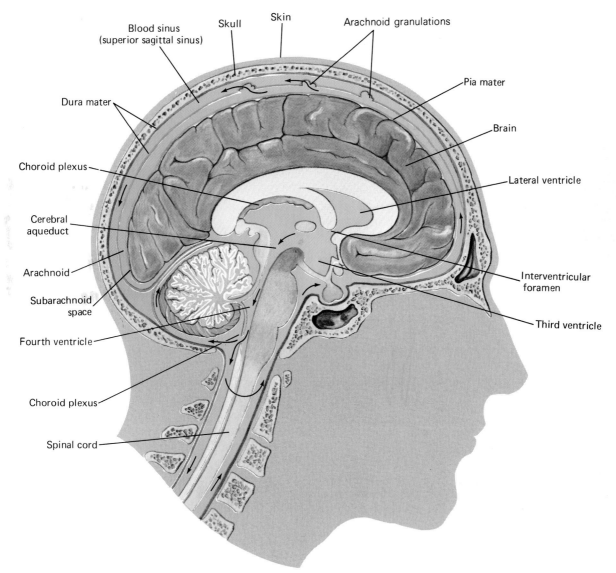

FIGURE 6–10 *Circulation of the cerebrospinal fluid in the brain and spinal cord. Cerebrospinal fluid is produced by the choroid plexuses located in the ventricles. The fluid circulates through the ventricles and subarachnoid space. It is continuously produced and continuously reabsorbed into the blood of the dural sinuses through the arachnoid granulations.*

tion of the brain itself. This more serious illness is encephalitis.

THE CEREBROSPINAL FLUID CUSHIONS THE CNS

The shock-absorbing **cerebrospinal fluid (CSF)** fills the ventricles, the cavities within the brain, and the spaces below the arachnoid layer (subarachnoid space) in the brain and spinal cord (Fig. 6–10). Most of the CSF is produced by clusters of capillaries, the **choroid plexuses (koe′**-royd), which project from the pia mater into the ventricles.

The CSF circulates through the ventricles, then passes into the subarachnoid space. Finally, it is reab-

sorbed into the blood through structures called arachnoid granulations. These structures project from the arachnoid layer into large blood sinuses within the dura mater.

The brain actually floats in the CSF. The CSF protects against mechanical injury. CSF also dissolves and transports substances filtered from the blood and serves as a medium for the exchange of nutrients and waste products between the blood and the brain.

A normal volume of CSF is essential to normal nervous system function. Blockage of CSF flow or abnormally rapid production can result in hydrocephalus, which means literally "water in the head." As CSF accumulates, the resulting pressure can cause enlargement of the skull in children and, eventually, brain damage; in severe cases, mental retardation may result. Hydrocephalus most commonly results from a birth defect in infants and children. Surgical placement of a shunt permits excess fluid to drain into a vein.

The dura mater and arachnoid extend below the level of the spinal cord. Thus, a needle can be safely inserted into the subarachnoid space at the level of the third and fourth lumbar vertebrae. A spinal tap (also called lumbar puncture) can be used to withdraw small amounts of CSF without damaging the cord itself. Analysis of this fluid can be helpful in diagnosing certain CNS disorders. For example, blood in the CSF may provide a clue in the diagnosis of cerebral (brain) hemorrhage. When indicated, lumbar puncture is often followed by CT scanning, which is now considered a more dependable method for diagnosing cerebral hemorrhage and brain tumors.

Injections of an anesthetic into the subarachnoid space block neural transmission from sensory neurons. This type of anesthesia is commonly called a "spinal" or, if administered very low in the subarachnoid space, a "saddle block." The patient remains awake but feels no pain in the lower part of the body.

A REFLEX ACTION IS A SIMPLE NEURAL RESPONSE

A simple example of a neural response is a **reflex action,** a predictable, automatic response to a specific stimulus. Most of the internal activities of the body are regulated by reflex actions. For example, body temperature is regulated by reflex actions. A change in body temperature stimulates the temperature-regulating center of the hypothalamus to mobilize homeostatic mechanisms that bring body temperature back to normal. Many responses to external stimuli, such as withdrawing from painful stimuli, are also reflex actions. Let us examine a withdrawal reflex as an example of a reflex action.

Like all neural responses, a reflex pathway depends on four processes: (1) reception of the stimulus; (2) transmission of information; (3) integration (interpretation and determination of an appropriate response); and (4) the actual response.

Withdrawal reflexes are protective. They require the participation of three sets of neurons (Fig. 6–11). Imagine that you accidentally rest your hand on a hot stove. Almost instantly, and before you become consciously aware of the pain, you jerk your hand away. Pain receptors (dendrites of sensory neurons) have sent messages through **afferent (sensory) neurons** to the spinal cord. There each neuron synapses with an **association neuron,** a neuron within the CNS that links sensory and motor neurons. Integration takes place. Then, impulses sent via **efferent (motor) neurons** to muscles in the arm and hand instruct these muscles to contract, jerking the hand away from the harmful stimulus.

At the same time that the association neuron sends a message to the motor neuron it may also dispatch a message up the spinal cord to the conscious areas of the brain. Almost at the same time you withdraw your hand you become aware of your plight and can make the conscious decision to hold your burned hand under cold water. None of this is part of the reflex action, however. Some reflex actions (e.g., the pupil reflex of the eye) do involve parts of the brain. However, these are the so-called lower parts that have nothing to do with conscious thought.

Reflex actions *are* sometimes affected by conscious thought. We can consciously inhibit or facilitate some reflexes. An example is the reflex that empties the urinary bladder when it fills with urine. In babies urination occurs by reflex action whenever the bladder becomes full. In early childhood we learn to facilitate the reflex by consciously stimulating it before the bladder pressure reaches the critical level. We also learn to inhibit the reflex consciously so that we do not urinate when the bladder becomes full at an inconvenient time or place.

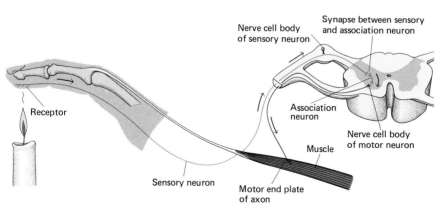

Nerve cell body of sensory neuron

Synapse between sensory and association neuron

Receptor

Association neuron

Nerve cell body of motor neuron

Muscle

Sensory neuron

Motor end plate of axon

FIGURE 6–11 The withdrawal reflex shown here involves a chain of three neurons. An afferent (sensory) neuron transmits the message from the receptor to the CNS, where it synapses with an association neuron. Then an appropriate efferent (motor) neuron (shown in color) transmits an impulse to the muscles that move the hand away from the flame (the response).

SUMMARY

I. The two principal divisions of the nervous system are the central nervous system (CNS) and the peripheral nervous system (PNS).
  A. The CNS consists of the brain and spinal cord.
  B. The PNS may be divided into somatic and autonomic systems; the two types of efferent nerves in the autonomic system are sympathetic and parasympathetic nerves.

II. Glial cells are the supporting cells of nervous tissue; neurons transmit messages.
  A. A neuron is made up of a cell body, an axon, and dendrites.
  B. Synaptic knobs at the ends of axons release neurotransmitters.
  C. Axons may be covered by both a cellular sheath and a myelin sheath.

III. Every neural response involves a sequence of several steps.
  A. Reception—a stimulus must be received by receptors.
  B. Transmission—information must be transmitted to the CNS.
  C. Integration—information must be sorted and interpreted so that an appropriate response can be determined.
  D. Transmission—a message must be delivered from the CNS to the appropriate muscle or gland.
  E. Actual response—the muscle contracts (or gland secretes), producing the actual response to the stimulus.

IV. The main divisions of the brain are the medulla, pons, midbrain, diencephalon, cerebellum, and cerebrum.
  A. The medulla is the lowest part of the brain stem. It contains nerve tracts passing from the spinal cord to the brain and tracts descending from the brain to the spinal cord. The medulla contains vital centers that control respiration, heart rate, and blood pressure.
  B. The pons serves as a bridge connecting various parts of the brain and helps to regulate respiration.
  C. The midbrain controls certain visual and auditory reflexes.
  D. The diencephalon includes the thalamus and hypothalamus.
    1. The thalamus is a major relay station for impulses going to and from the cerebrum.
    2. The hypothalamus serves as a link between the nervous and endocrine systems, serves as a link between the cerebrum and the lower autonomic centers, helps regulate temperature, helps maintain fluid balance, influences emotional and sexual behavior, and regulates appetite.
  E. The cerebellum makes movements smooth and coordinated; maintains posture; and maintains equilibrium.
  F. The cerebrum is divided into right and left hemispheres by the longitudinal fissure. The cerebral cortex consists of gyri separated by sulci or fissures.
    1. Each hemisphere is divided into six lobes—frontal, parietal, occipital, temporal, central, and limbic.
    2. The cerebrum has sensory, motor, and association functions.

V. The spinal cord is continuous with the medulla and extends to the level of the second lumbar vertebra.
  A. A cross section shows that the spinal cord has a central canal surrounded by gray matter and an outer portion of white matter.
  B. The spinal cord functions as a reflex control center and transmits information back and forth between the brain and the peripheral nerves.

VI. The brain and spinal cord are protected by bone, cerebrospinal fluid, and three connective tissue coverings called meninges—the dura mater, arachnoid, and pia mater.

VII. In a reflex pathway, a stimulus results in a predictable automatic response. A withdrawal reflex requires an afferent (sensory) neuron, association neuron, and an efferent (motor) neuron.

POST TEST

1. The CNS consists of the _____ and the _____ .

2. Sense receptors and nerves belong to the _____ nervous system.

3. The supporting cells of nervous tissue are called _____ cells.

4. Cells that are specialized to transmit nerve impulses are called _____ .

5. The nucleus of a neuron is located within the _____ _____ .

6. The fiber of a neuron specialized to transmit impulses away from the cell body is the _____ .

7. A mass of cell bodies outside the CNS is termed a _____ ; within the CNS it is called a _____ .

8. The first step in any type of neural action is _____ of a stimulus.

9. The junction between two neurons is called a _____ .

10. The cavities within the brain are called _____ .

11. The medulla, pons, and midbrain make up the _____ .

Match

Select the most appropriate match in Column B for each item in Column A.

Column A	Column B
12. Vital centers found here	a. cerebrum
13. Regulates visual reflexes	b. cerebellum
14. Helps maintain posture and equilibrium	c. midbrain
15. Controls voluntary movement	d. medulla
16. Link between nervous and endocrine systems	e. pons
	f. hypothalamus
	g. thalamus

Match

Column A	Column B
17. Contains Broca's speech area	a. occipital lobes
18. Contains auditory areas	b. frontal lobes
19. Contains visual areas	c. temporal lobes
	d. parietal lobe

20. The central canal of the spinal cord is surrounded by an area of _____ matter.

21. _____ tracts transmit sensory information up the spinal cord to the brain.

22. The outermost of the meninges is the tough _____ .

23. The ventricles of the brain contain _____ .

24. Three types of neurons that participate in a withdrawal reflex are afferent neurons, _____ neurons, and _____ neurons.

25. Label the diagram on the facing page.

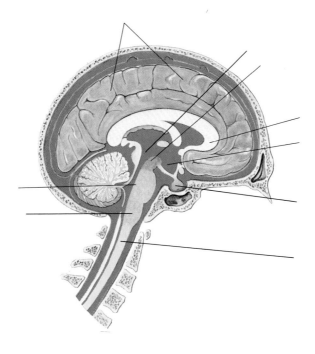

REVIEW QUESTIONS

1. What are the main divisions of the nervous system?
2. What is the main function of the nervous system?
3. How is a neuron adapted to perform its function?
4. What is a nerve? What is a tract?
5. Give examples of reception, transmission, integration, and response.
6. How are neural messages generally transmitted from one neuron to another?
7. List the main parts of the brain and give the functions of each.
8. Identify the part of the brain most closely associated with each of the following functions: (a) Regulation of body temperature; (b) Regulation of heart rate; (c) Reflex center for pupil constriction; (d) Link between nervous and endocrine systems; (e) Interpretation of language; (f) Maintaining posture.
9. In which part of the cerebrum would you find: (a) the basal ganglia; (b) Broca's speech area; (c) motor cortex; (d) primary visual area?
10. What are the functions of the spinal cord?
11. What structures protect the brain and spinal cord?
12. Imagine that you have just burned your finger with a match. Describe the events that occur. Draw a diagram of a withdrawal reflex pathway, label its parts, and relate the diagram to your description.

POST TEST ANSWERS

1. brain; spinal cord
2. peripheral nervous system (PNS)
3. glial
4. neurons
5. cell body
6. axon

7. ganglion; nucleus
8. reception
9. synapse
10. ventricles
11. brain stem
12. d
13. c
14. b
15. a
16. f
17. b
18. c
19. a
20. gray
21. Ascending
22. dura mater
23. cerebrospinal fluid (CSF)
24. association; efferent
25. see Figure 6–4

Seven

THE PERIPHERAL NERVOUS SYSTEM

CHAPTER OUTLINE

I. The somatic system responds to changes in the outside world
    A. Cranial nerves link the brain with sense receptors and muscles
    B. Spinal nerves link the spinal cord with various structures
        1. Each spinal nerve divides into branches
        2. The ventral branches form plexuses
II. The autonomic system maintains internal balance
    A. The sympathetic system mobilizes energy
    B. The parasympathetic system conserves and restores energy
    C. Sympathetic and parasympathetic nerves have opposite effects on many organs

LEARNING OBJECTIVES

After you have studied this chapter, you should be able to:
1. Contrast the somatic and autonomic divisions of the peripheral nervous system.
2. List the cranial nerves and give the functions of each.
3. Describe the structure of a typical spinal nerve.
4. Name and describe the major plexuses.
5. Describe the structures of a reflex pathway in the autonomic system.
6. Compare and contrast the sympathetic with the parasympathetic system.
7. Compare the effect of sympathetic with that of parasympathetic stimulation on specific organs such as heart and digestive tract.

The peripheral nervous system (PNS) is made up of the sense receptors, the nerves that link the sense organs with the central nervous system (CNS), and the nerves that link the CNS with the muscles and glands. That portion of the PNS that keeps the body in adjustment with the outside world is the somatic system. The nerves and receptors that maintain internal balance make up the autonomic system.

THE SOMATIC SYSTEM RESPONDS TO CHANGES IN THE OUTSIDE WORLD

The somatic system includes the sense receptors that react to changes in the outside world (see Chap. 8), the afferent neurons that keep the CNS informed of those changes, and the efferent neurons that tell

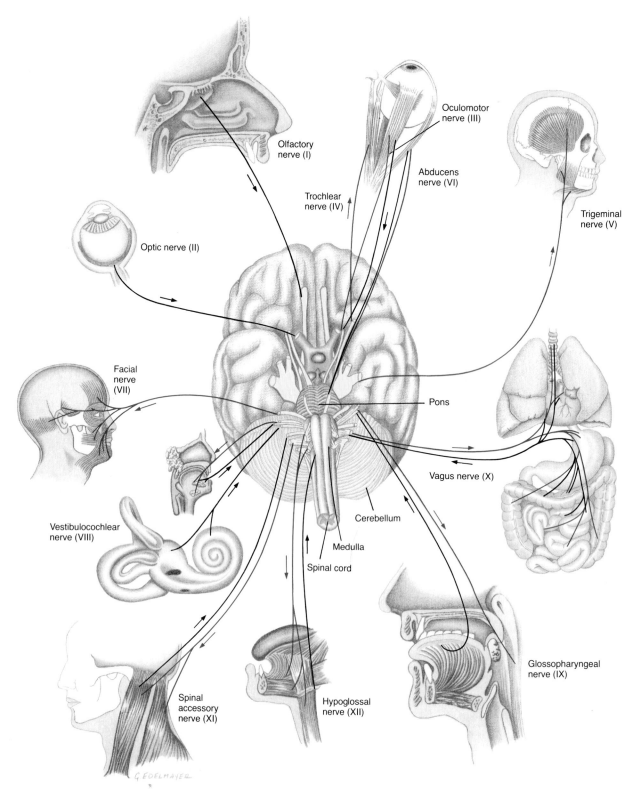

FIGURE 7–1 Base of the brain showing cranial nerves. Black indicates sensory; color indicates motor fibers.

the muscles how to respond. The afferent and efferent neurons of the somatic system, like those of the autonomic system, are part of the cranial and spinal nerves.

THE CRANIAL NERVES LINK THE BRAIN WITH SENSE RECEPTORS AND MUSCLES

Twelve pairs of nerves emerge from the brain (Fig. 7–1). These cranial nerves transmit information to the brain from sense receptors. Then they transmit orders from the CNS to muscles and glands.

Cranial nerves are designated by Roman numer-als as well as by name. The numbers indicate the sequence in which the nerves emerge from the brain. Table 7–1 lists the cranial nerves, their distributions, and their functions. Some cranial nerves consist only of sensory (afferent) fibers, but most are mixed nerves, consisting of both sensory and motor (efferent) neurons.

SPINAL NERVES LINK THE SPINAL CORD WITH VARIOUS STRUCTURES

Thirty-one pairs of spinal nerves emerge from the spinal cord. They are all mixed nerves, transmit-

TABLE 7–1

The cranial nerves

NAME	FUNCTION	DISTRIBUTION
I. Olfactory	Sensory: smell	Transmit messages from receptors in nose to cerebrum
II. Optic	Sensory: vision	Transmit messages from eye to brain
III. Oculomotor	Mixed, but mainly motor: movement of eyeball and eyelid; regulation of pupil size	Midbrain to eye muscles
IV. Trochlear	Mixed, but mainly motor: movement of eyeball	Midbrain to eye muscles
V. Trigeminal	Mixed. Sensory: sensations of head and face	Three branches; Face and scalp to pons
	Motor: chewing	Pons to muscles of mastication (chewing)
VI. Abducens	Mixed, but mainly motor: eye movement	Pons to muscles of eye
VII. Facial	Mixed. Sensory: taste	Taste buds on tongue to medulla
	Motor: facial expression, secretion of saliva and tears	Pons-medulla junction to muscles of the face and scalp, and to salivary and tear glands
VIII. Vestibulo-cochlear	Sensory: hearing and equilibrium	Cochlea and semicircular canals of inner ear to pons-medulla junction
Vestibular branch	Equilibrium	Organs of equilibrium of inner ear to brain
Cochlear (auditory) branch	Hearing	Organ of hearing in inner ear to brain
IX. Glossopharyn-geal	Mixed. Sensory: taste	Taste buds in tongue to medulla
	Motor: swallowing, saliva secretion	Medulla to muscles of pharynx; medulla to parotid salivary gland
X. Vagus	Mixed. Sensory: sensation from larynx, trachea, heart, and other thoracic and abdominal organs	Various organs to medulla *(Longest Nerve)*
XI. Spinal accessory	Mixed, but mainly motor: movement of shoulders and head	Medulla and spinal cord to muscles of shoulder and neck; and to muscles of pharynx and larynx
XII. Hypoglossal	Mixed, but mainly motor: tongue movement	Medulla to tongue muscles

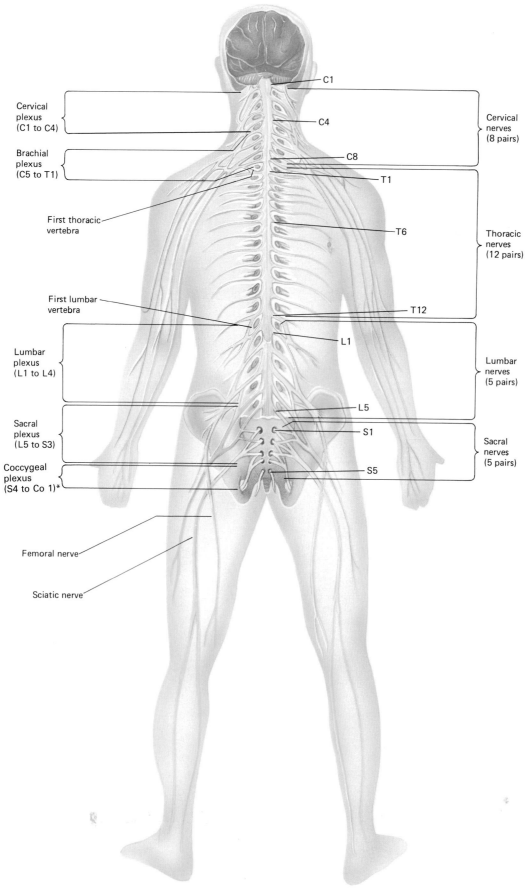

Cervical
plexus
(C1 to C4)

Brachial
plexus
(C5 to T1)

First thoracic
vertebra

First lumbar
vertebra

Lumbar
plexus
(L1 to L4)

Sacral
plexus
(L5 to S3)

Coccygeal
plexus
(S4 to Co 1)*

Femoral nerve

Sciatic nerve

C1

C4

C8

T1

T6

T12

L1

L5

S1

S5

Cervical
nerves
(8 pairs)

Thoracic
nerves
(12 pairs)

Lumbar
nerves
(5 pairs)

Sacral
nerves
(5 pairs)

*Co 1 is not shown in this figure.

FIGURE 7–2 Posterior view of the spinal cord showing the spinal nerves and some of their major branches and plexuses. Spinal nerves are named for the general region of the vertebral column from which they originate, and they are numbered in sequence.

ting sensory information to the cord through their afferent neurons and information from the central nervous system to the various parts of the body through their efferent neurons.

Spinal nerves are named for the general region of the vertebral column from which they originate and are numbered in sequence. There are 8 pairs of cervical spinal nerves, numbered C1 to C8; 12 pairs of thoracic spinal nerves, numbered T1 to T12; 5 pairs of lumbar spinal nerves, numbered L1 to L5; 5 pairs of sacral spinal nerves, numbered S1 to S5; and one pair of coccygeal spinal nerves (Fig. 7–2).

Each spinal nerve has two points of attachment with the cord. The **dorsal root** consists of sensory (afferent) fibers that transmit information from the sensory receptors to the spinal cord (Fig. 7–3). Just before the dorsal root joins the spinal cord it is marked by a swelling, the **spinal ganglion,** which consists of the cell bodies of the sensory neurons. The **ventral root** consists of motor (efferent) fibers leaving the cord. Cell bodies of the motor neurons are located within the gray matter of the cord. Dorsal and ventral roots join to form the spinal nerve (see Fig. 7–3).

Each Spinal Nerve Divides into Branches

Just after a spinal nerve emerges from the vertebral column, it divides into branches (Fig. 7–3). The dorsal branch of each nerve supplies the muscles and skin of the posterior part of the body in that region.

The dorsal branch divides and gives rise to various nerves. The ventral branch innervates the anterior and lateral body trunk in that area as well as the limbs.

The Ventral Branches Form Plexuses

The ventral branches of most of the spinal nerves do not pass directly to the body structures they innervate. Instead, the ventral branches of several spinal nerves interconnect forming networks called **plexuses.** Each plexus is a tangled network of fibers from all of the spinal nerves involved. The nerves that emerge from a plexus consist of neurons that originated in several different spinal nerves. Nerves that emerge from a plexus may be named for the region of the body that they innervate.

The main plexuses are the **cervical plexus,** the **brachial plexus,** the **lumbar plexus,** and the **sacral plexus** (see Fig. 7–2).

1. The cervical plexus receives sensory information from the back of the head, neck, shoulders, and upper chest. It sends impulses to the muscles of neck and shoulders. The phrenic nerve, which sends impulses to the diaphragm, arises from this plexus.

2. The brachial plexus supplies the shoulder, arm, and hand. Two of the nerves that emerge from this plexus are the ulnar (crazy bone) and radial.

3. The lumbar plexus supplies the lower abdominal wall, buttock, thigh, and genital structures. The femoral nerve is the largest nerve arising from this plexus.

4. The sacral plexus supplies the thigh, leg, and foot. The main branch of the sacral plexus is the sciatic nerve, which is the largest nerve in the body.

THE AUTONOMIC SYSTEM MAINTAINS INTERNAL BALANCE

The autonomic system works to maintain a steady state within the body. For instance, it functions to maintain a constant body temperature and to regulate the rate of the heartbeat. The autonomic system works automatically. It acts on smooth muscle, cardiac muscle, and glands.

Like the somatic system, the autonomic system is organized into reflex pathways (Fig. 7–4). Receptors within the organs relay information via afferent nerves to the CNS. The information is integrated at various levels. Then, the decision is transmitted along efferent nerves to the appropriate muscles or glands. The efferent portion of the autonomic system is subdivided into sympathetic and parasympathetic systems.

Recall that in the somatic system a single effer-

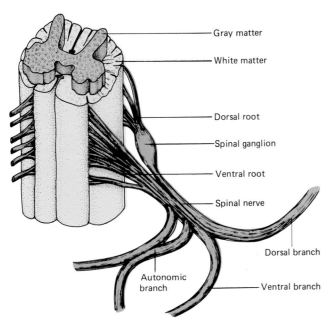

Gray matter

White matter

Dorsal root

Spinal ganglion

Ventral root

Spinal nerve

Dorsal branch

Autonomic branch

Ventral branch

FIGURE **7–3** Dorsal and ventral roots join to form a spinal nerve. The spinal nerve divides into several branches.

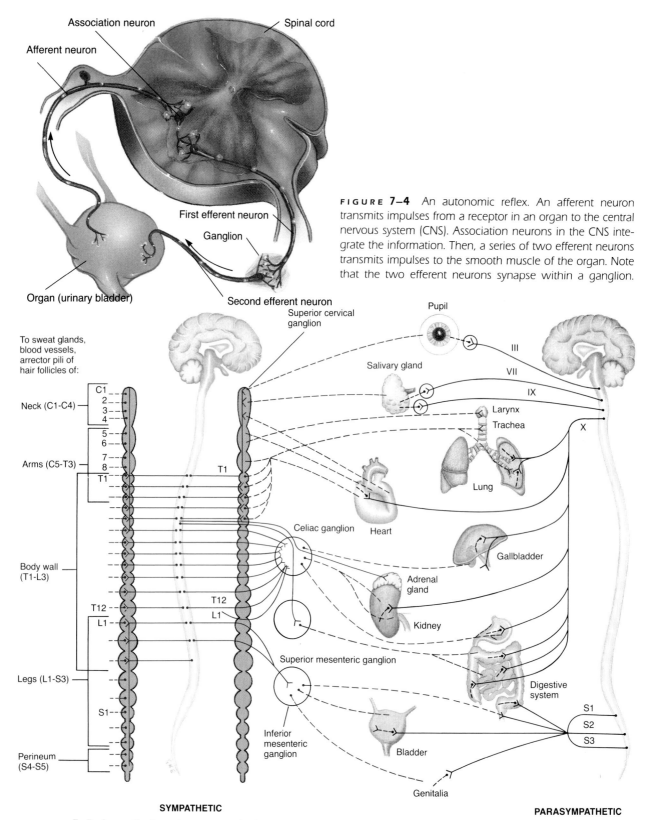

FIGURE 7–4 An autonomic reflex. An afferent neuron transmits impulses from a receptor in an organ to the central nervous system (CNS). Association neurons in the CNS integrate the information. Then, a series of two efferent neurons transmits impulses to the smooth muscle of the organ. Note that the two efferent neurons synapse within a ganglion.

FIGURE 7–5 Sympathetic and parasympathetic nervous systems. For clarity the sympathetic system has been divided. Nerves going to the body wall are shown on one side of the spinal cord and nerves going to the internal organs are shown on the other side. Complex as it appears, this diagram has been greatly simplified. Colored lines represent sympathetic nerves, black lines represent parasympathetic nerves, and dotted lines represent second efferent neurons.

ent neuron is found between the CNS and the muscle. In the autonomic system two efferent neurons are found between the CNS and the muscle it innervates. The first neuron synapses with the second within a ganglion.

THE SYMPATHETIC SYSTEM MOBILIZES ENERGY

The sympathetic system prepares the body for action. It is most active during stressful situations. For example, the sympathetic system dominates when you are rushing to class or taking a test.

Neurons of the sympathetic system emerge from the thoracic and lumbar regions of the spinal cord. Efferent sympathetic neurons pass through a branch of a spinal nerve, the autonomic branch. Then they pass into the ganglia of the paravertebral sympathetic ganglion chain. This chain is a series of ganglia located along the length of the vertebral column (Fig. 7-5). Most of the first efferent neurons end within the ganglia and synapse there with the second efferent neurons in the sequence.

Axons of some of the second efferent neurons leave the ganglion as various sympathetic nerves. They innervate blood vessels and organs in the head, neck, and thoracic region. Other sympathetic nerves innervate sweat glands.

Some of the first efferent neurons do not end in the ganglia of the paravertebral chain, but instead pass on to ganglia located in the abdomen. These ganglia are known as collateral ganglia. Efferent neurons emerging from the collateral ganglia innervate smooth muscles and glands of the abdominal and pelvic organs and their blood vessels. These include organs of the digestive, urinary, and reproductive systems.

THE PARASYMPATHETIC SYSTEM CONSERVES AND RESTORES ENERGY

The parasympathetic system is most active during periods of calm and physical rest. Your parasympathetic system is in control when you are relaxing in front of the television set. Its activities result in conserving and restoring energy.

Neurons of the parasympathetic system emerge from the brain (as part of cranial nerves) and from the sacral region of the spinal cord. About 75% of all parasympathetic fibers are in the vagus nerves.

The first efferent neurons synapse with the second efferent neurons in terminal ganglia located near or within the walls of the organs they innervate. Neurons from the cranial region innervate the eye, structures of the head, and thoracic and abdominal organs.

Branches of the vagus innervate the heart, lungs, liver, pancreas, esophagus, stomach, small intestine, and upper portion of the large intestine (Fig. 7-5).

The parasympathetic nerves that emerge from the sacral region form the pelvic nerves. They innervate the lower portion of the large intestine, urinary system, and reproductive system. The parasympathetic nerves do not innervate the blood vessels or sweat glands.

SYMPATHETIC AND PARASYMPATHETIC NERVES HAVE OPPOSITE EFFECTS ON MANY ORGANS

Many organs are innervated by both sympathetic and parasympathetic nerves. For example, sympa-

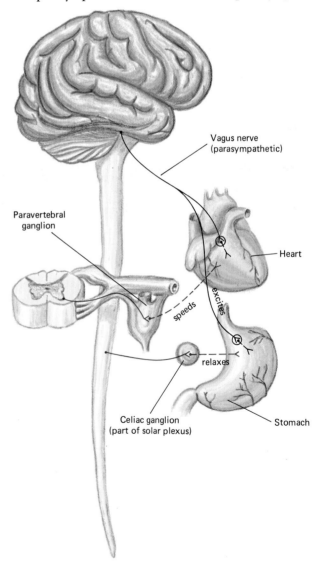

FIGURE 7-6 Dual innervation of the heart and stomach by sympathetic and parasympathetic nerves. Sympathetic nerves are shown in red. Second efferent neurons are indicated by dotted lines.

TABLE 7–2

Comparison of sympathetic and parasympathetic actions on selected effectors*

EFFECTOR	SYMPATHETIC ACTION	PARASYMPATHETIC ACTION
Heart	Increases rate and strength of contraction	Decreases rate; no direct effect on strength of contraction
Bronchial tubes	Dilates	Constricts
Iris of eye	Dilates (pupil becomes larger)	Constricts (pupil becomes smaller)
Sex organs	Constricts blood vessels; ejaculation	Dilates blood vessels; erection
Blood vessels	Generally constricts	No innervation for many
Sweat glands	Stimulates	No innervation
Intestine	Inhibits motility	Stimulates motility and secretion
Liver metabolism	Stimulates glycogen breakdown	No effect
Adipose tissue	Stimulates free fatty acid release from fat cells	No effect
Adrenal medulla	Stimulates secretion of epinephrine and norepinephrine	No effect
Salivary glands	Stimulates thick, viscous secretion	Stimulates profuse, watery secretion

*Refer to Figure 7–5 as you study this table. Note that many other examples could be added to this list.

thetic nerves increase both the rate and force of contraction of the heart. Parasympathetic (vagus) nerves have opposite effects, decreasing the heart's pumping effectiveness and allowing it some measure of rest (Fig. 7–5). The digestive system is mainly under parasympathetic control. Parasympathetic stimulation increases its activity. Sympathetic stimulation is not necessary for the normal function of the digestive system, but strong sympathetic stimulation does inhibit the movement of food through the digestive tract. Table 7–2 summarizes some autonomic effects on various organs (Fig. 7–6).

SUMMARY

I. The somatic system is the part of the PNS that keeps the body in adjustment with the external environment. It consists of sensory receptors and nerves.
II. Twelve pairs of cranial nerves link the brain with sensory receptors and effectors. Table 7–1 summarizes the cranial nerves.
III. Thirty-one pairs of spinal nerves link the spinal cord with sensory receptors and effectors.
    A. Each spinal nerve has a dorsal root consisting of sensory fibers and a ventral root consisting of motor fibers. The dorsal and ventral roots join to form a spinal nerve.
    B. Each spinal nerve branches. The dorsal branch supplies the skin and muscles of the dorsal part of the body; the ventral branch supplies the ventral and lateral body trunk.
    C. The ventral branches of several spinal nerves join to form a plexus. The principal plexuses are the cervical, brachial, lumbar, and sacral.
IV. The autonomic system of the PNS works to maintain a steady state within the internal environment.
    A. Afferent fibers of the autonomic system run through cranial and spinal nerves along with somatic fibers.
    B. The efferent portion of the autonomic system is divided into sympathetic and parasympathetic systems; their neurons also are part of certain spinal and cranial nerves.
    C. The sympathetic system emerges from the spinal cord at the thoracic and lumbar regions.

1. The sympathetic system regulates activities that mobilize energy and is especially important when the body is under stress.
2. A typical sympathetic pathway might consist of the following: An efferent neuron emerges from the spinal cord and ends in a sympathetic chain ganglion. It synapses with a second efferent neuron, which branches, forming a nerve that innervates smooth muscle or sweat glands.
   D. The parasympathetic system consists of nerves that emerge from the brain and from the sacral region of the spinal cord.
1. The parasympathetic system works to restore energy and is dominant during periods of relaxation.
2. The first efferent neuron in the chain synapses with the second in terminal ganglia located near or within the walls of the organs they innervate.
   E. Some organs are innervated by both sympathetic and parasympathetic nerves; e.g., the heart is stimulated by sympathetic nerves and its pumping effectiveness is decreased by parasympathetic (vagus) nerves.

POST TEST

1. The part of the PNS that keeps the body in adjustment with the external environment is the _____ system.
2. The second cranial nerve is the _____ nerve; the tenth cranial nerve is the _____ nerve.
3. The vestibulocochlear nerve is responsible for equilibrium and _____ .
4. There are _____ pairs of cervical spinal nerves and _____ pairs of thoracic spinal nerves.
5. The dorsal root of a spinal nerve consists of _____ fibers.
6. The ventral branches of several spinal nerves may interconnect to form a _____ .
7. The portion of the PNS that functions to maintain a steady state within the internal environment is the _____ system.
8. The rate and force of contraction of the heart are increased by its _____ nerves.
9. The digestive system is stimulated by _____ nerves.
10. An autonomic nerve that emerges from the brain or sacral region of the spinal cord would be a _____ nerve.
11. Label the diagram on the following page.

REVIEW QUESTIONS

1. Contrast the somatic and autonomic nervous systems.
2. List the cranial nerves and their principal functions.
3. What two structures join to form a spinal nerve?
4. Name the four main plexuses and identify the structures they innervate.
5. Contrast sympathetic and parasympathetic systems.
6. Give examples of how sympathetic and parasympathetic systems work together to maintain homeostasis.

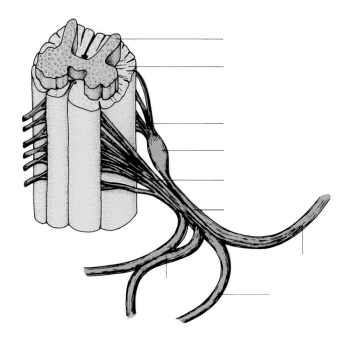

POST TEST ANSWERS

1. somatic
2. optic; vagus
3. hearing
4. 8; 12
5. sensory (afferent)
6. plexus

7. autonomic
8. sympathetic
9. parasympathetic
10. parasympathetic
11. see Figure 7–3

Eight

THE SENSE ORGANS

CHAPTER OUTLINE

   I. The eye contains visual receptors
      A. The retina contains the rods and cones
      B. The eye can be compared to a camera
      C. Vision involves several processes
  II. The ear functions in hearing and equilibrium
      A. The outer ear conducts sound waves to the middle ear
      B. The middle ear amplifies sound waves
      C. The inner ear contains receptors
         1. The cochlea contains the receptors for hearing
         2. The vestibule and semicircular canals help maintain equilibrium
 III. Smell is sensed by receptors in the nasal cavity
 IV. Taste is sensed by the taste buds
  V. The general senses are widespread through the body
      A. Tactile receptors are located in the skin
      B. Temperature receptors are nerve endings
      C. Pain sensation is a protective mechanism
      D. Proprioceptors inform us of our position

LEARNING OBJECTIVES

After you have studied this chapter, you should be able to:
1. Describe the structures of the eye and give their functions.
2. Describe the structures and functions of the three major parts of the ear.
3. Trace the transmission of sound through the ear.
4. Compare the receptors of taste and smell.
5. Describe the tactile receptors and temperature receptors
6. Explain how pain sensation is protective, and describe referred pain.
7. Locate proprioceptors in the body and describe their function.

We are continuously bombarded with sensory information about the internal environment and the world outside. Any detectable change in the environment—internal or external—is called a **stimulus.** We detect stimuli through our **sensory receptors.** Traditionally, the senses have been referred to as sight, hearing, taste, smell, and touch. In addition to these five senses, the body has many internal sensors that maintain homeostatic balance. For example, certain blood vessels have receptors that maintain a normal balance of oxygen and carbon dioxide. Thus, how we respond to changes in our environment depends both on receptors that sense changes in the *outside* world (cold versus hot, bitterness versus sweetness, pain versus pleasure) and on the internal receptors that sense changes *inside* the body.

THE EYE CONTAINS VISUAL RECEPTORS

Our eyes provide us with a great deal of information about our environment. The eye is an extremely delicate organ that is protected by its position in the body and by accessory structures. The eye and its muscles are set in the orbit formed by the skeletal bones of the face. They are cushioned by layers of fat. The eyelashes and eyelids help protect the eye anteriorly from foreign objects. The lids close by reflex action if danger is perceived. Frequent blinking lubricates and clears debris. Even though we are not aware of the process, tears flow at all times from the **lacrimal** (**lak′**-rih-mal) **glands.** They pass out through the lacrimal ducts to keep the eye moist and free of dust and minute objects.

The six **extrinsic muscles** of the eye originate from outside the eye and function in support and movement. The extrinsic muscles extend from the bony structure of the orbit or the covering of the eyeball. These muscles work in a coordinated, pre-

cise fashion enabling the two eyes to move together and focus on a single object.

The eyeball is formed by three layers of tissue: (1) the fibrous sclera and cornea; (2) the choroid layer; and (3) the retina. A lens, ciliary muscle, iris, and inner fluid-filled cavities make up the rest of the structure (Fig. 8–1).

The **sclera** (**sklay′**-rah), the "white of the eye," is opaque and white. It is a tough, fibrous tissue, generously supplied with nerve endings. It covers the entire eyeball except the anterior colored portion (iris and pupil). The sclera joins the **cornea** (**kor′**-nee-ah), the transparent layer that covers the iris and the pupil at the front of the eye. The cornea is frequently called the "window of the eye." The sclera is covered by the conjunctiva (kon-junk-**tie′**-vah), a moist mucus membrane that extends as a continuous lining of the inner layer of the eyelids.

The second layer of the eyeball is the choroid (**kow′**-royd). This layer is made of black pigment cells that absorb light rays so that they are not reflected back out of the eye. Blood vessels of the choroid nourish the retina.

The **iris,** the colored part of the eye, appears as blue, green, or brown. Its color is determined by the amount of pigment present. Composed of smooth muscle tissue, the iris regulates the amount of light entering the eye. The black spot, or opening in the

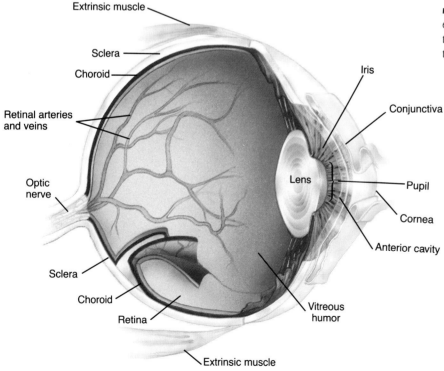

FIGURE 8–1 Structure of the eye. The eye is shown in cross section and has been partly dissected to show internal structure.

center of the circular muscles of the iris, is the **pupil** of the eye. When the eye is stimulated by bright light, the circular muscle of the iris contracts, decreasing the size of the pupil. In dim light, the iris increases the size of the pupil. Certain medications and levels of consciousness may also affect the size of the pupil.

The **lens** of the eye lies at the rear of the anterior cavity of the eyeball (Fig. 8–1). This cavity is filled with **aqueous humor,** a watery fluid, which helps to maintain an appropriate pressure within the eye. The lens is a clear, crystalline body that refracts (bends) light so that it can be focused on the retina. The lens is attached to the **ciliary muscles** by tiny fibers that make up the **suspensory ligament.**

Directly behind the lens is the posterior cavity of the eyeball, which contains a jellylike substance, the **vitreous humor.** The vitreous humor helps maintain the ball-like shape of the eye and also aids in refracting images.

THE RETINA CONTAINS THE RODS AND CONES

The **retina** (**ret′**-ih-nah) is the innermost layer of the eye. The retina contains sensory receptors called **rods** and **cones** that transmit signals through the retina to the optic nerve. Because of these specialized cells, the retina is the light-sensitive area of the eye. The cones are mainly responsible for color vision and vision during the daytime. The rods are mainly responsible for vision in dim light or darkness. Cones are most concentrated in the **fovea** (**foe′**-vee-ah), a small depression in the center of the posterior region of the retina. The fovea is the region of sharpest vision.

The image of an object is carried from the retina to the brain through the optic nerve (cranial nerve II). The optic nerve is formed by the union of individual axons of sensory neurons of the retina. The area where the optic nerve forms has no rods or cones. This area is known as the **optic disc,** or blind spot. Impulses of touch, pain, and temperature from the eye are transmitted to the brain by the trigeminal nerve (cranial nerve V).

THE EYE CAN BE COMPARED TO A CAMERA

Like a camera, the eye has an adjustable lens and a variable aperture system (pupil). The retina can be compared to the light-sensitive film used in a camera. Because of the ability of the eye to accommodate to different distances, the image is clearly focused on the retina unless there is some error in accommoda-tion. The choroid layer absorbs light rays like the interior dark surface of a camera.

VISION INVOLVES SEVERAL PROCESSES

For vision to occur, light must pass through the eye and form an image on the retina. Light passes through the transparent cornea, the aqueous humor, the lens, and the vitreous body before reaching the retina. After an image is formed on the retina, nerve impulses must be transmitted to the visual areas of the cerebral cortex.

Several processes are involved in focusing light rays on the retina. They include refraction (bending) of light rays by the cornea and lens, accommodation of the lens, adjustment of the size of the pupil, and positioning the two eyeballs so they are both directed toward the object. Positioning the eyeballs is the function of the six extrinsic eye muscles that control the movement of each eye.

The shape of the lens must be adjusted as we shift our focus on an object near or far from our position of viewing. Thus, the lens must be elastic so the ciliary muscles can control its shape as we change our focus on objects. **Accommodation** is an automatic process in which the curvature of the lens is increased to permit focusing on close objects. Accommodation is controlled by the autonomic nervous system. As we grow older, the lens loses some of its elasticity and can no longer adjust to bring objects into focus. This age-related change is called **presbyopia** (prez-bi-**oh′**-pee-ah).

THE EAR FUNCTIONS IN HEARING AND EQUILIBRIUM

The ear has three parts (Fig. 8–2):

1. The outer ear includes the part we see and a canal connecting with the middle ear.

2. The middle ear contains three small bones that conduct sound waves.

3. The inner ear contains sensory receptors for sound waves and for maintaining the equilibrium of the body.

THE OUTER EAR CONDUCTS SOUND WAVES TO THE MIDDLE EAR

The **pinna** (**pin′**-ah), the part of the ear that projects from the side of the head, surrounds the ear canal. The ear canal, or **external auditory canal,**

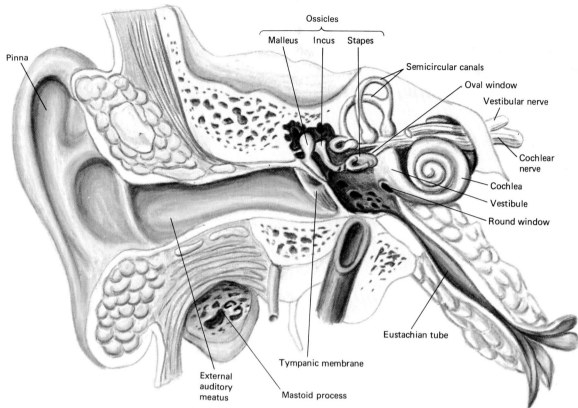

FIGURE 8-2 Structure of the ear.

leads to the middle ear. The lining of the canal contains **ceruminous** (se-**roo′**-mih-nus) **glands** that secrete earwax, more formally called **cerumen** (seh-**roo′**-men). Cerumen helps protect the lining of the canal from infection.

Separating the middle and external ear is a membrane, the **tympanic membrane** (tim-**pan′**-ik), or eardrum. Incoming sound waves cause this flexible membrane to vibrate, transmitting the sound waves to the middle ear.

THE MIDDLE EAR AMPLIFIES SOUND WAVES

The middle ear is a small, moist cavity in the temporal bone containing air and three small bones, or ossicles (**os′**-eh-kles). At the rear of the cavity the middle ear opens into the mastoid process of the temporal bone. This area is filled with air spaces that communicate with the middle ear and help equalize pressure. Under normal circumstances the air pressure is equalized on the two sides of the tympanic membrane by the **eustachian** (u-**stay′**-kee-an) **tube.** This tube connects the middle ear and the throat. Bacteria in the throat can pass through the eustachian

tube leading to painful middle ear infection with swelling of the tympanic membrane.

The three ossicles are the **malleus** (**mal′**-ee-us), **incus** (**ing′**-kus), and **stapes** (**stay′**-peez). These tiny bones form a chain from the tympanic membrane to the **oval window,** a small membrane between the middle and inner ear. Sound waves cause vibrations of the tympanic membrane. Then the vibrations of the tympanic membrane cause the malleus to vibrate. These vibrations are passed onto the incus and stapes. As the stapes rocks back and forth, it causes the oval window to bow in and out. As sound waves are transmitted from the tympanic membrane to the smaller oval window, they are amplified.

THE INNER EAR CONTAINS RECEPTORS

The inner ear contains sensory receptors that convert sound waves to nerve impulses. This part of the ear also contains receptors that enable us to maintain our equilibrium. The inner ear lies inside the temporal bone. It is a **bony labyrinth** (**lab′**-ih-rinth) composed of three compartments: (1) the ves-

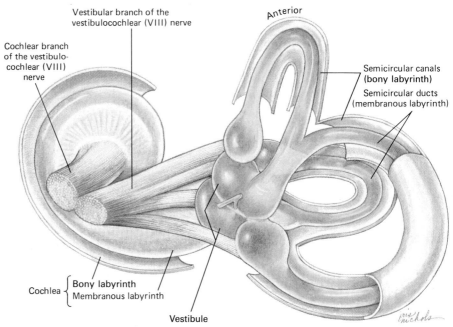

Cochlear branch
of the vestibulo-
cochlear (VIII)
nerve

Vestibular branch of the
vestibulocochlear (VIII) nerve

Anterior

Semicircular canals
(bony labyrinth)

Semicircular ducts
(membranous labyrinth)

Cochlea { Bony labyrinth
         Membranous labyrinth

Vestibule

FIGURE 8–3 *The structures of the inner ear. Outer white color shows bony labyrinth. Inner orange color shows the membranous labyrinth.*

tibule, which lies next to the oval window; (2) the cochlea; and (3) the semicircular canals (Fig. 8–3).

The bony labyrinth contains a fluid known as **perilymph (per′-ih-lymf)**. The perilymph surrounds the **membranous labyrinth,** a group of ducts and sacs that lie within the bony labyrinth. The membranous labyrinth contains a fluid called **endolymph.** The two fluids—perilymph and endolymph—are separated and have different chemical compositions. Both fluids carry vibrations through the system of canals within the inner ear.

The Cochlea Contains the Receptors for Hearing

The **cochlea (kok′-lee-ah)** is a snail-shaped portion of the inner ear that contains the organs of Corti, the sound receptors. The organs of Corti contain sensory cells that respond to sound waves by stimulating the **cochlear nerve.** The cochlear nerve then transmits the message to the brain.

We can summarize the steps in the physiology of hearing as follows:

Sound waves enter external auditory canal → stimulate vibration of tympanic membrane → stimulate the malleus, incus, and stapes → amplify the intensity of the sound waves → oval window vibrates → vibrations conducted through

the perilymph → vibrations transmitted to the endolymph → stimulate the sensory cells in the cochlea → transmission of neural impulses by the cochlear nerve to the brain.

The Vestibule and Semicircular Canals Help Maintain Equilibrium

The **vestibule** and **semicircular canals** make up the organ of equilibrium. These structures contain sensory cells that transmit information about the position of the body. The response of the sensory cells in the semicircular canals is produced by the flow of endolymph within the canals as the position of one's head changes. These responses in turn are transmitted to the **vestibular nerve,** which joins the cochlear nerve to form the **vestibulocochlear nerve** (cranial nerve VIII).

SMELL IS SENSED BY RECEPTORS IN THE NASAL CAVITY

Smell is sensed by receptor cells in the olfactory (smell) epithelium at the upper part of the nasal cavity (Fig. 8–4). The smells detected by the olfactory epithelium are transmitted to the olfactory center in

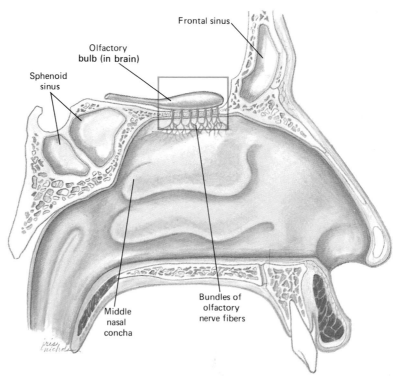

Frontal sinus

Olfactory
bulb (in brain)

Sphenoid
sinus

Middle
nasal
concha

Bundles of
olfactory
nerve fibers

FIGURE 8–4 Location and structure of the olfactory epithelium. Note that the receptor cells are located within the epithelium.

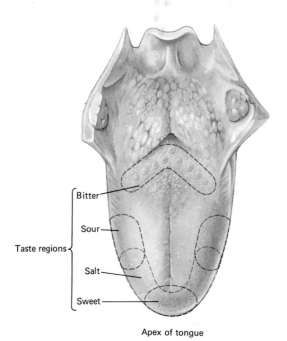

Bitter

Sour

Taste regions

Salt

Sweet

Apex of tongue

FIGURE 8–5 The sense of taste. Taste buds are most numerous on the tongue. Certain regions of the tongue respond more strongly than other regions to specific tastes.

the brain through the olfactory nerve (cranial nerve I). Olfactory cells are not replaced, so when they are damaged, our sense of smell is impaired.

TASTE IS SENSED BY THE TASTE BUDS

The sense of taste (gustation) is the job of the taste buds on the tongue and various parts of the mouth. The normal adult mouth has an average of 10,000 taste buds. As an individual gets older, the number of taste buds gradually decreases. Taste buds respond only if the material to be tasted is in solution.

The taste buds sense four main tastes: (1) sweet; (2) sour; (3) salty; and (4) bitter. Sweet and salty tastes are sensed mainly at the tip of the tongue (Fig. 8–5). Sour taste is detected mainly at the sides of the tongue, and bitter taste at the posterior part of the tongue. Three cranial nerves—the facial (cranial nerve VII), the glossopharyngeal (cranial nerve IX), and the vagus (cranial nerve X)—transmit impulses from the taste buds to the brain.

Both smell and taste are important in stimulating appetite and digestive juices. Much of what we think is taste is actually smell. A bad head cold decreases appetite partly because the efficiency of the olfactory receptors is reduced by inflammation.

THE GENERAL SENSES ARE WIDESPREAD THROUGH THE BODY

The general senses include the receptors that respond to touch, pressure, vibration, pain, changes in temperature, and muscle stretch. Some of these receptors are illustrated in Figure 8–6.

TACTILE RECEPTORS ARE LOCATED IN THE SKIN

Tactile receptors respond to pressure, touch, and vibration. They are located in the skin and are especially concentrated in some areas such as the fingers and lips.

FIGURE **8–6** Receptors in the skin sense touch, pressure, vibration, temperature change, and pain.

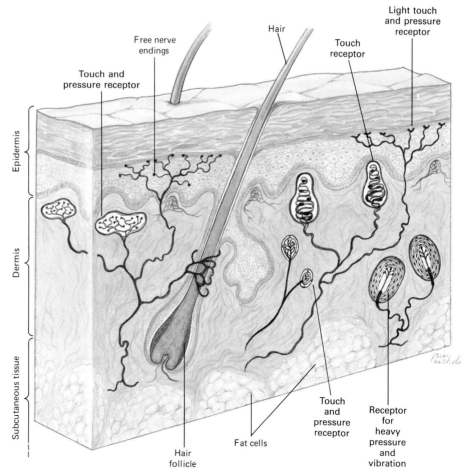

TEMPERATURE RECEPTORS ARE NERVE ENDINGS

We can sense changes in temperature from freezing cold to burning hot. The temperature receptors are thought to be free nerve endings. They are widely distributed and are especially concentrated in the lips, mouth, and anus.

PAIN SENSATION IS A PROTECTIVE MECHANISM

The sensation of pain is a protective mechanism that makes us aware of tissue injury. Pain receptors are sensory nerve endings found in the skin and certain internal tissues.

Most internal organs are poorly supplied with pain receptors. For this reason pain from internal organs is often difficult to locate. In fact, the pain is often *referred* to a superficial area that may be some distance away. A headache is sometimes **referred pain** from the blood vessels or meninges beneath the surface of the skull. A person with angina who feels cardiac pain in his left arm is experiencing referred pain. The pain originates in the heart as a result of ischemia (insufficient oxygen), but it is felt in the arm. Neurons from both the heart and the arm connect with the same neurons in the spinal cord. The brain interprets the incoming message as coming from the body surface. This is because pain from the body surface is far more common than internal pain. The brain acts on the basis of its past experience. When internal pain is felt both at the site of the distress and as referred pain it may seem to spread, or *radiate* from the organ to the superficial area.

Through the ages humans have developed methods for relieving pain. Acupuncture is one of the oldest techniques still in use. For thousands of years acupuncture has been used to relieve pain, but how it works has remained a mystery. Some biologists think that endorphins (chemicals in the CNS that affect pain perception) may explain how acupuncture works. Acupuncture needles stimulate nerves deep within the muscles, which in turn stimulate the pituitary gland and parts of the brain to release endorphins. The endorphins may inhibit neurons in the brain that normally fire in response to pain.

A more recent method for relieving pain is transcutaneous electrical nerve stimulation. In this procedure a battery-powered device called a TENS (transcutaneous electric nerve stimulator) unit is used. Electrodes attached to the skin over a painful area stimulate the skin, producing a mild tingling or massaging sensation. The stimulation may interrupt pain impulses being transmitted to the spinal cord or may increase endorphin production. Stimulation of the area may also increase circulation, which facilitates healing.

PROPRIOCEPTORS INFORM US OF OUR POSITION

Proprioceptors (pro-pree-o-**sep**'-tors) help us maintain the position of the body and its parts. These receptors are located within muscles, tendons, and joints. Impulses are carried rapidly to the brain so that the central nervous system is aware of the location of the parts of the body at all times. The brain coordinates the information from the vestibule and semicircular canals in the inner ear to maintain equilibrium and coordination of muscular activities. This provides us with a conscious awareness of body position and movement (known as the kinesthetic sense).

SUMMARY

I. The sensory receptors help us maintain contact with the environment and thus help maintain homeostasis.

II. The eye is protected by its position in the orbit and by the eyelids, eyelashes, and tears.

  A. The cornea is continuous with the sclera, a tough membrane that envelops the rest of the eyeball.

  B. The iris regulates the amount of light entering the eye. In bright light it contracts, narrowing its opening, the pupil; in weak light it dilates the pupil, permitting more light to enter.

  C. The internal surface of the eye is covered by a black coat, the choroid, which prevents light rays from scattering.

  D. Light passes through the lens and is received by light receptors in the retina.

    1. Rods are sensory cells in the retina sensitive to dim light, but not to color.

    2. Cones are sensory cells in the retina sensitive to color.

  E. Accommodation is an automatic process in which the curvature of the lens is increased in order to clearly focus on a close object.

F. In vision the image is focused on the retina. Then the image is conducted from the retina to the brain by the optic nerve.

III. The ear functions in hearing and equilibrium.
    A. The outer ear is separated from the middle ear by the tympanic membrane.
    B. The middle ear contains three small bones—the malleus, incus, and stapes—that amplify sound waves. They extend from the tympanic membrane to the oval window.
    C. The inner ear contains the cochlea, vestibule, and semicircular canals.
        1. The cochlea contains the organs of Corti, which convert sound waves to nerve impulses for transmission to the brain.
        2. The vestibule and semicircular canals make up the organ of equilibrium.

IV. Smell is sensed by the olfactory receptors, which transmit impulses to the brain through the olfactory nerve (cranial nerve I).

V. Taste is sensed through the taste buds on the tongue and is transmitted by cranial nerves to the brain.

VI. The general senses include receptors that respond to touch, pressure, vibrations, change in temperature, pain, and muscle stretch.
    A. Tactile receptors located in various parts of the skin respond to touch, pressure, and vibration.
    B. Temperature receptors are free nerve endings.
    C. Pain serves as a protective mechanism for the body.
    D. Proprioceptors are position receptors that help us maintain the position of the body and its parts.

POST TEST

Match
Select the most appropriate match in Column B for each item in Column A.
The same answer can be used more than once or not at all.

Column A	*Column B*
1. Opening	a. pupil
2. Colored part of the eye	b. cornea
3. Area of sharpest vision	c. ciliary body
4. Function in dim light	d. iris
5. Senses color vision	e. fovea
6. Window of the eye	f. lens
7. Crystalline body that adjusts for accommodation	g. rods
	h. cones

Match

Column A	*Column B*
8. Between middle and inner ear	a. pinna
9. Porous bone that connects with middle ear	b. malleus
10. Surrounds membranous labyrinth	c. eustachian tube
11. Outer portion of ear	d. mastoid process
12. Connects middle ear with throat	e. bony labyrinth
13. Bone in middle ear	f. cochlear nerve
14. Transmits neural impulses from organ of Corti to brain	g. oval window

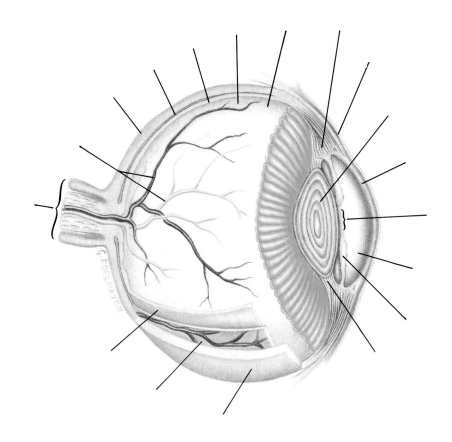

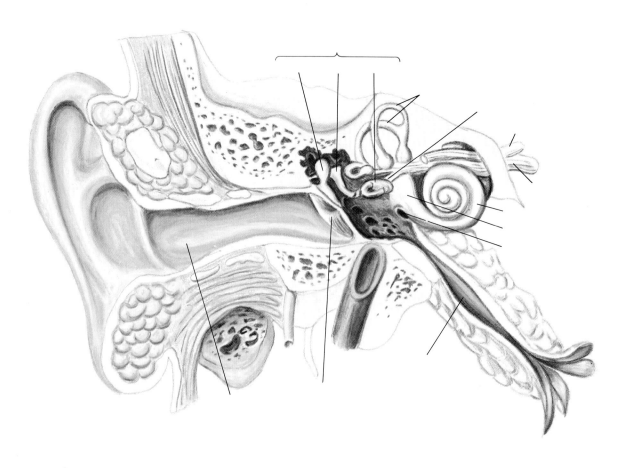

15. Receptors in the olfactory epithelium sense _____ .

16. The four main tastes are _____ , _____ , _____ , and _____ .

17. A headache is sometimes _____ pain.

18. Proprioceptors help us maintain _____ .

19. Label each of the diagrams on the facing page.

REVIEW QUESTIONS

1. How do sensory receptors help us maintain homeostasis?

2. What are the layers of the eyeball?

3. What are the functions of: (a) the pupil; (b) the iris; (c) the lens; (d) rods and cones?

4. Summarize the steps in the physiology of hearing.

5. What are the functions of: (a) the malleus, incus, and stapes; (b) cochlea; (c) organ of Corti; (d) eustachian tube?

6. What is the function of the semicircular canals?

7. Compare the function of the auditory and vestibular branch of cranial nerve VIII.

8. What are the four tastes recognized by the taste buds and how are these transmitted to the brain?

9. Where are the proprioceptors located?

POST TEST ANSWERS

1. a
2. d
3. e
4. g
5. h
6. b
7. f
8. g
9. d
10. e

11. a
12. c
13. b
14. f
15. smell
16. sweet, salty, sour, bitter
17. referred
18. the position of the body and its parts
19. see Figures 8–1 and 8–2

Nine

ENDOCRINE CONTROL

CHAPTER OUTLINE

I. Hormones act on target cells
   A. Many hormones act through second messengers
   B. Steroid hormones activate genes
   C. Prostaglandins are local hormones
II. Endocrine glands are regulated by feedback control
III. The hypothalamus and pituitary gland work closely together
   A. The posterior lobe releases two important hormones
   B. The anterior lobe secretes seven different hormones
      1. Tropic hormones stimulate other endocrine glands
      2. Prolactin stimulates secretion of milk
      3. Growth hormone stimulates protein synthesis
IV. The thyroid gland is located in the neck
V. Parathyroid glands are located on the thyroid
VI. The islets of Langerhans are the endocrine portion of the pancreas
   A. Insulin and glucagon regulate the concentration of glucose in the blood
   B. In diabetes mellitus, glucose accumulates in the blood
VII. The adrenal glands function in metabolism and stress
   A. The adrenal medulla secretes epinephrine and norepinephrine
   B. The adrenal cortex secretes steroid hormones
VIII. Stress threatens homeostasis
IX. Several other tissues secrete hormones

LEARNING OBJECTIVES

After you have studied this chapter, you should be able to:

1. Define the term hormone and describe the functions of hormones.
2. Identify the principal endocrine glands and locate them in the body.
3. Describe how hormones work.
4. Describe how endocrine glands are regulated by feedback mechanisms.
5. Justify describing the hypothalamus as the link between nervous and endocrine systems. (Describe the mechanisms by which the hypothalamus exerts its control.)
6. Identify the hormones released by the anterior and posterior lobes of the pituitary, give their origin, and describe their actions.
7. Identify the hormones secreted by the thyroid gland and summarize their actions.
8. Describe how thyroid hormone secretion is regulated, and describe the effects of hyposecretion and hypersecretion.
9. Describe how the parathyroid and thyroid glands regulate calcium levels.
10. Contrast the actions of insulin and glucagon.
11. Describe the role of the adrenal medulla in the body's responses to stress. (Give the actions of epinephrine and norepinephrine.)
12. Identify the hormones secreted by the adrenal cortex and give the actions of glucocorticoids and mineralocorticoids.

The endocrine system works with the nervous system to maintain the steady state of the body. The endocrine system helps regulate growth, reproduction, use of nutrients by cells, salt and fluid balance, and metabolic rate. This system is also important in helping us cope with stress.

The endocrine system consists of tissues and glands that secrete chemical messengers called **hormones.** Recall from Chapter 2 that endocrine glands lack ducts. They release their hormones into the surrounding tissues. The hormones diffuse into capillaries and are transported by the blood. Hormones affect the activity of their **target tissues,** the tissues upon which they act.

Hormones can have widespread effects throughout the body. Responses to nervous system stimulation tend to be rapid and brief. In contrast, responses to hormones may require several hours or even longer and effects may be long lasting. Sometimes the

target tissue may be very specific, as in the case of the male hormone testosterone, which causes hair to grow on the face but not on the scalp. In other cases the entire body can be the target. For example, the thyroid hormones stimulate metabolic rate in most cells. Many hormones have more than one effect.

The study of endocrine function, called **endocrinology,** is a very exciting field of biological research. The principal endocrine glands are illustrated in Figure 9–1 and are described in Table 9–1.

HORMONES ACT ON TARGET CELLS

A hormone may pass through many tissues "unnoticed" until it reaches its target tissue. How does the target tissue "recognize" its hormone? Specialized proteins on or in the target cell act as receptors and bind the hormone. This process is highly specific. The receptor site is like a lock, and the hormones are like different keys. Only the hormone that fits the lock can influence the metabolic machinery of the cell.

When the hormone combines with the receptor, a series of reactions is activated. Because the hormone turns on the system, it is referred to as the **first messenger.**

MANY HORMONES ACT THROUGH SECOND MESSENGERS

Hormones that are large molecules combine with receptors on the plasma membrane of the target cell. Then a message is relayed to the appropriate site within the cell by a **second messenger.** (One compound that acts as a second messenger is **cyclic AMP** (adenosine monophosphate or cAMP).) The second messenger activates enzymes that trigger a chain of reactions leading to a certain metabolic effect.

STEROID HORMONES ACTIVATE GENES

Steroid hormones and thyroid hormones are relatively small molecules that pass easily through the plasma membrane of a target cell. They pass through the cytoplasm and into the nucleus. Specific protein receptors in the nucleus combine with the hormone. This hormone-receptor complex then interacts with the DNA. Appropriate genes are activated, leading to the manufacture of needed proteins. These proteins may stimulate changes in cell activities.

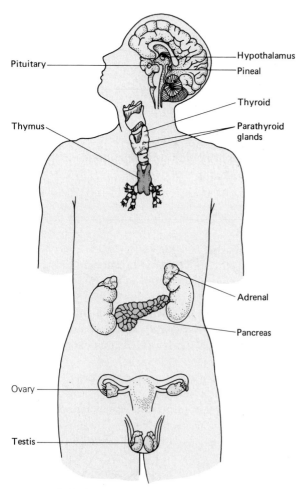

Pituitary
Hypothalamus
Pineal
Thyroid
Thymus
Parathyroid glands
Adrenal
Pancreas
Ovary
Testis

FIGURE 9–1 Location of the principal endocrine glands. Both male and female gonads are shown.

TABLE 9–1
Principal endocrine glands and their hormones*

ENDOCRINE GLAND AND HORMONE	TARGET TISSUE	PRINCIPAL ACTIONS
Hypothalamus		
Releasing and inhibiting hormones	Anterior lobe of pituitary gland	Stimulates or inhibits secretion of specific hormones
Hypothalamus (Production) and Posterior Lobe of Pituitary (Storage and release)		
Oxytocin	Uterus	Stimulates contraction
	Mammary glands	Stimulates ejection of milk into ducts
Antidiuretic hormone (ADH)	Kidneys (collecting ducts)	Stimulates reabsorption of water; conserves water
Anterior Lobe of Pituitary		
Growth hormone (GH)	General	Stimulates growth by promoting protein synthesis
Prolactin	Mammary gland	Stimulates milk secretion
Thyroid-stimulating hormone (TSH)	Thyroid gland	Stimulates secretion of thyroid hormones; stimulates increase in size of thyroid gland
Adrenocorticotropic hormone (ACTH)	Adrenal cortex	Stimulates secretion of adrenocortical hormones
Gonadotropic hormones (FSH, LH)	Gonads	Stimulate gonad function
Thyroid Gland		
Thyroxine (T_4) and triiodothyronine (T_3)	General	Stimulate metabolic rate; essential to normal growth and development
Calcitonin	Bone	Lowers blood-calcium level by inhibiting removal of calcium from bone
Parathyroid Glands		
Parathyroid hormone (PTH)	Bone, kidneys, digestive tract	Increases blood-calcium level by stimulating bone breakdown; stimulates calcium reabsorption in kidneys; activates vitamin D.
Islets of Pancreas		
Insulin	General	Lowers blood-glucose level by facilitating glucose uptake and utilization by cells; stimulates glycogen production
Glucagon	Liver, adipose tissue	Raises blood-glucose level by stimulating manufacture of glucose from glycogen and noncarbohydrate nutrients
Adrenal Medulla		
Epinephrine and norepinephrine	Skeletal muscle, cardiac muscle, blood vessels, liver, adipose tissue	Help body cope with stress; increase heart rate, blood pressure, metabolic rate; reroute blood; mobilize fat; raise blood-sugar level

Table continued on following page

TABLE 9–1 *Continued*

Principal endocrine glands and their hormones*

ENDOCRINE GLAND AND HORMONE	TARGET TISSUE	PRINCIPAL ACTIONS
Adrenal Cortex		
Mineralocorticoids (aldosterone)	Kidney tubules	Maintain sodium and phosphate balance
Glucocorticoids (cortisol)	General	Help body adapt to long-term stress; raise blood-glucose level
Ovary†		
Estrogens	General	Stimulate development of secondary sex characteristics
	Reproductive structures	Stimulate growth of sex organs at puberty; prompt monthly preparation of uterus for pregnancy
Progesterone	Uterus	Completes preparation of uterus for pregnancy
	Breasts	Stimulates development
Testis		
Testosterone	General	Stimulates development of secondary sex characteristics and growth spurt at puberty
	Reproductive structures	Stimulates development of sex organs; stimulates sperm production
Pineal Gland		
Melatonin	Gonads	May help control onset of puberty in humans

*The digestive hormones are described in Chapter 15; the thymus gland are discussed in Chapter 13.
†The reproductive hormones are discussed in Chapter 18.

PROSTAGLANDINS ARE LOCAL HORMONES

Prostaglandins (pros-tah-**glan'**-dins) are a group of closely related lipids that are manufactured by many different tissues in the body. These include the prostate gland (where they were first identified), lungs, liver, and digestive tract. They are sometimes referred to as *local* hormones because they act on nearby cells. Prostaglandins interact with other hormones to regulate various metabolic activities. Some prostaglandins reduce blood pressure; others raise it. Certain prostaglandins cause capillaries to constrict; others dilate capillaries. Some stimulate smooth muscle to contract, whereas others cause muscle to relax. Various prostaglandins dilate the air respiratory passageways, inhibit secretion in the stomach, and stimulate contraction of the uterus.

Because prostaglandins are involved in the regulation of so many metabolic processes, they have great potential for a variety of clinical uses. At present, prostaglandins are used to induce labor in pregnant women, to induce abortion, and to promote healing of ulcers in the stomach and duodenum. Their use as a birth-control drug is being investigated. Some investigators think that these substances may someday be used to treat such illnesses as asthma, arthritis, nasal congestion, and perhaps cancer.

ENDOCRINE GLANDS ARE REGULATED BY FEEDBACK CONTROL

Endocrine glands are regulated by feedback control. Information about hormone levels or their effect is fed back to the gland. The gland then responds in a homeostatic manner. The parathyroid glands of the neck, which help regulate calcium level in the blood, provide a good example of negative feedback.

Parathyroid hormone helps regulate the calcium concentration in the blood. Even a slight decrease in

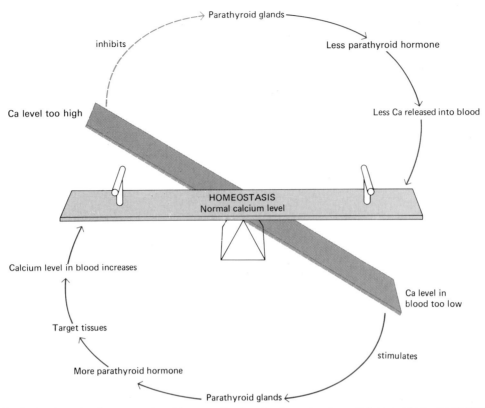

FIGURE 9–2 Endocrine glands are regulated by negative feedback mechanisms. When calcium concentration decreases below normal limits, the parathyroid glands secrete more parathyroid hormone. This hormone activates processes that increase calcium level, thus restoring homeostasis. An abnormally high calcium level inhibits the parathyroid hormones so that less hormone is secreted.

calcium concentration is sensed by the parathyroid glands. They respond by increasing their secretion of parathyroid hormone (Fig. 9–2). Parathyroid hormone increases the calcium concentration in the blood and tissues.

When calcium concentration rises above normal limits, the parathyroid glands are inhibited and slow their output of hormone. Note that both responses are negative-feedback mechanisms because, in both cases, the effects are opposite (negative) to the stimulus.

A few examples of positive-feedback regulation are known. In positive feedback, the output increases the hormone secretion, rather than turning it off.

When an endocrine gland is not regulated effectively, the rate of secretion becomes abnormal. In **hyposecretion,** the gland decreases its hormone output. This condition deprives target cells of needed stimulation. In **hypersecretion,** a gland increases its output to abnormal levels. This condition overstimulates target cells.

THE HYPOTHALAMUS AND PITUITARY GLAND WORK CLOSELY TOGETHER

Endocrine activity is controlled by the **hypothalamus,** which links the nervous and endocrine systems. In response to input from other areas of the brain and from hormones in the blood, the hypothalamus secretes several releasing and inhibiting hormones. These hormones act on the pituitary gland, regulating secretion of several pituitary hormones. The hypothalamus also produces two hormones—oxytocin and antidiuretic hormone—that are stored in the pituitary gland.

The **pituitary gland** is a remarkable organ only about the size of a pea. Connected to the hypothalamus by a stalk of tissue, the pituitary gland lies in a bony cavity (the sella turcica) of the sphenoid bone. Sometimes called the master gland of the body, the pituitary secretes at least nine distinct hormones

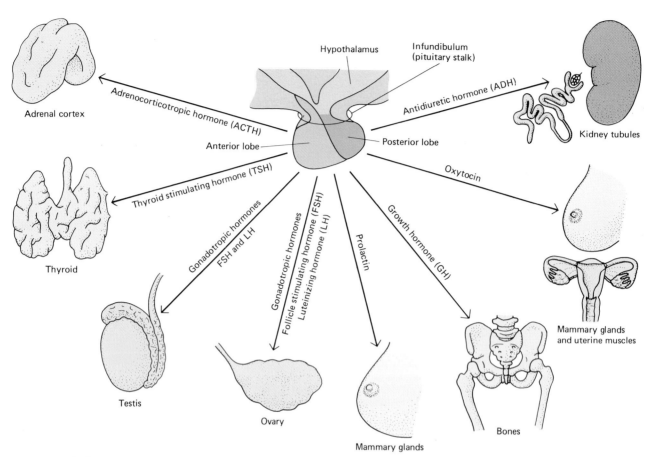

FIGURE 9–3 The pituitary gland is suspended from the hypothalamus by a stalk of neural tissue. The hormones secreted by the pituitary gland and the target tissues they act upon are shown.

(Fig. 9–3). These hormones control the activities of several other endocrine glands and influence many body processes. The pituitary gland consists of two main lobes, the anterior and posterior lobes.

THE POSTERIOR LOBE RELEASES TWO IMPORTANT HORMONES

The **posterior lobe** of the pituitary gland secretes two hormones, **oxytocin** (ox″-see-**tow′**-sin) and **antidiuretic** (an″-tie-die″-you-**ret′**-ik) **hormone (ADH).** These hormones are actually produced in certain neurons in the hypothalamus. The hormones are enclosed within little sacs (vesicles). They pass slowly down the axons of these neurons into the posterior lobe where they are stored.

Oxytocin stimulates contraction of smooth muscle in the wall of the uterus. This hormone also stimulates release of milk from the breast. Toward the end of pregnancy, oxytocin levels rise, stimulating the strong contractions of the uterus needed to expel the baby. Oxytocin is sometimes administered clinically (under the name Pitocin) to initiate or speed labor.

ADH regulates fluid balance in the body and indirectly helps control blood pressure. ADH helps the body conserve water by increasing water reabsorption from the collecting ducts in the kidney (see Chap. 16). The result is a decrease in urine output and an increase in tissue fluid. Nicotine, barbiturates, anxiety, trauma, and some anesthetics increase ADH secretion. You might have wondered why alcohol consumption increases urine output: Alcohol inhibits ADH secretion. The resulting increase in urine output dehydrates the body and causes the feeling of thirst.

ADH deficiency can lead to the condition called **diabetes insipidus** in which enormous quantities of urine may be excreted. This fluid loss must be replaced or serious dehydration rapidly develops.

THE ANTERIOR LOBE SECRETES SEVEN DIFFERENT HORMONES

The **anterior lobe** of the pituitary gland secretes six important hormones, including growth hormone, prolactin, and several hormones that stimulate other endocrine glands. Each of the anterior pituitary hormones is regulated in some way by a **releasing hormone** and in some cases also by an **inhibiting hormone** produced in the hypothalamus.

Tropic Hormones Stimulate Other Endocrine Glands

The anterior lobe of the pituitary gland secretes four **tropic hormones,** hormones that stimulate other endocrine glands. The tropic hormones are: (1) thyroid-stimulating hormone (TSH), which stimulates the thyroid gland; (2) adrenocorticotropin (ACTH), which stimulates the adrenal cortex; and the gonadotropins, (3) follicle-stimulating hormone (FSH) and (4) luteinizing hormone (LH), which control the activities of the gonads (sex glands).

Prolactin Stimulates Secretion of Milk

During lactation (milk production), **prolactin** (pro-**lak′**-tin) stimulates the cells of the mammary glands to secrete milk.

Growth Hormone Stimulates Protein Synthesis

Whether one will be tall or short depends upon many factors, including genes, diet, hormonal balance, and even emotional nurturance. **Growth hormone (GH)** (also called **somatotropin**) stimulates body growth mainly by stimulating protein synthesis.

Circus midgets are **pituitary dwarfs,** individuals whose pituitary gland did not produce enough growth hormone during childhood. Though miniature, a pituitary dwarf has normal intelligence and is usually well proportioned. If the growth centers in the long bones are still open when this condition is diagnosed, it can be treated by injection with growth hormone. Circus giants and other abnormally tall individuals develop when the anterior pituitary secretes too much growth hormone during childhood.

THE THYROID GLAND IS LOCATED IN THE NECK

Shaped somewhat like a shield, the **thyroid gland** is located in the neck. It lies anterior to the trachea and just below the larynx (see Fig. 9–1). Its two lobes of dark red glandular tissue are connected by a bridge of tissue, the isthmus. The thyroid gland secretes two thyroid hormones and a hormone called calcitonin (which will be discussed in connection with the parathyroid glands).

The main thyroid hormone is **thyroxine** (thy-**rok′**-sin), or **T_4** (because it has four iodine atoms in its structure). (A second hormone, T_3, has three iodine atoms in its structure.) The protein-bound iodine, or PBI, is an index of the amount of circulating thyroid hormones and is sometimes measured clinically for that purpose.

The thyroid hormones stimulate metabolic rate and promote growth. The regulation of thyroid hormone secretion depends on a feedback system between the anterior pituitary and the thyroid gland. The anterior pituitary secretes **thyroid-stimulating hormone (TSH),** which promotes synthesis and secretion of thyroid hormones. When the normal concentration of thyroid hormones in the blood falls, the anterior pituitary secretes more TSH.

Low concentration of thyroid hormones → stimulates anterior pituitary → secretes more TSH → stimulates thyroid gland → secretes more thyroid hormones → thyroid hormone concentration increases

When the level of thyroid hormones in the blood rises above normal, the anterior pituitary is inhibited and slows its release of TSH. Too much thyroid hormone in the blood also affects the hypothalamus, inhibiting secretion of TSH-releasing hormones.

Concentration of thyroid hormones increases ---→ inhibits anterior pituitary ---→ secretes less TSH ---→ inhibits thyroid gland ---→ secretes less thyroid hormones ---→ concentration decreases

Extreme **hypothyroidism** during childhood results in low metabolic rate and retarded mental and physical development. This condition is called **cretinism.** (A cretin is very different from a pituitary dwarf.) Any abnormal enlargement of the thyroid gland is termed a **goiter** and may be associated with either hypo- or hypersecretion. One cause is iodine deficiency. Without iodine the gland cannot make thyroid hormones, so their concentration in the blood decreases. In response, the anterior pituitary secretes large amounts of TSH, and the thyroid gland enlarges. Thanks to iodized salt, goiter is no longer common in the United States. In other parts of the world, however, an estimated 200 million persons still suffer from this easily preventable disorder.

PARATHYROID GLANDS ARE LOCATED ON THE THYROID

The **parathyroid glands** are embedded in the connective tissue that surrounds the thyroid gland (see Fig. 9–1). Usually there are four glands, but the number may vary from two to ten. The parathyroid glands secrete **parathyroid hormone (PTH),** a small protein that regulates the calcium level of the blood and tissue fluid.

Appropriate concentrations of calcium are essential for normal nerve and muscle function, bone metabolism, cell-membrane permeability, and blood clotting. PTH increases calcium levels by stimulating release of calcium from the bones. PTH also stimulates calcium reabsorption by the kidney tubules. This action raises the calcium level in the blood while preventing loss in the urine. PTH also activates vitamin D, which then increases the amount of calcium absorbed from the intestine.

The parathyroid glands are regulated by the concentration of calcium in the blood and tissue fluid (see Fig. 9–2). When the calcium concentration rises above normal, the parathyroid glands slow their secretion of PTH.

> Calcium concentration too high - - -→ inhibits parathyroid glands - - -→ secrete less PTH - - -→ calcium concentration decreases

When calcium concentration becomes very high, **calcitonin** (kal″-sih-**tow**′-nin) is released from the thyroid gland. This hormone quickly inhibits removal of calcium from bone.

When the level of calcium in the tissue fluid falls even slightly, parathyroid hormone secretion increases.

> Calcium concentration too low → stimulates parathyroid glands → secrete more PTH → calcium level increases

When PTH secretion is too low, the calcium level falls. Nerve fibers become more excitable and may discharge spontaneously. This causes muscles to twitch and to go into spasms, a condition called tetany. Spasm of the muscles of the larynx interferes with respiration and may lead to death.

Too much PTH results in too much calcium being removed from the bones. The bones are weakened and may fracture easily. The kidneys attempt to excrete the excess calcium removed from the bones.

So much calcium may be present in the urine that crystals of calcium form kidney stones.

THE ISLETS OF LANGERHANS ARE THE ENDOCRINE PORTION OF THE PANCREAS

Usually thought of as a digestive organ, the pancreas lies in the abdomen posterior to the stomach. The pancreas has both exocrine and endocrine functions. Its exocrine cells produce digestive enzymes (see Chap. 15).

More than a million small clusters of cells known as the **islets of Langerhans** are scattered throughout the pancreas. About 70% of the islet cells are **beta cells** that produce the hormone insulin. **Alpha cells** secrete the hormone glucagon.

INSULIN AND GLUCAGON REGULATE THE CONCENTRATION OF GLUCOSE IN THE BLOOD

The main action of **insulin** (**in**′-suh-lin) is to stimulate the storage of glucose. By stimulating cells to take up glucose from the blood, insulin *lowers* the blood-glucose level. Cells store glucose by converting it into glycogen.

Glucagon (**gloo**′-kuh-gon) *raises* the blood-sugar level. It does this by stimulating liver cells to convert glycogen to glucose. It also stimulates the liver cells to make glucose from noncarbohydrates. The actions of glucagon are opposite to those of insulin.

Secretion of insulin and glucagon is directly controlled by the blood-sugar level. After a meal, the concentration of glucose in the blood rises. This stimulates the beta cells to increase insulin secretion. Then, as the cells remove glucose from the blood, its concentration decreases. Insulin secretion decreases accordingly.

> Glucose concentration too high → stimulates beta cells → increased insulin secretion → glucose concentration decreases

When one has not eaten for several hours, the blood-sugar level begins to fall. When it falls from its normal fasting level of about 90 mg/100 ml to about 70 mg/100 ml, the alpha cells of the islets secrete glucagon. Glucose is taken out of storage in the liver and the blood-sugar level returns to normal.

Glucose concentration too low →
stimulates alpha cells → increased
glucagon secretion → glucose
concentration increases

Insulin and glucagon work together but in opposite ways to keep the blood-sugar level within normal limits. When glucose level rises, insulin release brings it back to normal; when it falls, glucagon acts to raise it again (Fig. 9–4). The insulin-glucagon system is a powerful, fast-acting mechanism for keeping the blood-sugar level normal. Can you think of reasons why it is important to maintain a constant blood-sugar level? Perhaps the most important one is that brain cells are completely dependent upon a continuous supply of glucose because they are normally unable to use any other nutrient as fuel.

IN DIABETES MELLITUS, GLUCOSE ACCUMULATES IN THE BLOOD

The main disorder associated with pancreatic hormones is **diabetes mellitus** (die-ah-**be′**-teez mel-**lie′**-tus). Insulin-dependent diabetes, referred to as **type I diabetes,** usually develops before age 20. In

this disorder there is a marked decrease in the number of beta cells in the pancreas. This loss of beta cells results in insulin deficiency. Type I diabetes is clinically treated with insulin injections.

More than 90% of all cases of diabetes are noninsulin dependent, or **type II.** This type develops gradually, usually in overweight persons over age 40. In many cases of type II diabetes, sufficient insulin is released by the islets of Langerhans. The problem is that the target cells are not able to take up the insulin and use it.

In diabetes mellitus, cells cannot take in enough glucose. Glucose remains in the blood, and the blood-glucose level rises (hyperglycemia). Instead of the normal fasting level of about 90 mg/100 ml, the diabetic may have from 300 to more than 1000 mg/100 ml. Glucose does not normally appear in the urine. However, in diabetics, the blood-glucose concentration is so high that sugar spills out into the urine.

THE ADRENAL GLANDS FUNCTION IN METABOLISM AND STRESS

The paired **adrenal glands** are small, yellow masses of tissue located above the kidneys (Fig. 9–5).

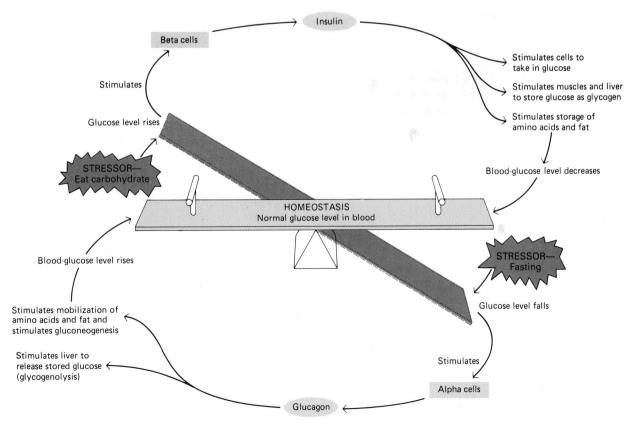

FIGURE 9–4 Regulation of blood-glucose (sugar) level by insulin and glucagon.

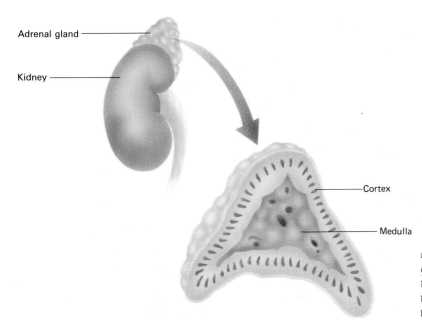

Adrenal gland

Kidney

Cortex

Medulla

FIGURE 9–5 *The paired adrenal glands are small, yellow masses of tissues that lie in contact with the upper ends of the kidneys. Each gland consists of a central medulla and an outer cortex.*

Each gland consists of a central portion, the **adrenal medulla,** and a larger outer region, the **adrenal cortex.** These regions function as distinct glands. Both secrete hormones that help to regulate metabolism, and both help the body to deal with stress.

THE ADRENAL MEDULLA SECRETES EPINEPHRINE AND NOREPINEPHRINE

The adrenal medulla develops from nervous tissue and is sometimes considered part of the sympathetic nervous system. The adrenal medulla secretes two hormones, **epinephrine** (ep″-ih-**nef′**-rin) (also called adrenaline) and **norepinephrine** (nor″-ep-ih-**nef′**-rin) (also called noradrenaline). Norepinephrine is the same substance secreted as a neurotransmitter by sympathetic neurons and by some neurons in the central nervous system.

The adrenal medulla is called the emergency gland of the body because it prepares us to cope with threatening situations. If a monster were suddenly to appear before you, hormone secretion from this gland would initiate an alarm reaction enabling you to think quickly, then fight harder or run much faster than normally. Some of the actions of epinephrine and norepinephrine are to:

1. Increase metabolic rate as much as 100%.
2. Increase the heart rate and stimulate the heart to contract with greater strength.
3. Increase blood pressure.
4. Increase alertness.
5. Dilate the airways so that breathing is more effective. (Epinephrine and related drugs are used clinically to relieve nasal congestion and asthma.)

6. Reroute the blood so that more flows to the organs essential for emergency action. Blood vessels to the skin and most internal organs are constricted; those to the brain, muscles, and heart are dilated. Constriction of the blood vessels to the skin has the added advantage of decreasing blood loss from superficial wounds. (It also explains the sudden paleness that comes with fear or rage.)

7. Increase strength of contraction of skeletal muscles.

8. Raise glucose and fatty acid levels in the blood, so that there is enough fuel to provide the extra energy needed.

Under normal conditions, both epinephrine and norepinephrine are secreted continuously in small amounts. Their secretion is under nervous control. When anxiety is aroused, neural messages are sent through sympathetic nerves to the adrenal medulla. Secretion of these hormones then increases.

Anxiety → affects hypothalamus → sends messages over sympathetic nerves → stimulate adrenal medulla → secrete more epinephrine and norepinephrine

THE ADRENAL CORTEX SECRETES STEROID HORMONES

The **adrenal cortex** secretes three different types of hormones. These hormones are all steroids:

1. **Glucocorticoids** (gloo″-ko-**kor**′-tih-koids) help the body cope with stress. The main glucocorticoid is **cortisol** (also called **hydrocortisone**). The principal action of the glucocorticoids is to promote production of glucose from other nutrients. This action provides the excess nutrients needed by the cells when the body is under stress. Thus, the adrenal cortex provides an important backup system for the adrenal medulla. The physiology of stress will be discussed in further detail later in this chapter.

Glucocorticoids also reduce inflammation and are used clinically in allergic reactions, infections, arthritis, and certain other disorders. When present in large amounts over long periods of time, glucocorticoids can cause serious side effects. They depress the immune system and so decrease one's ability to fight infections.

2. **Mineralocorticoids** (min″-er-al-o-**kor**′-tih-koids) regulate water and salt balance. **Aldosterone** (**al**′-doe-stee-rone) is the principal mineralocorticoid. Its main function is to maintain homeostasis of sodium and potassium ions. It does this mainly by stimulating the kidneys to conserve sodium and to excrete potassium.

3. **Sex hormones.** Very small amounts of both **androgens** (hormones that have masculinizing effects) and **estrogens** (hormones that have feminizing effects) are secreted by the adrenal cortex in both sexes. The amounts of these hormones released are so small that they have little effect on the body.

Secretion of hormones by the adrenal cortex is regulated by ACTH from the pituitary. In turn, ACTH secretion is controlled by a releasing hormone from the hypothalamus. Almost any type of stress is reported to the hypothalamus, which activates the system, so ACTH is released. When the body is not under stress, high levels of these hormones in the blood inhibit both the hypothalamus and the pituitary.

STRESS THREATENS HOMEOSTASIS

Good health and survival depend upon maintaining homeostasis. **Stressors,** stimuli that disrupt the steady state of the body, must be dealt with swiftly and effectively. Stressors, whether in the form of infection, disease, arguments, or even the anxiety of taking a test for which one is not fully prepared, may threaten homeostasis, putting the body in a state of **stress.** The brain sends messages activating the sympathetic nervous system and the adrenal glands. Epinephrine and norepinephrine are released, and the body prepares for fight or flight. The hypothalamus

also signals the anterior pituitary hormonally to secrete ACTH, which increases cortisol secretion, thereby adjusting metabolism to meet the increased demands of the stressful situation (Fig. 9–6).

Some stressors are short-lived. We react to the situation and quickly resolve it. Other stressors may last for days, weeks, or even years. A chronic disease or an unhappy marriage or job situation is an example of a long-term stressor.

Physiologist Hans Selye introduced the term **general-adaptation syndrome (GAS)** to describe the body's response to stress. This syndrome has three phases:

1. The **alarm reaction,** in which the adrenal medulla prepares the body for fight or flight. The heart beats faster, pulse and blood pressure rise, blood is rerouted, metabolic rate increases, and all the other physiological changes take place that help in coping with an emergency situation.

2. If stress continues over a long period, the body enters the second stage, the **resistance reaction.** During this stage blood pressure remains abnormally high and metabolism is geared to help the body resist the effects of the stressor, whether fighting infection or dealing with an emotional problem. Protein breakdown is characteristic of the resistance stage. Levels of many hormones, including cortisol, aldosterone, thyroxine, and growth hormone, are elevated.

3. The final phase of the GAS is the **stage of exhaustion,** in which the body seems to wear out and death may occur.

It has been suggested that in our stressful society, many persons remain in the resistance stage of the GAS almost continuously. Chronic stress is harmful because of the side effects of long-term elevated levels of cortisol. Although glucocorticoids are helpful in reducing inflammation, they can also interfere with normal immune responses, so that infection spreads. Chronic high blood pressure may contribute to heart disease. Among the diseases linked to excessive amounts of these hormones are ulcers, high blood pressure, atherosclerosis, and arthritis.

SEVERAL OTHER TISSUES SECRETE HORMONES

Many other tissues of the body secrete hormones. Some of these will be discussed in other chapters. For example, the hormones secreted by the ovary and testis will be discussed in Chapter 18. The digestive tract secretes hormones that help regulate digestion (see Chap. 15).

The **pineal gland,** located in the brain, secretes

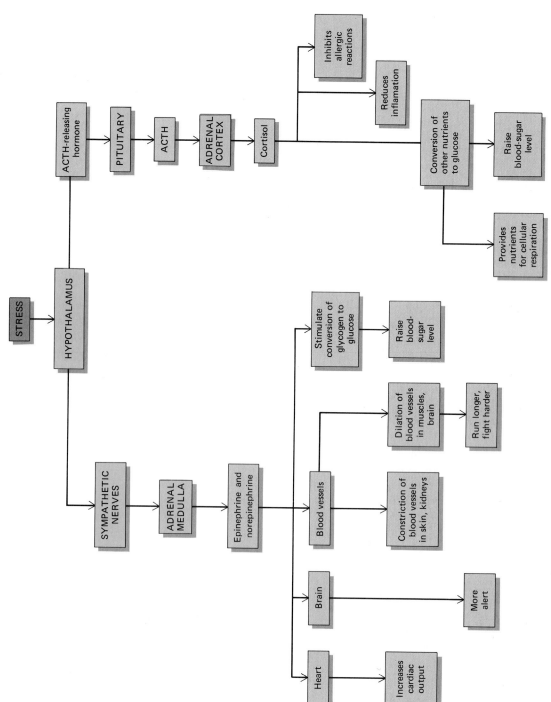

FIGURE 9–6 The adrenal medulla and the adrenal cortex both play important roles in helping the body to cope with stress. Some of the effects of their hormones are shown here.

melatonin. This hormone may help control the onset of puberty (period of sexual maturation) in the male.

The kidneys secrete a hormone that stimulates red blood cell production. The thymus gland secretes the hormone **thymosin,** important in immune function. A hormone known as **atrial natriuretic factor (ANF)** is released by stretched cardiac muscle fibers in response to increased blood volume. ANF helps reduce blood pressure.

SUMMARY

I. The endocrine system regulates homeostasis of many metabolic processes; it consists of endocrine glands and tissues that release hormones.
   A. Endocrine glands are ductless glands that secrete hormones into the tissue fluid.
   B. Hormones are chemical messengers secreted by endocrine glands. They are transported to target tissues by the blood and stimulate the target tissue to change some metabolic activity.
II. Several mechanisms of hormone action are known.
   A. Many hormones bind to receptors on the plasma membrane of target cells. This activates a second messenger, such as cyclic AMP, which triggers the chain of events leading to the actual response.
   B. Steroid hormones enter target cells and combine with receptors within the nucleus. The steroid-receptor complex moves into the nucleus and activates specific genes.
III. Endocrine glands are regulated by feedback controls.
IV. The hypothalamus is the link between the nervous and endocrine systems.
   A. The hypothalamus secretes releasing and inhibiting hormones that regulate the anterior pituitary gland.
   B. The hypothalamus also produces the hormones oxytocin and ADH, which are released by the posterior pituitary gland.
V. The posterior pituitary gland releases the hormones oxytocin and ADH.
   A. Oxytocin stimulates the uterus to contract and stimulates release of milk from the lactating breast.
   B. ADH (antidiuretic hormone) promotes reabsorption of water by the kidney ducts.
VI. The anterior pituitary gland releases growth hormone, prolactin, and several tropic hormones.
   A. Growth hormone promotes growth by promoting protein synthesis.
   B. Prolactin stimulates milk production in the lactating breast.
   C. The tropic hormones include thyroid-stimulating hormone (TSH), ACTH, and the gonadotropic hormones.
VII. The thyroid hormones T_3 and T_4 stimulate the rate of metabolism.
   A. A rise in thyroid hormone level in the blood inhibits secretion of TSH by the pituitary; a decrease stimulates TSH secretion.
   B. Extreme hypothyroidism in childhood may result in cretinism.
VIII. The parathyroid glands secrete PTH (parathyroid hormone), which increases calcium levels in the blood and tissue fluid.
   A. PTH stimulates release of calcium from bones, stimulates calcium conservation by the kidneys, and helps activate vitamin D.
   B. An increase in calcium level inhibits PTH secretion; a decrease in calcium level stimulates secretion.
IX. The islets of Langerhans secrete insulin and glucagon, hormones that regulate the glucose level in the blood.
   A. Insulin lowers the blood-sugar level by stimulating uptake and storage of glucose by the cells.
   B. Glucagon raises the blood-sugar level by stimulating release of glucose from storage and manufacture of glucose from other nutrients.
X. The adrenal glands consist of the adrenal medulla and the adrenal cortex; both release hormones that help the body cope with stress.
   A. The adrenal medulla releases epinephrine and norepinephrine. These hormones increase heart rate, metabolic rate, and strength of muscle contraction and reroute the blood to organs that need more blood in time of stress.

B. The adrenal cortex releases cortisol, which promotes manufacture from other nutrients, thereby raising the blood-sugar level; this hormone provides backup to the adrenal medullary hormones.

C. The adrenal cortex also releases aldosterone, which helps maintain sodium and potassium balance.

XI. In response to stress the adrenal medulla initiates an alarm reaction that prepares the body to cope with stress. Secretion of cortisol by the adrenal cortex ensures a steady supply of needed nutrients for the rapidly metabolizing cells.

POST TEST

1. Endocrine glands lack _____ and release

   _____ .

2. A hormone may be defined as a _____ .

3. Hormones combine with receptors on _____ cells.

4. The _____ serves as the link between nervous and endocrine systems.

5. The hormone _____ stimulates contraction of the uterus.

6. The hormone _____ stimulates milk production in the lactating breast.

7. Growth hormone is produced by the _____ .

8. Oxytocin is produced by the _____ .

9. Oxytocin is stored and released by the _____ when needed.

10. Hypersecretion of growth hormone during childhood may result in

    _____ .

11. The action of the thyroid hormones is to stimulate _____ .

12. In addition to the thyroid hormones, the thyroid gland produces a hormone called _____ , which acts to _____ .

13. A hormone that raises the level of sodium in the blood is

    _____ .

14. Blood-sugar level is lowered by the hormone _____ released from the pancreas.

15. Glucagon acts to _____ blood-sugar level.

16. The adrenal medulla releases _____ and

    _____ .

17. Beta cells in the islets of Langerhans produce _____ .

18. Label the diagram on the facing page.

REVIEW QUESTIONS

1. How do hormones recognize their target tissues? How do hormones work?

2. List the hormones released by the anterior pituitary gland and give their actions.

3. How is the thyroid gland regulated? Draw a diagram to illustrate your answer.

4. What are the actions of parathyroid hormone?

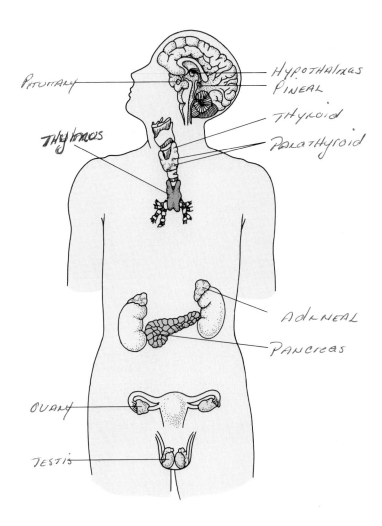

PITUITARY

HYPOTHALAMUS
PINEAL

THYROID
PARATHYROID

THYMUS

ADRENAL
PANCREAS

OVARY

TESTIS

5. How are the parathyroid glands regulated?

6. What is cyclic AMP? What are prostaglandins?

7. What are the symptoms associated with an imbalance in calcium metabolism?

8. How is blood-sugar level regulated? Describe the role of insulin and glucagon in maintaining a steady blood-sugar level.

9. How do the adrenal glands help the body adjust to stress?

POST TEST ANSWERS

1. ducts; hormones
2. chemical messenger that stimulates a change in some metabolic activity
3. target
4. hypothalamus
5. oxytocin
6. prolactin
7. anterior pituitary
8. hypothalamus
9. posterior pituitary
10. abnormally tall individuals
11. the rate of metabolism
12. calcitonin; lower calcium level in the blood
13. aldosterone
14. insulin
15. increase (raise)
16. epinephrine; norepinephrine
17. insulin
18. see Figure 9–1

Ten

THE CIRCULATORY SYSTEM: BLOOD

CHAPTER OUTLINE

 I. Blood consists of cells and platelets suspended in plasma
 II. Plasma is the fluid component of blood
 III. Red blood cells transport oxygen
 IV. White blood cells defend the body against disease
 V. Platelets function in blood clotting
 VI. Successful blood transfusions depend on blood groups
    A. The ABO system consists of antigens A and B
    B. The Rh system consists of several Rh antigens

LEARNING OBJECTIVES

After you have studied this chapter, you should be able to:
1. List the functions of the circulatory system.
2. Describe the composition of blood plasma and describe the functions of plasma proteins.
3. Describe the structure and function of red blood cells.
4. Describe the structure and function of white blood cells.
5. Describe the structure and function of platelets and summarize the chemical events of blood clotting.
6. Identify the antigen and antibody associated with each ABO blood type, and explain why blood types must be carefully matched in transfusion therapy.
7. Identify the cause and importance of Rh incompatibility.

The circulatory system is the transportation system of the body. It also protects the body against disease organisms. Substances transported by the circulatory system are carried by the blood. The circulatory system:

1. Transports nutrients from the digestive system to all parts of the body.
2. Transports oxygen from the lungs to all the cells of the body.
3. Transports carbon dioxide and other metabolic wastes from the cells to the excretory organs.

4. Transports hormones from the endocrine glands to target tissues.
5. Helps maintain normal body temperature.
6. Helps maintain fluid balance.
7. Protects the body against disease-causing organisms.

The circulatory system consists of two subsystems—the **cardiovascular** (kar-dee-o-**vas'**-ku-lar) **system** and the **lymphatic** (lim-**fat'**-ik) **system.** In the cardiovascular system the heart pumps blood through a vast system of blood vessels. The lymphatic system helps preserve fluid balance and protects the body against disease. In this chapter we will focus on the blood.

BLOOD CONSISTS OF CELLS AND PLATELETS SUSPENDED IN PLASMA

Blood consists of red blood cells, white blood cells, and cell fragments called platelets, all suspended in a pale yellowish fluid called **plasma** (**plaz′**-muh) (Fig. 10–1). In an adult weighing about 70 kg (154 lb), blood volume is normally about 5.6 liters (about 6 qt). The normal pH (a measure of acidity/alkalinity) of blood is slightly alkaline (ranging between 7.35 and 7.45).

PLASMA IS THE FLUID COMPONENT OF BLOOD

Plasma consists of 92% water, about 7% protein, a sprinkling of salts, and many materials being transported, including oxygen and other dissolved gases, glucose and other nutrients, metabolic wastes, and hormones (Fig. 10–2). When the proteins involved in clotting have been removed, the remaining liquid is called **serum.**

Plasma proteins may be divided into three groups, or fractions: (1) **albumins;** (2) **globulins;** and (3) **fibrinogen** (fye-**brin′**-o-jin). One of their homeostatic functions is to maintain blood volume. As blood flows through the tiny blood vessels called capillaries, some of the plasma seeps through the capillary walls and passes into the tissues. However, large protein molecules have difficulty passing through the capillary walls, so most of them remain in the blood. There they exert an osmotic force that helps pull plasma back into the blood.

Aside from their general functions, some plasma proteins perform specific jobs. One group of the globulins, the **gamma globulins,** serves as **antibodies,** substances that provide immunity (protection) against disease. Fibrinogen and several other plasma proteins are important in the process of blood clotting. The gamma globulins are produced in the lymph tissues. The other plasma proteins are manufactured in the liver.

RED BLOOD CELLS TRANSPORT OXYGEN

An adult male has about 30 trillion **red blood cells (RBCs),** or **erythrocytes** (ee-**rith′**-row-sites), circulating in his blood. This amounts to about 5.4 million per cubic millimeter (mm^3). (Females have slightly fewer.) Red blood cells are one of the most specialized cell types in the body. They are adapted for producing and packaging hemoglobin, the red pigment that transports oxygen. Red blood cells are very small (about 7 μm in diameter and about 2 μm thick). About 3000 lined up end to end would span only about 1 inch!

A mature red blood cell is a tiny, flexible, biconcave disc. (Biconcave means thinner in the center than around the edge.) When viewed under an ordinary light microscope, the center portion of the red blood cell appears relatively clear because the cytoplasm is thinnest there. A mature red blood cell lacks a nucleus as well as most other organelles.

As blood circulates through the lungs, oxygen diffuses into the blood and into the red blood cells, where it combines weakly with hemoglobin to form **oxyhemoglobin.** When blood circulates through the brain or some other tissue where cells are low in oxygen, the reverse reaction occurs. The oxygen then diffuses out of the capillaries and into the cells.

Oxyhemoglobin is bright red. It is responsible for the color of the oxygen-rich blood that flows through arteries. Hemoglobin that is not combined with oxygen is bluish in color and accounts for the darker appearance of venous blood.

Each second about 2.4 million red blood cells must be manufactured to replace a similar number that wear out and are destroyed. In children, red blood cells are produced in the red bone marrow of almost all bones. Recall that red bone marrow is a type of connective tissue found in spongy bone. In adults, red bone marrow is found only in certain bones such as the vertebrae, sternum, skull, and ribs.

The red bone marrow has **stem cells,** which multiply, giving rise to the blood cells. After a 3- to 5-day maturation period, red blood cells squeeze through the walls of capillaries within the bone marrow and enter the circulation.

Without a nucleus and other organelles, a red blood cell is unable to manufacture proteins. When its proteins break down they cannot be replaced. The cell becomes fragile and may rupture as it squeezes through a tight channel in the circulation. Old or

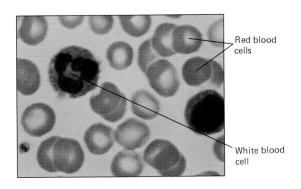

Red blood
cells

White blood
cell

F I G U R E **10–1** Photomicrograph of blood. The cells shown are red blood cells except for two white blood cells (approximately × 1200).

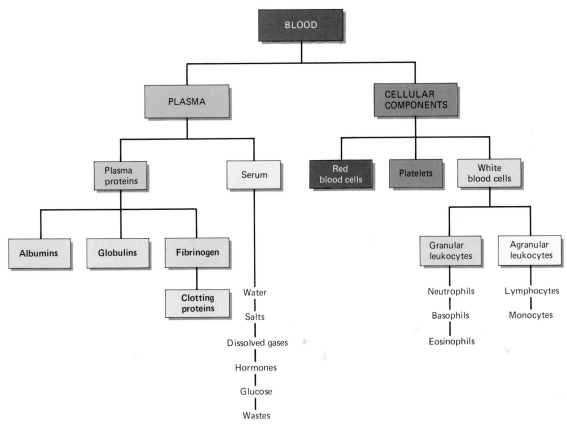

F I G U R E **10–2** Components of blood.

damaged cells are phagocytized in the liver, spleen, or bone marrow. The average circulating life span of a red blood cell is about 120 days.

When production of new red blood cells does not match the rate of red blood cell destruction, the number of red blood cells becomes deficient. With too few red blood cells, there is a deficiency of hemoglobin. This condition is called **anemia** (a-**nee'**-me-ah). With decreased amounts of hemoglobin, oxygen transport is reduced and cells do not receive enough oxygen. The most common cause of anemia is a deficiency of iron in the diet. Iron is an essential ingredient of hemoglobin. The body cannot synthesize hemoglobin without iron. That would be like trying to make a chocolate cake without chocolate; an essential ingredient would be missing.

WHITE BLOOD CELLS DEFEND THE BODY AGAINST DISEASE

White blood cells (WBCs), or **leukocytes** (**loo'**-koe-sites), defend the body against agents that cause disease. White blood cells develop from stem cells in the red bone marrow, but some types complete their maturation elsewhere in the body. While red blood cells function within the blood, many white cells leave the circulation and perform their duties in various tissues. They move through the tissues, flowing along like amebas. As they wander through the body, the white blood cells phagocytize bacteria, dead cells, and foreign matter.

Five different types of white blood cells are found in the circulating blood. Three types have granules containing powerful enzymes. These enzymes can destroy bacteria that enter the body. The kinds of white blood cells that contain granules are **neutrophils** (**noo'**-trow-fils), **basophils** (**bay'**-so-fils), and **eosinophils** (ee-oh-**sin'**-oh-fils) (Fig. 10–3). Two types of white blood cells have no specific granules in their cytoplasm. These are the **lymphocytes** (**lim'**-foe-sites) and **monocytes** (**mon'**-oh-sites). Lymphocytes are very important in immunity; one type produces antibodies. Monocytes migrate into the connective tissues and develop into macrophages, the large scavenger cells of the body.

White blood cells are far less numerous than the red blood cells (only about 1 white cell to every 700 red blood cells). Normally, an adult has about 7000 white blood cells/mm^3 of blood. A white blood cell count elevated above 10,000/mm^3 may indicate the presence of bacterial infection. Leukemia is a form of cancer in which white blood cells multiply wildly

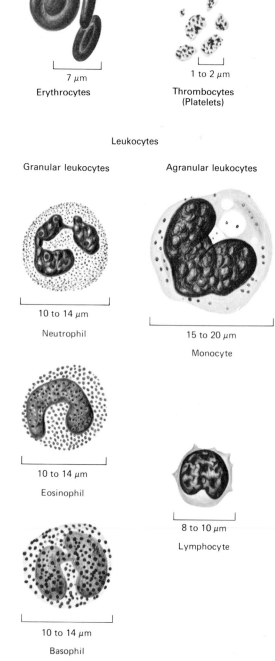

Erythrocytes — 7 μm

Thrombocytes (Platelets) — 1 to 2 μm

Leukocytes

Granular leukocytes

Agranular leukocytes

Neutrophil — 10 to 14 μm

Monocyte — 15 to 20 μm

Eosinophil — 10 to 14 μm

Lymphocyte — 8 to 10 μm

Basophil — 10 to 14 μm

FIGURE 10–3 Main types of blood cells in the circulating blood.

within the bone marrow. They crowd out developing red blood cells and platelets, leading to anemia and impaired blood clotting.

Viral infections can cause lowered white cell counts. Depressed white cell counts are also found in patients with rheumatoid arthritis, cirrhosis of the liver, and certain other disorders. Exposure to radiation and certain drugs, including those used in cancer chemotherapy, may severely lower white cell production. Because bacterial infections tend to increase the white blood cell count, while viral infections tend to decrease the white cell count, physicians often consider the results of blood tests before prescribing antibiotics. Such drugs (e.g., penicillin and streptomycin) are effective against bacteria but do not kill viruses.

PLATELETS FUNCTION IN BLOOD CLOTTING

Platelets, also called thrombocytes (**throm'**-bow-sites), are not actually cells. They are tiny fragments of cytoplasm that become detached from certain very large cells in the bone marrow. There are about 300,000 platelets/mm³ of circulating blood! These cell fragments prevent blood loss. When you cut your finger, platelets gather and seal the hole in the blood vessel wall. A complex series of chemical reactions produces tiny fibers that reinforce the platelets, forming a strong clot.

Although the process of blood clotting is quite complex, we can summarize its three main steps (Fig. 10–4):

1. When tissue is damaged, a series of reactions takes place involving certain proteins in the blood. These proteins are called **clotting factors.** One of the clotting factors is released by platelets. The reactions result in formation of a complex of substances known as **prothrombin activator.**

2. Prothrombin activator is an enzyme. It catalyzes the conversion of **prothrombin** to its active form, **thrombin.** Prothrombin is a globulin found in

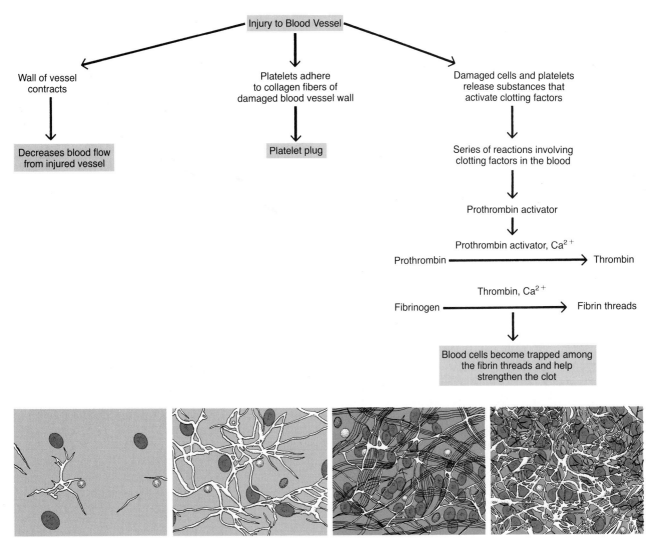

FIGURE 10–4 Overview of blood clotting. Fibrin threads form the webbing of the clot. Blood cells, platelets, and plasma become trapped among the fibrin threads and help to strengthen the clot.

the plasma. This protein is manufactured in the liver with the help of vitamin K. Calcium ions must be present for prothrombin to be converted to thrombin.

3. Thrombin acts as an enzyme to convert the plasma protein fibrinogen to **fibrin,** a fibrous protein that forms long threads. These fibrin threads form the webbing of the clot. They trap blood cells, platelets, and plasma, which help to strengthen the clot (Fig. 10–4).

Within a few minutes after clot formation, the clot begins to contract and squeezes out serum, that is, plasma containing neither fibrinogen nor clotting factors. As the clot contracts, the ends of the damaged blood vessel are pulled closer together, and the clot itself becomes smaller and harder. The clotting process may be summarized as follows:

$$\text{Prothrombin} \xrightarrow[\text{calcium ions}]{\text{prothrombin activator,}} \text{thrombin}$$

$$\text{Fibrinogen} \xrightarrow{\text{thrombin}} \text{fibrin threads}$$

SUCCESSFUL BLOOD TRANSFUSIONS DEPEND ON BLOOD GROUPS

Transfusing blood from a healthy person to a patient is a routine, lifesaving procedure. During surgery or after hemorrhage, whole blood can be transfused to restore an adequate volume of circulating blood. Blood components can be separated by centrifuging (spinning the blood at high speed so the heavier components settle at the bottom of a tube). (See the figure in Table 10–1). Then, components of blood can be transfused. For example, plasma itself can be used to expand blood volume in patients who are in circulatory shock (discussed in Chap. 13). Whole blood or blood components can be stored in blood banks and withdrawn as needed.

In transfusing blood, the blood of the donor must be carefully matched with the blood of the recipient. If the blood is not compatible, a transfusion reaction will occur. This is a serious allergic reaction in which antibodies in the recipient's blood attack the foreign red blood cells in the transfused blood, causing them to **agglutinate** (clump). Red blood cells may break, releasing hemoglobin into the plasma, a process known as **hemolysis** (he-**mol'**-ih-sis).

THE ABO SYSTEM CONSISTS OF ANTIGENS A AND B

Although several blood typing systems are used, the most important clinically are the ABO and Rh systems. Each of us has type A, B, AB, or O blood (Table 10–2). Red blood cells have specific proteins called **antigens** on their surfaces. These antigens are different in persons with different blood types (Fig. 10–5). Those with type A blood have red cells coated with type A antigen. Individuals with type B blood have type B antigen, and those with type AB blood have both kinds of antigen—A and B. Individuals with type O blood have neither type of antigen on their red cells. They are referred to as universal donors because theoretically they can donate blood to patients with any blood type.

Certain **antibodies** (also proteins) are found in

TEST	DESCRIPTION
Complete blood count (CBC)	Consists of four separate tests: (1) measurement of hemoglobin; (2) hematocrit; (3) white blood cell count and differential (percentage of each white cell type); (4) examination of red blood cells and platelets. (Sometimes a red blood cell count is also made.)
Hemoglobin	Hemoglobin and hematocrit tests are used to check for anemia and to follow the progress of an anemic patient. Normal adult value: 12 to 15 g/100 ml for women; 14 to 17 g/100 ml for men. Whole blood is treated chemically so that the hemoglobin forms a stable pigment (cyanmethemoglobin); then the optical density of the solution is measured in a photometer. (Optical density is directly proportional to concentration of hemoglobin.)

TABLE 10–1
Routine blood tests

TABLE 10–1 *Continued*

Routine blood tests

TEST	DESCRIPTION
Hematocrit	Hematocrit is an indication of percentage of red cells per unit of blood volume. Normal adult values: 36 to 46% for women; 42 to 54% for men. Blood is centrifuged. Then the volume of red cells is read off a scale on the tube; expressed as percentage of whole blood volume.

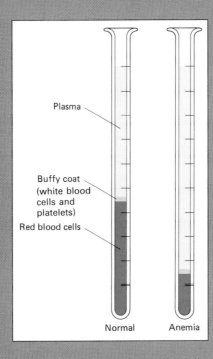

Plasma

Buffy coat (white blood cells and platelets)

Red blood cells

Normal   Anemia

Hematocrits in the normal and in the anemic individual. Blood is separated into its components by spinning it at high speed, a process called centrifugation.

TEST	DESCRIPTION
White blood cell count (WBC)	Used in diagnosis of bacterial infection and in certain diseases such as leukemia. Used to monitor the effects of radiation or drug therapy that may depress WBC to dangerous levels. Whole blood is mixed with a weak acid solution for the purpose of diluting the blood and hemolyzing the red cells. The diluted blood is placed in a counting chamber (hemocytometer: a microscope slide with a well and a grid marking off tiny squares) and the white cells are counted. Then the number per cubic millimeter can be calculated.
Red blood cell count (RBC)	May be counted manually as in WBC, or an electronic cell counter may be used.
Differential cell count	Used to determine the relative number of each type of white cell in the blood. The differential cell count can be made by analysis of a stained blood smear.
Platelet count	Used in diagnosis of bleeding disorders and in evaluating effects of chemotherapy or radiation therapy on platelet production. Blood is diluted and stained; then platelets are counted in a counting chamber.
Prothrombin time (PT)	Used when clotting disorder is suspected and when monitoring response to oral anticoagulant therapy. Plasma is isolated from drawn blood. Calcium is added to plasma in the presence of tissue thromboplastin. Time elapsed between Ca^{2+} addition and clot formation is prothrombin time (normal plasma clotting time is about 11 seconds).

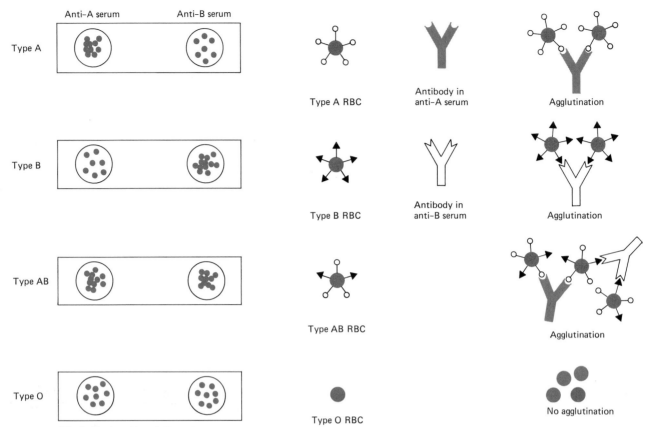

F I G U R E **10–5** Typing blood. Each blood type has a different combination of antigen and antibody. In typing blood, serum containing antibody to type A blood is placed on one area of a slide and serum containing antibody to type B is placed on another area of the slide. A drop of blood is mixed with each type of serum. If the blood contains A antigen, it will agglutinate with the anti-A serum. If the blood contains B antigen, it will agglutinate with the anti-B serum.

the plasma. Individuals with type A blood have anti-B antibodies circulating in their blood. Those with type B blood have anti-A antibodies. Persons with type AB blood have neither type of antibody, and those with type O blood have both. Each type of antibody recognizes a specific type of antigen. For example, if a patient with type A blood is accidentally given type B blood, his antibodies will combine with the type B antigens on the surfaces of the donated red blood cells. This causes the donated cells to agglutinate and produces hemolysis. Such mismatching can be fatal, especially if the mistake should ever be repeated. Blood typing is routinely carried out by mixing a sample of a person's blood with serum containing different types of antibodies to determine whether agglutination occurs.

THE RH SYSTEM CONSISTS OF SEVERAL RH ANTIGENS

The Rh system consists of at least eight different kinds of Rh antibodies, each referred to as an Rh factor. By far the most important is antigen D. Most persons of Western European descent are Rh positive, which means that they have antigen D on the surfaces of their red blood cells (as well as the antigens of the ABO system appropriate to their blood type). The 15% or so of the population who are Rh negative have no antigen D and will produce antibodies against that antigen when exposed to Rh-positive blood.

TABLE 10–2

ABO blood types

BLOOD TYPE	ANTIGEN ON RBC	ANTIBODIES IN PLASMA
O	—	Anti-A, anti-B
A	A	Anti-B
B	B	Anti-A
AB	A, B	—

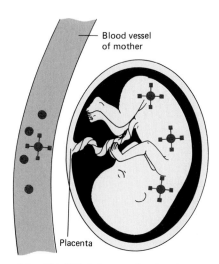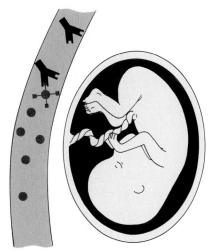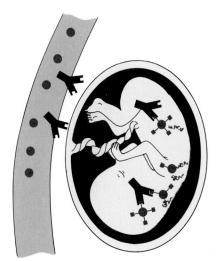

A few Rh+ RBCs leak across the placenta from the fetus into the mother's blood

(a)

The mother produces anti-Rh antibodies in response to Rh antigen on Rh+ RBCs

(b)

Anti-Rh antibodies cross the placenta and enter the blood of the fetus. Hemolysis of Rh+ blood occurs. The fetus may develop erythroblastosis fetalis.

(c)

● Rh− RBC of mother

Rh+ RBC of fetus with Rh antigen on surface

Anti-Rh antibody made against Rh+ RBC

Hemolysis of Rh+ RBC

FIGURE **10–6** Rh incompatibility can cause serious problems when an Rh-negative woman and an Rh-positive man produce an Rh-positive offspring. *(a)* Some Rh red blood cells leak across the placenta from the fetus into the mother's blood. *(b)* The woman produces antibodies in response to the antigens on the Rh⁺ RBCs. *(c)* Some of the antibodies cross the placenta and enter the blood of the fetus, causing hemolysis. The fetus may develop erythroblastosis fetalis.

Unlike the antibodies of the ABO system, antibody D does not occur in the blood of Rh-negative persons unless they have been exposed to the D antigen. However, once antibodies to Rh blood have been produced, they remain in the blood.

Although several kinds of maternal-fetal blood-type incompatibilities are known, Rh incompatibility is probably the most important. Rh incompatibility can cause serious problems when an Rh-negative woman and an Rh-positive man produce an Rh-positive baby. At the time of birth, a small amount of the baby's blood may mix with the mother's, stimulating her body to produce antibodies against the Rh-positive blood. If she should carry an Rh-positive child in a subsequent pregnancy, her antibodies can cross the placenta (the organ of exchange between mother and developing baby) and cause hemolysis of the baby's red blood cells (Fig. 10–6). Breakdown products of the hemoglobin released into the circulation damage many organs, including the brain. This type of hemolytic disease is known as **erythroblastosis fetalis** (ee-rith″-row-blas-**tow**′-sis fee-**tal**′-is).

SUMMARY

I. The circulatory system transports nutrients, oxygen, wastes, and hormones; helps maintain body temperature; helps maintain fluid balance; and protects the body against disease.
II. Blood consists of red blood cells, white blood cells, and platelets suspended in plasma.
III. Blood plasma consists of water, plasma proteins, salts, nutrients, oxygen and other gases, hormones, and wastes. Three fractions of plasma proteins are albumins, globulins, and fibrinogen.
IV. Red blood cells, or erythrocytes, are tiny, biconcave discs that transport hemoglobin.
V. White blood cells, or leukocytes, defend the body against pathogens and other foreign substances.
  A. Granular leukocytes include the neutrophils, basophils, and eosinophils.
  B. Nongranular leukocytes include the lymphocytes and monocytes.

VI. Platelets are cell fragments formed from large cells in the bone marrow; they function in blood clotting.
   A. Platelets patch tears in blood vessel walls by forming a platelet plug.
   B. Platelets also release clotting factors that help produce prothrombin activator. This enzyme converts prothrombin to thrombin, which, in turn, converts fibrinogen to fibrin.
VII. Blood is typed on the basis of specific antigens on the surfaces of red blood cells.
   A. Individuals with type A blood have type A antigen and anti-B antibodies.
   B. People with type B blood have type B antigen and anti-A antibodies.
   C. People with type AB blood have both types of antigens, and no antibodies to A or B blood; those with type O blood have neither type of antigen but both types of antibodies.
   D. People with Rh-positive blood have antigen D on the surface of their red blood cells, as well as the antigens of the appropriate ABO type. Rh-negative individuals may produce antibody D when exposed to antigen D.

POST TEST

1. The function of red blood cells is to transport _____ .

2. The liquid portion of the blood is called _____ .

3. Some of the gamma globulins serve as _____ .

4. Fibrinogen functions in blood _____ .

5. Red blood cells are produced in the _____ .

6. A deficiency of hemoglobin is called _____ .

7. The function of white blood cells is to _____ .

8. _____ gather and patch damaged blood vessels.

9. Fibrinogen is converted to _____ by an enzyme called _____ .

10. A person with type B blood has type _____ antigens on the surfaces of his red blood cells and anti- _____ antibodies in his plasma.

11. Erythroblastosis fetalis may occur when there is _____ incompatibility. This may occur when a woman with _____ blood produces a baby with _____ blood.

REVIEW QUESTIONS

1. List five functions of the circulatory system and identify which specific blood components carry out each job.

2. What are the functions of the plasma proteins as a group? Of globulins specifically?

3. In what ways are mature red blood cells specifically adapted to their function?

4. What are the functions of platelets? Explain.

5. Imagine that a patient with type AB blood is accidentally given type A blood in a transfusion. What, if any, ill effects may occur? What if a patient with type O blood is given type A blood?

6. What is Rh incompatibility?

POST TEST ANSWERS

1. oxygen
2. plasma
3. antibodies
4. clotting
5. red bone marrow
6. anemia

7. defend the body against disease
8. Platelets
9. fibrin; thrombin
10. B; A
11. Rh; Rh-negative; Rh-positive

Eleven

THE CIRCULATORY SYSTEM: THE HEART

CHAPTER OUTLINE

    I. The heart wall consists of three layers
   II. The heart has four chambers
  III. Valves prevent backflow of blood
  IV. The heart has its own blood vessels
   V. The conduction system consists of specialized cardiac muscle
  VI. The cardiac cycle includes contraction and relaxation phases
 VII. Heart sounds result from closing of the valves
VIII. The heart is regulated by the nervous system

LEARNING OBJECTIVES

After you have studied this chapter, you should be able to:
1. Describe the structure of the wall of the heart.
2. Identify the chambers of the heart and compare their functions.
3. Locate the atrioventricular and semilunar valves and compare their structure.
4. Identify the principal blood vessels that serve the heart wall.
5. Identify the components of the conduction system and trace the path of a muscle impulse through the heart.
6. Describe the events of the cardiac cycle. Define systole and diastole, and correlate normal heart sounds with the events of the cardiac cycle.
7. Define cardiac output and explain how the heart is regulated.

The heart is a hollow, muscular organ not much bigger than a fist. It weighs less than a pound. In an average lifetime, the heart pumps about 300 million liters (80 million gal) of blood through the vast complex of blood vessels that bring oxygen and nourishment to the cells of the body. Depending on the body's changing needs, the heart can vary its output from 5 to 35 liters of blood per minute.

The heart is located in the thorax between the lungs. About two thirds of this cone-shaped organ lies to the left of the body's midline. When you place your fingers on the left side of the chest between the fifth and sixth ribs, you can feel the heart pulsate each time it beats.

THE HEART WALL CONSISTS OF THREE LAYERS

The wall of the heart is richly supplied with nerves, blood vessels, and lymph vessels. From the inside out, the layers of the heart are the endocardium, myocardium, and pericardium.

1. The **endocardium** (en″-doe-**kar**′-dee-um) consists of a smooth endothelial lining resting upon connective tissue.

2. By far the greatest bulk of the heart wall consists of **myocardium** (my″-o-**kar**′-dee-um), the cardiac muscle that contracts to pump the blood.

3. The outer layer of the heart is the **pericardium** (per-ih-**kar**′-dee-um). The pericardium consists of two layers that are separated by a potential space, the pericardial cavity. The outer layer (the parietal pericardium) forms a strong sac for the heart and helps to anchor it within the thorax.

THE HEART HAS FOUR CHAMBERS

The heart is a double pump. The right and left sides of the heart are completely separated by a wall or **septum.** The heart has four chambers: an atrium and ventricle on each side (Figs. 11–1 to 11–3). The atria receive blood returning to the heart from the veins and act as reservoirs between contractions of the heart. The ventricles pump blood into the great arteries leaving the heart.

The right side of the heart receives oxygen-poor blood—blood somewhat depleted of its oxygen supply—returning from the tissues and pumps it into the pulmonary circulation. Pulmonary arteries carry blood to the lungs, where gases are exchanged. Pulmonary veins then return oxygen-rich blood to the left side of the heart. The left side of the heart pumps oxygen-rich blood into the systemic circulation, the network of blood vessels that serves all the body systems. The sequence of blood flow through the heart is:

Right atrium → right ventricle → through pulmonary circulation → left atrium → left ventricle → through systemic circulation

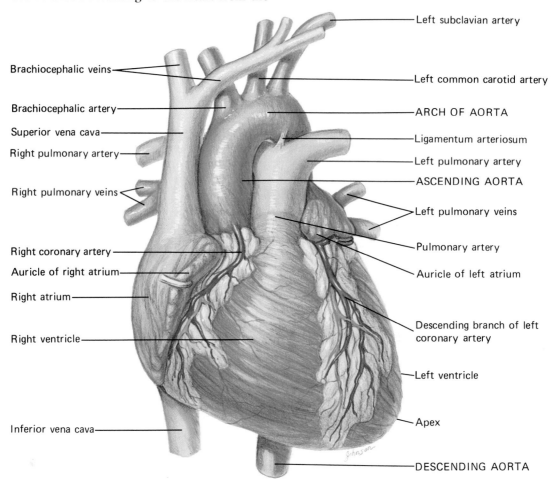

FIGURE 11–1 Anterior view of the heart. Note the great blood vessels that carry blood to and from the heart. *(From Guyton, A.C.: Anatomy and Physiology. Philadelphia, Saunders College Publishing, 1985.)*

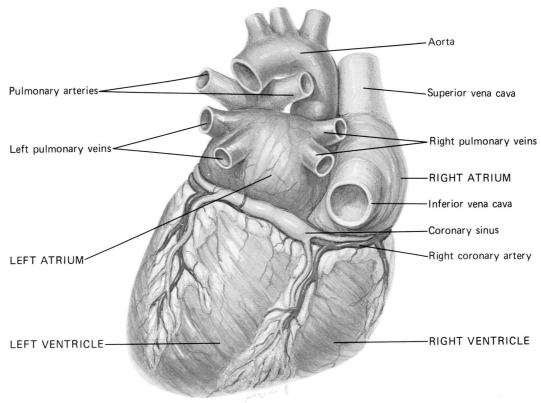

Aorta

Pulmonary arteries

Left pulmonary veins

LEFT ATRIUM

LEFT VENTRICLE

Superior vena cava

Right pulmonary veins

RIGHT ATRIUM

Inferior vena cava

Coronary sinus

Right coronary artery

RIGHT VENTRICLE

F I G U R E 11–2 Posterior view of the heart. *(From Guyton, A.C.: Anatomy and Physiology. Philadelphia, Saunders College Publishing, 1985.)*

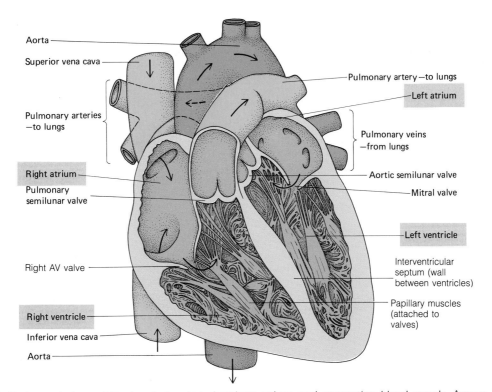

Aorta

Superior vena cava

Pulmonary arteries
—to lungs

Right atrium

Pulmonary
semilunar valve

Right AV valve

Right ventricle

Inferior vena cava

Aorta

Pulmonary artery—to lungs

Left atrium

Pulmonary veins
—from lungs

Aortic semilunar valve

Mitral valve

Left ventricle

Interventricular
septum (wall
between ventricles)

Papillary muscles
(attached to
valves)

F I G U R E 11–3 Internal view of the heart showing chambers, valves, and connecting blood vessels. Arrows indicate the direction of blood flow.

The wall between the atria is the **interatrial septum.** The wall between the ventricles is the **interventricular septum.** A small, muscular pouch called the **auricle** (**aw'**-reh-kle) increases the surface area of each atrium. It can be seen at the upper surface of each atrium in Figure 11–3. Irregular muscle columns project from the inner surface of both ventricles. One set of these, the **papillary** (**pap'**-il-ler"-ee) **muscles,** is continuous with cords of connective tissue attached to the edges of the valves between the atria and ventricles. These connective tissue cords are popularly referred to as the "heart strings."

VALVES PREVENT BACKFLOW OF BLOOD

When blood is pumped from either atrium into the corresponding ventricle, pressure in the ventricle becomes greater than in the atrium. When the atrium relaxes, blood must be prevented from flowing backward into it. To prevent such backflow of blood, an **atrioventricular (AV)** (a"-tree-o-ven-**trik'**-u-lar) **valve** guards the passageway between each atrium and ventricle (Figs. 11–4 and 11–6). The AV valves consist of flaps or cusps of fibrous tissues that project from the heart wall.

The AV valve between the right atrium and the right ventricle has three cusps and is known as the **tricuspid** (tri-**kus'**-pid) **valve.** The left AV valve, with only two cusps, is the **bicuspid** (bi-**kus'**-pid) **valve,** but it is commonly known as the **mitral** (**mi'**-tral) **valve.** A common valve deformity is mitral stenosis, a narrowing of the opening of the mitral valve. In this condition, the valve is thickened and slows the flow of blood from the left atrium into the left ventricle. Mitral stenosis is usually the result of rheumatic fever inflammation. Diseased valves can now be surgically removed and replaced with artificial valves.

The three cusps of each **semilunar** (sem"-ee-**loo**-nar) **valve** are shaped like half-moons. The semilunar valves guard the exits from the ventricles. The semilunar valve between the left ventricle and the aorta is known as the **aortic** (a-**or'**-tik) **valve,** and the one between the right ventricle and the pulmonary artery is the **pulmonary valve.**

THE HEART HAS ITS OWN BLOOD VESSELS

Although the heart is filled with blood, it needs blood vessels to bring blood to all its cells. This is because its wall is so thick that oxygen and nutrients

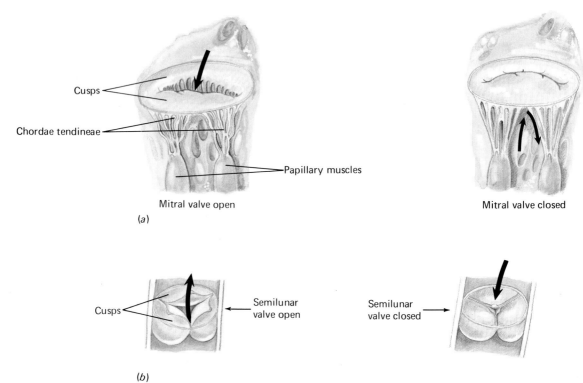

Cusps

Chordae tendineae

Papillary muscles

Mitral valve open

(a)

Mitral valve closed

Cusps

Semilunar valve open

Semilunar valve closed

(b)

F I G U R E **11–4** How the valves of the heart work. (a) An AV valve—the mitral valve—in the open and closed positions. (b) A semilunar valve in the open and closed positions.

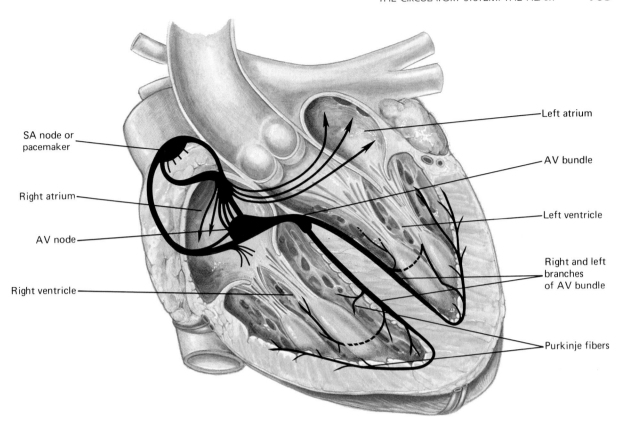

FIGURE 11–5 *The conduction system of the heart.*

cannot effectively diffuse to all the cells. Two **coronary arteries** branch off from the aorta (the artery that receives blood from the left ventricle) as it leaves the heart (Fig. 11–1). Branches of the coronary arteries bring blood to all the tissue of the heart. Blood leaving the heart wall flows through **coronary veins.** These veins join to form a large vein, the **coronary sinus,** that empties into the right atrium.

THE CONDUCTION SYSTEM CONSISTS OF SPECIALIZED CARDIAC MUSCLE

You may have viewed horror films in which a heart beats spookily after being separated from the body of its owner. Some script writers may have rooted their fantasies in a knowledge of cardiac physiology. When removed from the body, the heart can continue to beat for many hours if it is provided with appropriate nutrients and salts. This is possible because the heart has its own specialized conduction system and can beat independently of its nerve supply.

The heart's conduction system is composed of specialized cardiac muscle. This system includes the sinoatrial node, the atrioventricular node, and the atrioventricular bundle (Fig. 11–5). The **sinoatrial (SA) node** is a small mass of specialized muscle in the posterior wall of the right atrium. The SA node is known as the pacemaker of the heart because it automatically excites itself and starts each heartbeat.

The ends of the fibers of the SA node fuse with surrounding ordinary muscle fibers of the atrium so the muscle impulse spreads through the atria, producing atrial contraction. One group of atrial muscle fibers conducts the impulse directly to the **atrioventricular (AV) node,** located in the right atrium along the lower part of the septum. Here, transmission of the impulse is delayed briefly. This delay allows the atria to complete their contraction before the ventricles begin to contract.

From the AV node the muscle impulse spreads into specialized muscle fibers that form the **atrioventricular (AV) bundle** (also called the bundle of His). These large fibers conduct impulses about six times faster than ordinary cardiac muscle fibers. The AV bundle divides into right and left bundles, which extend into the right and left ventricles.

Fibers of the AV bundle end on fibers of ordinary cardiac muscle within the myocardium, so the impulse spreads through the ordinary muscle fibers of the ventricles. Cardiac muscle fibers are joined at their ends by dense bands (intercalated discs). These tight junctions between the muscle cells allow the muscle impulse to pass rapidly from cell to cell. The entire atrium or ventricle contracts as if it were one giant cell.

In summary, the pathway taken by a muscle impulse through the heart is:

SA node → cardiac muscle of atria → AV node → AV bundle → muscle of ventricles

THE CARDIAC CYCLE INCLUDES CONTRACTION AND RELAXATION PHASES

The events that occur during one complete heartbeat make up the cardiac cycle. Each complete cycle lasts for about 0.8 second and occurs about 72 times per minute. It consists of a contraction in which blood is forced out of the heart and then a relaxation in which the heart fills with blood. The period of contraction is known as **systole** (sis′-tow-lee); the period of relaxation is **diastole** (dye-**as**′-tow-lee).

Each cardiac cycle begins with a muscle impulse that spreads from the SA node throughout the atria, resulting in the contraction of the atria. As the atria contract, the AV valves are open, and blood is forced from the atria into the ventricles. As this happens, the semilunar valves are closed (Fig. 11–6).

As the atria relax, they are filled with blood from the veins. During this time, the AV valves are closed and the ventricles are contracting, forcing blood through the semilunar valves into the arteries. Then, as the ventricles begin to relax, the semilunar valves close and the AV valves open. Blood flows into the ventricles and the cycle begins again.

While the atria are contracting, the ventricles are relaxed. Then the atria relax while the ventricles contract and remain relaxed during the first part of ventricular relaxation.

HEART SOUNDS RESULT FROM CLOSING OF THE VALVES

When you listen to the heart through a stethoscope, you can hear certain characteristic sounds,

usually described as a "lub-dup." These sounds are produced each time the valves close. The first sound, the "lub," marks the beginning of ventricular systole (contraction). Heard as a low-pitched, relatively long sound, it is caused by the closure of the AV valves as the ventricles begin to contract.

The second sound marks the beginning of ventricular diastole and is caused by the closing of the semilunar valves. Because these valves close very rapidly, the "dup" sound is heard as a quick snap. Diastole is longer than systole, so when the heart is beating at a normal rate there is a slight pause after the second sound. Thus, one hears "lub-dup" pause, "lub-dup" pause.

Abnormal heart sounds called heart murmurs indicate the possibility of valve disorders. When a valve does not close properly, some blood may flow backward. This can result in a hissing sound. Murmurs can also be detected when a valve becomes narrowed (stenosis) and rough.

THE HEART IS REGULATED BY THE NERVOUS SYSTEM

The normal heart rate is about 70 beats per minute. Although the heart is capable of beating rhythmically on its own, it cannot by itself change the strength and rate of contraction to meet the changing needs of the body. This kind of control is the job of the autonomic nervous system. Under conditions of stress, sympathetic nerves can increase the strength of contraction as much as 100%. Under more calm conditions, the vagus nerve, a parasympathetic nerve, slows the heart. The balance between sympathetic and parasympathetic nerve stimulation determines the heart rate.

The endocrine system also helps regulate heart rate. During stress, epinephrine and norepinephrine released from the adrenal medulla speed the heartbeat. Increased body temperature, whether it results from strenuous exercise or fever, also increases heart rate. A fast heart rate—more than 100 beats per minute—is called **tachycardia** (tak″-ee-**kar**′-dee-ah).

A slow heart rate—less than 60 beats per minute—is referred to as **bradycardia** (brad″-ee-**kar**′-dee-ah). Heart rate decreases when the body temperature is lowered. This is why a patient's temperature is sometimes deliberately lowered during heart surgery.

The **cardiac output,** the volume of blood pumped by one ventricle in 1 minute is about 5 liters (about 5 quarts). This amount is approximately equal to the total volume of blood in the body. Cardiac

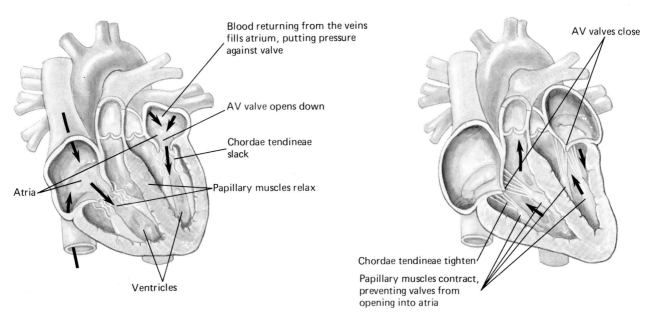

Blood returning from the veins fills atrium, putting pressure against valve

AV valve opens down

Chordae tendineae slack

Atria

Papillary muscles relax

Ventricles

(a) Blood flows from atria to ventricles

Atria contract forcing additional blood into ventricles

AV valves close

Chordae tendineae tighten

Papillary muscles contract, preventing valves from opening into atria

(b) Ventricles contract, forcing blood against valve cusps

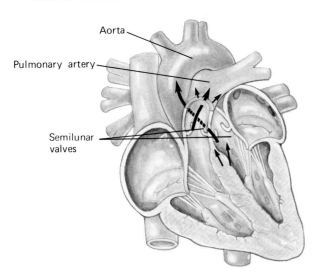

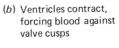

Aorta

Pulmonary artery

Semilunar valves

(c) When ventricles contract, blood is pushed up against semilunar valves, forcing them open

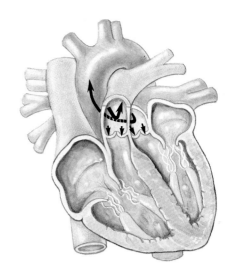

(d) As ventricles relax, blood starts to flow back from arteries

Blood fills cusps of semilunar valves, forcing them to close

FIGURE 11-6 Blood flow through the heart during the cardiac cycle.

output depends mainly on **venous return,** the amount of blood delivered to the heart by its veins. The greater the amount of blood delivered to the heart by the veins, the more blood the heart pumps (within limits).

During vigorous exercise, the normal heart can beat as many as 200 times per minute and increase its output 4 to 5 times. In a trained athlete, the heart enlarges and is capable of pumping a greater quantity of blood per beat. An athlete's heart is thus more efficient.

SUMMARY

I. The heart is a hollow, muscular organ that lies in the thorax between the lungs.
II. The bulk of the heart wall consists of myocardium, the middle muscular layer. The inner layer of the heart wall is the endocardium, and the outer layer is the pericardium.
III. The heart has four chambers—the right and left atria, which receive blood returning to the heart, and the right and left ventricles, which pump blood out into the great arteries.
IV. The entrance and exit of each ventricle is guarded by a valve that prevents backflow of blood.
   A. The entrance of each ventricle has an atrioventricular (AV) valve—the tricuspid valve between the right atrium and ventricle and the mitral valve between the left atrium and ventricle.
   B. The semilunar valves are located between each ventricle and the artery into which it pumps blood. The semilunar valve between the left ventricle and aorta is the aortic valve. The semilunar valve between the right ventricle and pulmonary artery is the pulmonary valve.
V. The coronary arteries deliver blood to the heart wall; the coronary veins return blood to the coronary sinus, which empties into the right atrium.
VI. The heart has its own conduction system and can beat independently of its nerve supply.
   A. Each heartbeat begins in the SA node. The muscle impulse spreads through the atria, causing atrial contraction. One group of fibers conducts the impulse to the AV node.
   B. From the AV node the impulse spreads through the AV bundle and finally reaches the ordinary fibers of the ventricles.
VII. The sequence of events that occurs during one complete heartbeat is a cardiac cycle. The contraction phase is systole; the relaxation phase is diastole.
   A. Each cardiac cycle begins with the generation of an impulse in the SA node that produces atrial systole (contraction).
   B. As the atria contract, additional blood is forced into the ventricles.
   C. Ventricular systole occurs next, forcing blood through the semilunar valves into the systemic and pulmonary circulations. At the same time the atria have returned to diastole and are again filling with blood.
VIII. When listening to the heart through a stethoscope, one can hear a "lub" sound when the AV valves close, followed by a "dup" sound when the semilunar valves snap shut.
IX. The nervous and endocrine systems regulate the heartbeat so that its rate and strength of contraction adjusts to the changing needs of the body.
   A. Cardiac output is the amount of blood pumped by one ventricle in 1 minute.
   B. The more blood returned to the heart by the veins, the greater the volume of blood that will be pumped during the next systole.

POST TEST

1. The heart is enclosed by a tough sac formed by its outer layer, the
_____ .
2. The bulk of the heart wall consists of _____ .
3. The wall separating the ventricles of the heart is called the
_____ .

4. The left AV valve is often called the _____ valve.

5. Aortic and pulmonary valves are _____ valves.

6. Blood is delivered to the heart wall by the _____ arteries.

7. The _____ is called the pacemaker of the heart.

8. From the AV node, the muscle impulse spreads into specialized muscle fibers that form the AV _____ .

9. In the cardiac cycle the period of contraction is called _____ and the period of relaxation is called _____ .

10. At the time the atria are contracting, the ventricles are _____ .

11. The volume of blood pumped by one ventricle in 1 minute is the _____ _____ .

12. Heart rate is slowed by _____ nerves and speeded by _____ nerves.

13. The amount of blood delivered to the heart by the veins is called _____ _____ .

14. Label the diagram.

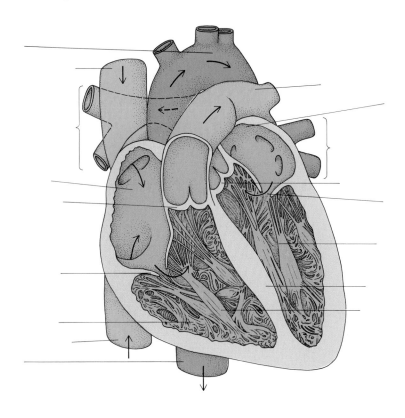

REVIEW QUESTIONS

1. Relate the structure of the heart wall to the heart's function.

2. List each chamber of the heart and give its function.

3. Trace a drop of blood through the heart, listing each structure through which it passes in sequence.

4. Name and locate the four valves of the heart and give the function of each.

5. Why does the heart wall require its own blood supply? Name the blood vessels that bring blood to and from the heart wall.

6. Trace a muscle impulse through the heart.

7. Why is the SA node called the pacemaker of the heart?

8. Define systole and diastole, and describe the cardiac cycle.

9. What causes each of the heart sounds?

10. Define cardiac output and explain how it is influenced by venous return.

11. Describe the regulation of the heart by sympathetic and parasympathetic nerves.

POST TEST ANSWERS

1. pericardium
2. myocardium (cardiac muscle)
3. interventricular septum
4. mitral
5. semilunar
6. coronary
7. sinoatrial node (SA node)
8. bundle
9. systole; diastole
10. relaxed
11. cardiac output
12. parasympathetic (vagus); sympathetic
13. venous return
14. see Figure 11–3

Twelve

CIRCULATION OF BLOOD AND LYMPH

CHAPTER OUTLINE

   I. Three main types of blood vessels are arteries, capillaries, and veins
  II. The blood vessel wall consists of layers
 III. Blood circulates through two circuits
     A. The pulmonary circulation carries blood to and from the lungs
     B. The systemic circulation carries blood to the tissues
        1. The aorta has four main regions
        2. The superior and inferior vena cavas return blood to the heart
        3. Four arteries supply the brain
        4. The liver has an unusual circulation
  IV. Several factors influence blood flow
     A. The alternate expansion and recoil of an artery is its pulse
     B. Blood pressure depends on blood flow and resistance to blood flow
     C. Pressure changes as blood flows through the systemic circulation
     D. Several mechanisms regulate blood pressure
     E. Blood pressure is expressed as systolic pressure over diastolic pressure
   V. The lymphatic system is a subsystem of the circulatory system
     A. Lymph nodes filter lymph
     B. Tonsils filter tissue fluid
     C. The spleen is the largest lymphatic organ
     D. The thymus gland plays a role in immune function

LEARNING OBJECTIVES

After you have studied this chapter, you should be able to:

1. Compare the structure and functions of arteries, capillaries, and veins.
2. Trace a drop of blood through the pulmonary and systemic circulations, listing the principal vessels and heart chambers through which it must pass on its journey from one part of the body to another. (For example, trace a drop of blood from the inferior vena cava to an organ such as the brain and then back to the heart.)
3. Identify the main divisions of the aorta and its principal branches.
4. Trace a drop of blood through the hepatic portal system.
5. Give the physiological basis for arterial pulse, and describe how pulse is measured.
6. Define blood pressure and give its relationship to blood flow and resistance.
7. Compare blood pressure in the different types of blood vessels of the systemic circulation.
8. Describe the homeostatic mechanisms that regulate blood pressure, and explain how blood pressure is measured.

The blood vessels carry blood into the tissues of the body. Some of the plasma leaves the blood vessels bringing with it nutrients, oxygen, and other materials needed by the cells. This tissue fluid bathes the cells and keeps them moist. In this chapter we will first examine the various types of blood vessels and some of their pathways through the body. Then we will look at the physiology of blood circulation. Finally, we will examine the lymphatic system that returns fluid to the blood.

THREE MAIN TYPES OF BLOOD VESSELS ARE ARTERIES, CAPILLARIES, AND VEINS

The main types of blood vessels are the arteries, capillaries, and veins (Fig. 12–1). These different types of blood vessels vary with respect to their structure and functions.

1. **Arteries** carry blood from the ventricles of the heart to each of the organs of the body. All arteries except the pulmonary arteries carry blood rich in oxygen. Arteries are strong vessels built to carry blood under high pressure. The smallest branches of an artery, called **arterioles** (ar-**teer'**-ee-olz), are important in regulating blood pressure.

2. From the arterioles blood flows through **capillaries** (**cap'**-ih-lar-ees). These tiny vessels form extensive networks within each tissue. Capillaries permit materials to be exchanged between the blood and tissues. Their walls are so thin that oxygen and nutrients easily diffuse through them. The capillary wall is also somewhat porous, so plasma itself can leave the circulation through it.

3. Blood passes from the capillaries into **veins.** (The smallest veins are called venules.) Veins conduct blood back toward the heart. All veins except the pulmonary vein carry blood that is poor in oxygen.

THE BLOOD VESSEL WALL CONSISTS OF LAYERS

The wall of an artery or vein has three layers, or tunics (Fig. 12–2). The inner layer consists of **endothelium** (en-doe-**theel'**-ee-um) (a simple epithelium) that forms a smooth surface for the blood. The middle layer consists of connective tissue and smooth muscle. In large arteries, this is the thickest layer and contains several layers of elastic fibers. The

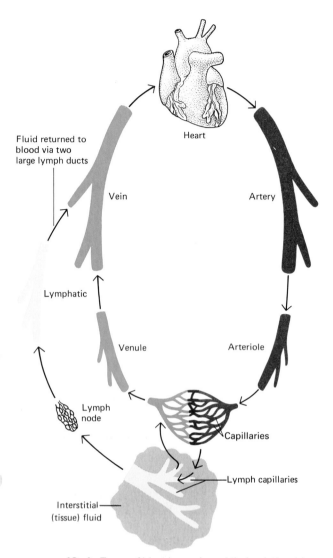

FIGURE 12–1 *Types of blood vessels and their relationship to one another. Lymphatic vessels return excess tissue fluid to the blood.*

outer layer is a relatively thin layer in arteries, but is the thickest layer in the walls of large veins. It consists of connective tissue rich in elastic and collagen fibers.

In general, veins have thinner walls than arteries. Most large veins have valves that permit the vein to conduct blood toward the heart even against the force of gravity. A vein valve usually consists of two cusps formed by inward extensions of the endothelium. These cusps prevent blood from flowing backward.

The capillary wall consists mainly of endothelium. At the point where a capillary branches from an arteriole, a smooth muscle cell surrounds the vessel.

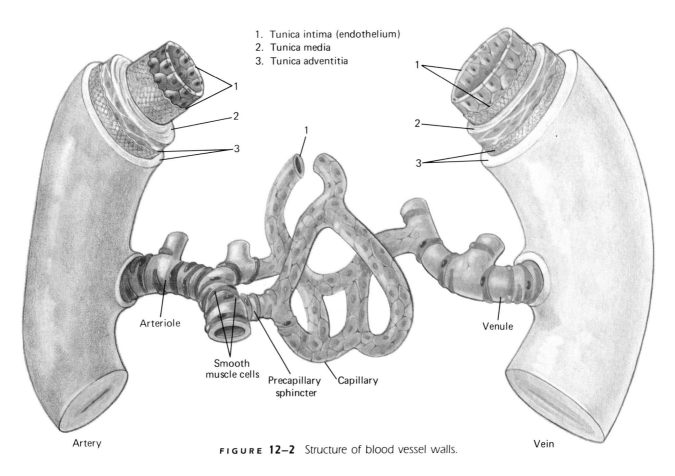

1. Tunica intima (endothelium)
2. Tunica media
3. Tunica adventitia

Arteriole

Smooth
muscle cells
Precapillary
sphincter

Capillary

Venule

Artery

Vein

FIGURE 12–2 Structure of blood vessel walls.

By contracting or relaxing, this muscle regulates the flow of blood into the capillaries.

In the liver, spleen, and bone marrow, arterioles and venules are connected by capillary-like vessels called **sinusoids** rather than by typical capillaries. The endothelial cells lining a sinusoid do not all come into contact with one another, leaving gaps in the wall. For this reason sinusoids are very leaky. Macrophages lie along the outer walls of sinusoids. They reach into the vessels to remove worn-out blood cells and foreign matter from the circulation.

BLOOD CIRCULATES THROUGH TWO CIRCUITS

Blood flows through a continuous network of blood vessels that forms a double circuit: (1) the **pulmonary circulation** connects heart and lungs; and (2) the **systemic circulation** connects the heart and all the organs and tissues. The left ventricle pumps blood into the systemic circulation, which brings oxygen-rich blood to all the different organs and tissues. Blood returns to the right atrium of the heart

poor in oxygen but loaded with carbon dioxide wastes. Then the blood is pumped by the right ventricle into the pulmonary circulation, where gases are exchanged.

From the pulmonary circulation, blood is returned to the left atrium. It is pumped into the left ventricle, which pumps it back out into the systemic circulation. This general pattern of circulation is shown in Figure 12–3. A more detailed view is shown in Figure 12–4.

THE PULMONARY CIRCULATION CARRIES BLOOD TO AND FROM THE LUNGS

Blood that is poor in oxygen returns from the systemic circulation to the right atrium. It is pumped into the right ventricle and then into the **pulmonary arteries.** These blood vessels deliver blood to the lungs. In the lungs, blood flows through extensive networks of capillaries. Carbon dioxide diffuses out of the blood and oxygen diffuses into it.

The **pulmonary veins** return the blood, rich in oxygen once more, to the left atrium. Blood then passes into the left ventricle and is pumped into the

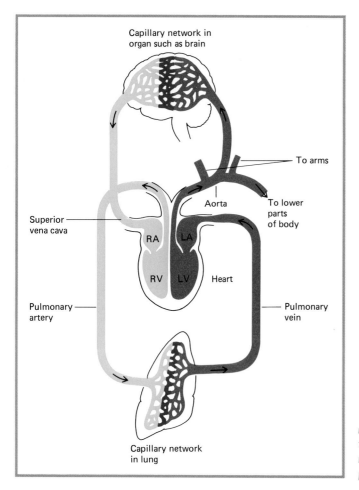

FIGURE 12-3 *Simplified diagram of circulation through the systemic and pulmonary circuits. Red represents oxygen-rich blood. Blue represents oxygen-poor blood.*

systemic circulation again. Note that the pulmonary veins are the only veins that carry oxygen-rich blood, and the pulmonary arteries are the only arteries that transport blood that is poor in oxygen.

In summary, blood flows through the pulmonary circulation in the following sequence:

> Right atrium → right ventricle → pulmonary artery → pulmonary capillaries → pulmonary veins → left atrium

THE SYSTEMIC CIRCULATION CARRIES BLOOD TO THE TISSUES

Blood returning from the pulmonary circulation enters the left atrium and is pumped into the left ventricle. The left ventricle pumps the blood into the largest artery in the body, the **aorta** (ay-**or**'-tah).

Branches of the aorta deliver blood to all the organs and tissues of the body.

The Aorta Has Four Main Regions

We can identify four regions of the aorta (Fig. 12-5):

1. The **ascending aorta** is the first part of the aorta. It travels upward (superiorly).

2. The **aortic arch** curves from the ascending aorta and makes a U-turn.

3. The **thoracic** (thow-**ras**'-ik) **aorta** descends from the aortic arch passing through the thorax. It lies posterior to the heart.

4. The **abdominal aorta** is the region of the aorta below the diaphragm. It is the longest region of the aorta. The abdominal aorta descends downward through the abdominal cavity. The thoracic and abdominal aortae are referred to as the descending aorta.

The principal branches of each region of the aorta are given in Table 12-1.

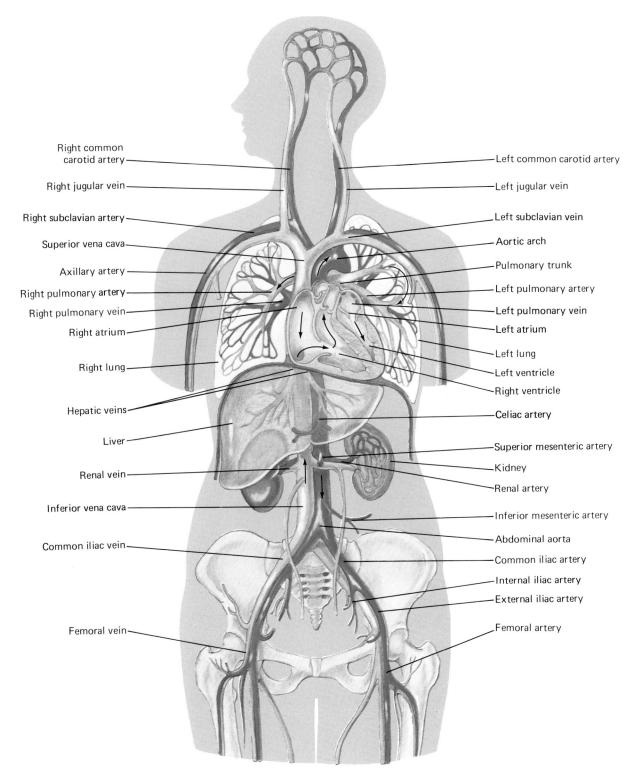

Right common carotid artery

Right jugular vein

Right subclavian artery

Superior vena cava

Axillary artery

Right pulmonary artery

Right pulmonary vein

Right atrium

Right lung

Hepatic veins

Liver

Renal vein

Inferior vena cava

Common iliac vein

Femoral vein

Left common carotid artery

Left jugular vein

Left subclavian vein

Aortic arch

Pulmonary trunk

Left pulmonary artery

Left pulmonary vein

Left atrium

Left lung

Left ventricle

Right ventricle

Celiac artery

Superior mesenteric artery

Kidney

Renal artery

Inferior mesenteric artery

Abdominal aorta

Common iliac artery

Internal iliac artery

External iliac artery

Femoral artery

FIGURE 12–4 Circulation of blood through some of the principal arteries and veins. Blood vessels carrying oxygen-rich blood are red; those carrying blood low in oxygen are blue.

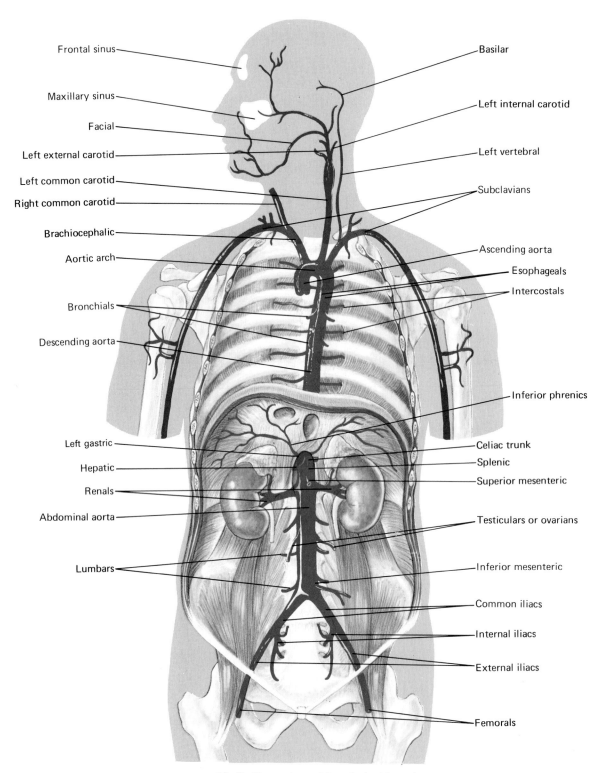

Frontal sinus

Maxillary sinus

Facial

Left external carotid

Left common carotid

Right common carotid

Brachiocephalic

Aortic arch

Bronchials

Descending aorta

Left gastric

Hepatic

Renals

Abdominal aorta

Lumbars

Basilar

Left internal carotid

Left vertebral

Subclavians

Ascending aorta

Esophageals

Intercostals

Inferior phrenics

Celiac trunk

Splenic

Superior mesenteric

Testiculars or ovarians

Inferior mesenteric

Common iliacs

Internal iliacs

External iliacs

Femorals

FIGURE 12–5 The aorta and its principal branches.

TABLE 12–1

The aorta and its principal branches

DIVISION OF AORTA	ARTERIAL BRANCH	REGION SUPPLIED
Ascending aorta	Coronary arteries	Wall of heart
Aortic arch	Brachiocephalic (innominate)	
	Right common carotid	Branches into external carotid (supplying head and neck) and internal carotid (supplying brain and head)
	Right subclavian	Sends branches to neck and right upper limb
	Left common carotid	Branches into external carotid (supplying head and neck) and internal carotid (supplying brain and head)
	Left subclavian	Sends branches to neck and left upper limb
Thoracic aorta	*Visceral Branches*	
	Bronchial	Bronchi of lungs
	Esophageal	Esophagus
	Parietal Branches	
	Several pairs of posterior intercostal arteries	Intercostal and other chest muscles, and pleurae; join with other arteries that serve chest wall
	Subcostal	Last pair of arteries to branch from thoracic aorta; serve chest wall
Abdominal aorta	*Visceral Branches*	
	Celiac	Branches to supply the liver (hepatic artery), stomach (gastric artery), and spleen, pancreas, and stomach (splenic artery)
	Superior mesenteric	Small intestine and first part of large intestine
	Suprarenal	Adrenal glands
	Renal	Kidneys
	Ovarian (in female)	Ovaries
	Testicular (in male)	Testes
	Inferior mesenteric	Colon, rectum
	Common iliac	
	External	Lower limbs
	Internal	Branches supply gluteal muscles, urinary bladder, uterus, vagina
	Parietal Branches	
	Inferior phrenic	Diaphragm
	Lumbar	Spinal cord and lumbar region of back
	Middle sacral	Sacrum, coccyx, gluteus maximus, and rectum

The Superior and Inferior Vena Cavas Return Blood to the Heart

Veins bringing blood back from the tissues drain into two large veins that return the blood to the right atrium of the heart. These veins are the **superior vena cava** and the **inferior vena cava.** The superior vena cava receives blood from the upper portions of the body (Table 12–2). The inferior vena cava receives blood returning from below the level of the diaphragm.

Four Arteries Supply the Brain

Four arteries bring blood to the brain. The two **internal carotid arteries** enter the cranial cavity in

TABLE 12–2

Veins draining into the vena cavas

VEIN	FORMED FROM	AREA(S) DRAINED
Into Superior Vena Cava		
Internal jugular	Sinuses of dura mater	Brain, skull
External jugular	Veins of face	Muscles and skin of face and scalp
Subclavian	Axillary, cephalic, basilic and their tributaries, scapular, and thoracic veins	Upper limb, chest, mammary glands
Brachiocephalic (innominate)	Internal jugular, external jugular, and subclavian	Brain, face, neck
Azygos	Lumbar and intercostal veins	Posterior aspect of thorax and abdominal cavities
Into Inferior Vena Cava		
Hepatics	Sinusoids of liver	Liver
Renals	Veins of kidney	Kidney
Ovarians or testiculars	Veins of gonads	Ovaries or testes
Common iliac	External iliac (extension of the femoral vein)	Lower limbs
	Internal iliac	Organs of lower abdomen

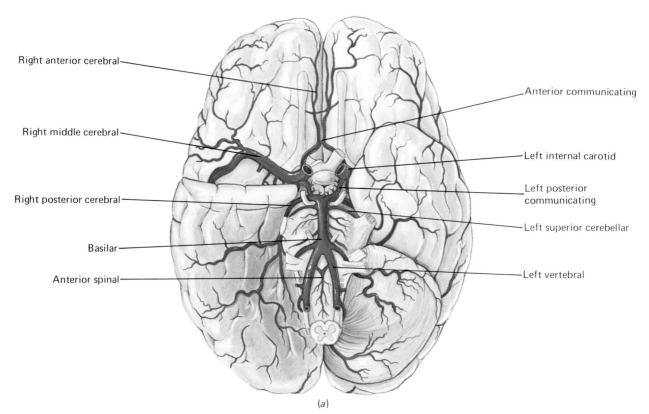

Right anterior cerebral

Right middle cerebral

Right posterior cerebral

Basilar

Anterior spinal

Anterior communicating

Left internal carotid

Left posterior communicating

Left superior cerebellar

Left vertebral

(a)

FIGURE 12–6 *Circulation in the brain. (a) Arterial circulation in the brain. Note the circle of Willis, which is an arterial anastomosis. It provides alternative circulatory pathways to ensure an adequate blood supply to the brain cells.*

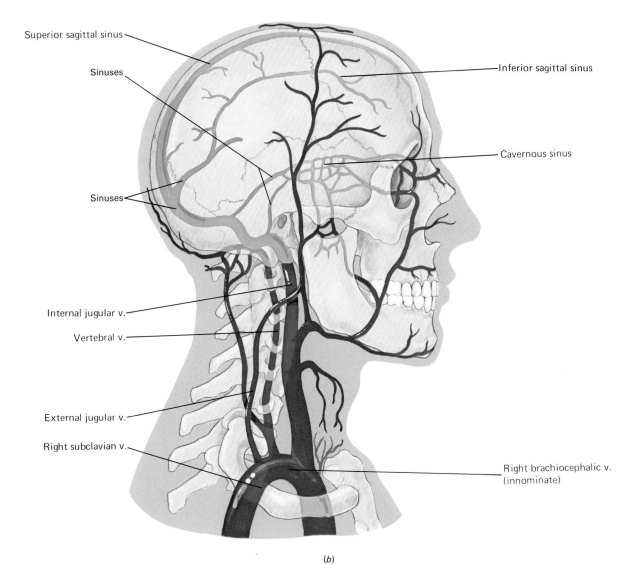

Superior sagittal sinus

Sinuses

Sinuses

Internal jugular v.

Vertebral v.

External jugular v.

Right subclavian v.

Inferior sagittal sinus

Cavernous sinus

Right brachiocephalic v. (innominate)

(b)

FIGURE 12–6 *Continued (b)* Large sinuses receive blood from brain capillaries and deliver it to veins that leave the brain and return blood to the heart.

the midregion of the cranial floor. The two **vertebral arteries** (branches of the subclavian arteries) pass through the foramen magnum and join on the ventral surface of the brain stem. Together they form the **basilar artery.** Branches of the internal carotid arteries and basilar artery form a circle of arteries at the base of the brain. This circle is called the **circle of Willis.** The joining of two or more arteries is called an arterial **anastomosis** (ah-nas-tow-**mow′**-sis). If one of the arteries serving the brain becomes blocked or damaged in some way, this arterial circuit helps ensure that the brain cells will continue to receive an adequate blood supply through other vessels.

From the brain capillaries, blood drains into large **venous sinuses** located in the folds of the dura mater (the outer covering of the brain) (Fig. 12–6).

A venous sinus is a specialized vein that has no smooth muscle in its wall. Blood from the venous sinuses empties into the **internal jugular veins** at either side of the neck. The blood passes through the **brachiocephalic** (bray-kee-o-seh-**fal′**-ik) **veins** and into the superior vena cava, which returns it to the heart.

A simplified summary of blood flow to and from the brain follows:

Aorta → common carotid artery →
internal carotid artery → circle of Willis
→ capillaries in brain → venous sinus →
internal jugular vein → brachiocephalic
vein → superior vena cava

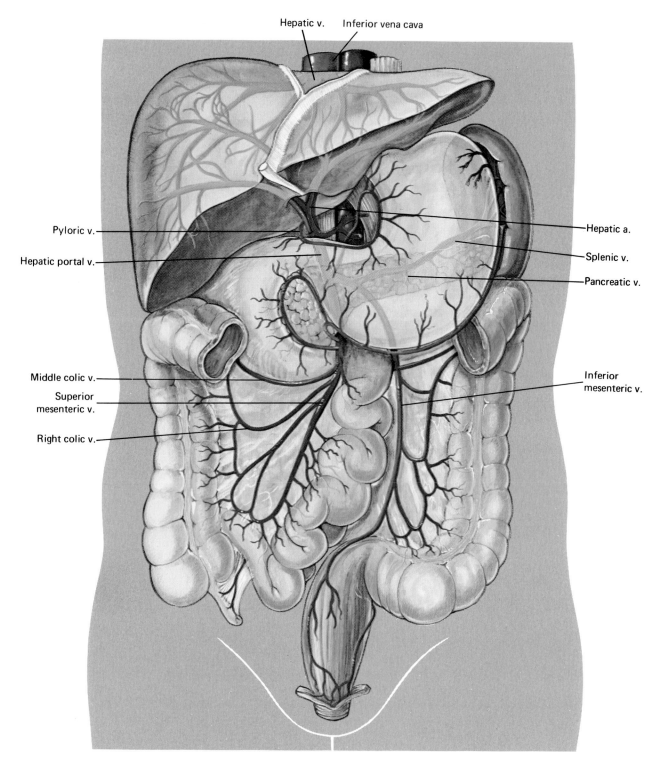

Hepatic v.   Inferior vena cava

Pyloric v.

Hepatic portal v.

Hepatic a.

Splenic v.

Pancreatic v.

Middle colic v.

Superior mesenteric v.

Right colic v.

Inferior mesenteric v.

FIGURE 12–7 The hepatic portal system. Blood circulating through the hepatic portal vein has passed through capillaries in the intestine and is partly depleted of its oxygen supply. Oxygen-rich blood is delivered to the liver by the hepatic arteries. Its branches deliver blood to the hepatic sinuses where it mixes with the venous blood from the hepatic portal vein.

The Liver Has an Unusual Circulation

As you have seen, blood generally flows from arteries to capillaries and then to veins. The veins conduct the blood back toward the heart. However, the body has a few veins that carry blood to a second set of exchange vessels. Such veins are called **portal veins.** The **hepatic portal vein** delivers blood from the organs of the digestive system to the liver.

Blood is delivered to the intestines by the **mesenteric** (mes″-en-**ter**′-ik) **arteries** and enters capillaries in the intestinal wall. Nutrients are absorbed into these capillaries. Then the blood, rich in nutrients, flows into the **superior mesenteric vein.** This vein empties into the hepatic portal vein, which also receives blood returning from the lower portion of the intestine and from the spleen (Fig. 12–7). The hepatic portal vein conducts blood to the liver, where it gives rise to an extensive network of hepatic sinusoids, exchange vessels somewhat like capillaries.

As blood flows through the sinusoids, liver cells remove nutrients whose concentrations are above homeostatic levels. The hepatic sinusoids deliver blood to the hepatic veins, which leave the liver and empty into the inferior vena cava.

SEVERAL FACTORS INFLUENCE BLOOD FLOW

In Chapter 11 we discussed some of the factors that influence the flow of blood through the heart. Here we will focus on the movement of blood through the blood vessels.

THE ALTERNATE EXPANSION AND RECOIL OF AN ARTERY IS ITS PULSE

Each time the left ventricle pumps blood into the aorta, the elastic wall of the aorta stretches. This expansion moves down the aorta and its branches in a wave that is faster than the flow of the blood itself. As soon as the wave has passed, the elastic wall of the artery snaps back to its normal size. This alternate expansion and recoil of an artery is the arterial pulse.

The ability of the large arteries to expand and then snap back to their original diameter is important in maintaining a continuous flow of blood. As the left ventricle forces a large volume of blood into the aorta during systole, the aorta expands to accommodate it. During diastole, as the walls of the aorta recoil to normal size, the blood is kept flowing into the cap-

illaries. Without this mechanism, blood would rush through the arteries and into the arterioles and capillaries in enormous gushes each time the ventricle contracted. This would damage the delicate walls of the capillaries.

When you place your finger over an artery near the skin surface, you can feel the pulse. The **radial artery** in the wrist is most frequently used to measure pulse. However, the common carotid artery in the neck region or any other superficial artery that lies over a bone or other firm structure may be used (Fig. 12–8). These locations are sometimes referred to as pressure points because pressure applied directly on the vessel at these points may stop arterial bleeding if a wound is distal to the pressure point.

The number of pulsations counted per minute indicates the number of heartbeats per minute. This is because every time the heart contracts a pulse wave is initiated. Because it takes time for the pulse wave to pass from the ventricle to the artery, the pulse is felt just after the ventricles contract.

BLOOD PRESSURE DEPENDS ON BLOOD FLOW AND RESISTANCE TO BLOOD FLOW

Blood pressure is the force exerted by the blood against the inner walls of the blood vessels. It is determined by: (1) the flow of blood; and (2) by the resistance to that flow. The flow of blood depends directly upon the pumping action of the heart. When

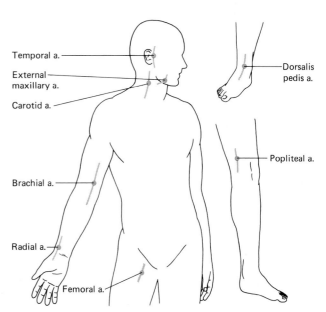

FIGURE 12–8 The pulse may be felt at any of the locations indicated in the diagram. All of the arteries indicated lie near the body surface over a bone or other firm structure.

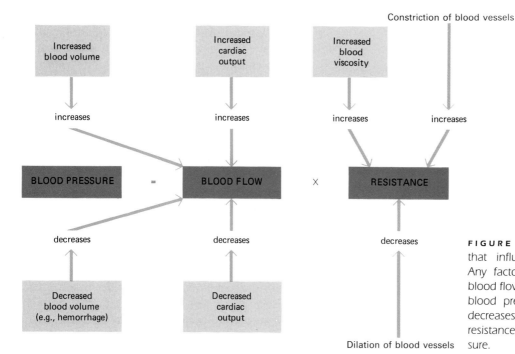

FIGURE 12–9 *Some factors that influence blood pressure. Any factor that increases either blood flow or resistance increases blood pressure. Any factor that decreases either blood flow or resistance decreases blood pressure.*

cardiac output increases, blood flow increases, causing a rise in blood pressure (Fig. 12–9). When cardiac output decrease, blood flow decreases, causing a fall in blood pressure.

The volume of blood flowing through the body also affects blood pressure. The normal volume of blood in the body is about 5 liters. If blood volume is reduced by hemorrhage or by chronic bleeding, the blood pressure drops. On the other hand, an increase in blood volume causes an increase in blood pressure. For example, a high dietary intake of salt causes water to be retained in the body. This may result in an increase in blood volume and lead to an increase in blood pressure.

Blood flow is slowed by resistance. When the resistance to flow increases, blood pressure increases. An important source of resistance is the friction between the blood and the wall of the blood vessel. The diameter of a blood vessel is especially important. A small change in the diameter of a blood vessel causes a big change in blood pressure.

PRESSURE CHANGES AS BLOOD FLOWS THROUGH THE SYSTEMIC CIRCULATION

Because arteries are large, their walls do not present much resistance to blood flow. Arterioles, however, have a much smaller diameter and so they offer a great deal of resistance to blood flow. This permits relatively high pressures to build up in the blood behind them. More important, arterioles can dilate and constrict, thereby changing the amount of

resistance to blood flow. Changes in resistance affect the blood pressure and the rate of blood flow. In fact, the amount of blood pressure within the arteries is regulated mainly by the degree of constriction or dilation of the arterioles.

The diameter of a capillary is very small, so individual capillaries offer great resistance to blood flow. However, blood has so many capillaries through which to pass that the *total* resistance, when all the capillaries are considered together, is far less than that of the arterioles.

As blood flows through capillaries, most of the pressure caused by the action of the heart is spent. By the time the blood passes into the veins its pressure is very low. However, even this small pressure is usually sufficient to push blood through the veins to the heart.

Very little pressure is needed to force the blood through the veins because veins offer little resistance to blood flow. Their diameters are large, and vein walls are thin and can easily be stretched. They can hold large volumes of blood. Indeed, at any moment more than half of all the blood in the circulation may be found within the veins. Thus, veins serve as a kind of blood reservoir.

When blood is lost during hemorrhage, arterial pressure begins to fall. Special receptors (baroreceptors) respond, causing the veins to constrict; large amounts of blood leave the veins and enter the heart. This response prevents the heart from failing and may keep the circulation going even when large amounts of blood are lost. In severe hemorrhage, **circulatory shock** may occur. In this condition blood pressure may fall so drastically that blood flow to the tissues is not adequate and tissue damage may occur.

When the body is in an upright position, gravity offers a great deal of resistance to venous blood flow. It is really quite remarkable that blood in the feet manages to make its way back to the heart. How is this accomplished? Recall that a system of valves prevents backflow of blood within the veins. Blood is pushed along by the pressure of blood behind it and by compression of veins when skeletal muscle contracts.

During exercise, increased muscle contraction results in increased flow of blood through the veins and into the heart. Cardiac output increases. On the other hand, when one stands perfectly still for a long period of time (for example, when a soldier stands at attention) blood pools in the veins. Within a few moments, pressure also increases in the capillaries (veins are not accepting blood from them because they are already dammed up with blood), and plasma is lost to the tissue fluid. Arterial blood pressure falls and blood supply to the brain decreases. This sometimes results in fainting.

SEVERAL MECHANISMS REGULATE BLOOD PRESSURE

Whenever you change position, blood pressure fluctuates. It is kept within normal limits by the interaction of several complex homeostatic mechanisms. Specialized receptors, called **baroreceptors** (bar″-o-re-**sep′**-tors), are present in the walls of certain arteries and in the heart wall. When blood pressure increases, the walls of the baroreceptors stretch, and messages are sent to cardiac centers in the medulla. Then parasympathetic nerves signal the heart to slow, thus lowering blood pressure.

Low blood pressure stimulates the kidneys to release the hormone **renin.** Then renin converts a plasma protein to **angiotensins,** a group of hormones that act as powerful constrictors. Their action raises blood pressure. The kidneys also act indirectly to maintain blood pressure by helping to regulate blood volume. Hormones signal the kidneys to excrete more or less water or salts; this, in turn, affects blood volume.

BLOOD PRESSURE IS EXPRESSED AS SYSTOLIC PRESSURE OVER DIASTOLIC PRESSURE

In arteries, blood pressure rises during systole and falls during diastole. A blood pressure reading is expressed as **systolic pressure** over **diastolic pressure.** For example, normal blood pressure for a young adult would be about 120/80. (The numbers refer to millimeters of mercury.) Systolic pressure is represented by the numerator, diastolic by the denominator. The systolic pressure may vary greatly with physical exertion and emotional stress.

Clinically, blood pressure is measured with a **sphygmomanometer** (sfig″-mow-mah-**nom′**-eh-ter) and stethoscope. The sphygmomanometer consists of a column of mercury connected by a rubber tube to an inflatable rubber cuff. An air pump with a valve is attached to the cuff.

To measure the pressure, the cuff is wrapped around a patient's arm over the brachial artery. Air is pumped into the cuff until the air pressure is great enough to compress the artery so that no pulse is heard on the anterior surface of the elbow joint (using the stethoscope). Then the valve is opened slightly so that the pressure in the cuff begins to fall. Soon, a distinct sound is heard as blood spurts into the artery again. The pressure at that instant is read as the systolic pressure.

The sound gets louder and then changes in quality, and finally becomes inaudible. Pressure at the instant the sound is no longer heard is read as the diastolic pressure.

High blood pressure (a diastolic pressure that is consistently over 95 mmHg) is referred to as **hypertension.** This condition is a risk factor for heart disease.

THE LYMPHATIC SYSTEM IS A SUBSYSTEM OF THE CIRCULATORY SYSTEM

The **lymphatic system** is a subsystem of the circulatory system. Its three principal functions are:

1. To collect and return tissue fluid (interstitial fluid), including plasma proteins, to the blood, and thus help maintain fluid balance.

2. To defend the body against disease by producing lymphocytes.

3. To absorb lipids from the intestine and transport them to the blood.

The lymphatic system consists of the clear, watery **lymph** formed from tissue fluid, the lymphatic vessels that conduct the lymph, lymph tissue organized in lymph nodules and nodes, the tonsils, spleen, and thymus (Fig. 12–10). The lymph system has nei-

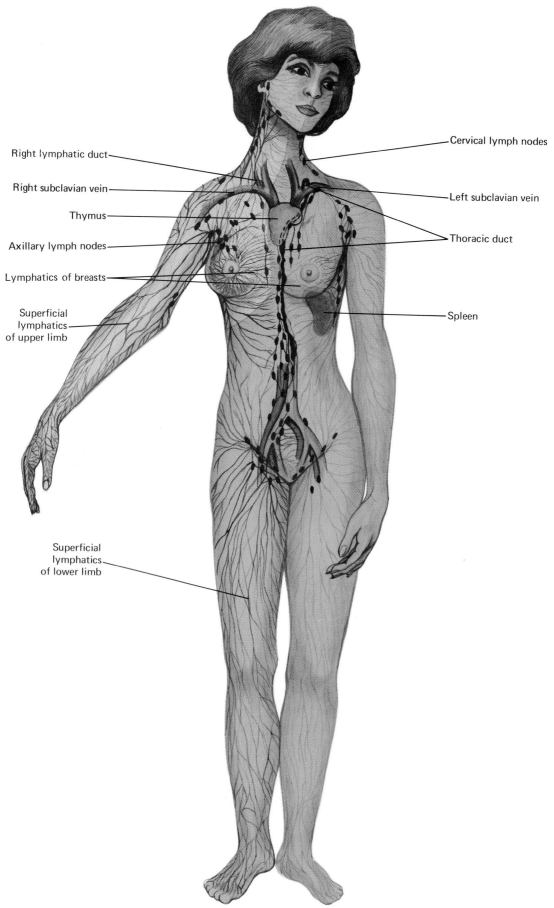

Right lymphatic duct

Right subclavian vein

Thymus

Axillary lymph nodes

Lymphatics of breasts

Superficial
lymphatics
of upper limb

Superficial
lymphatics
of lower limb

Cervical lymph nodes

Left subclavian vein

Thoracic duct

Spleen

182   FIGURE 12-10 *See legend on opposite page*

ther a heart nor arteries. Its microscopic dead-end capillaries extend into most tissues, alongside the blood capillaries. The lymph circulation is a drainage system. Its job is to collect excess tissue fluid and to return it to the blood.

Three types of lymphatic vessels are lymph capillaries, lymphatics, and lymph ducts. Lymph capillaries conduct lymph to larger vessels called **lymphatics** (lim-fat'-iks). At strategic locations, lymphatics enter lymph nodes. As the lymph flows slowly through the lymph sinuses within the tissue of the lymph node, it is filtered. Macrophages remove bacteria and other foreign matter as well as debris.

Lymphatics that leave the lymph nodes conduct lymph toward the shoulder region. Lymphatic vessels from all over the body except the upper right quadrant drain into the **thoracic duct.** This duct delivers the lymph into the base of the left subclavian vein. Lymph from the lymphatic vessels in the upper right quadrant of the body drain into the **right lymphatic duct,** which empties lymph into the base of the right subclavian vein. In this way lymph is continuously emptied into the blood, where it mixes with the plasma.

An example of the pattern of lymph circulation is:

> Lymph capillaries → lymphatic →
> lymph node → lymphatic → thoracic duct

LYMPH NODES FILTER LYMPH

Lymph nodes, sometimes called lymph glands, are masses of lymph tissue surrounded by a connective tissue capsule. Their two main functions are: (1) to filter the lymph; and (2) to produce lymphocytes. Lymph nodes are distributed along the main lymphatic routes. As illustrated in Figure 12–10, they are most numerous in the axillary and groin regions, and many are located in the thorax and abdomen.

By filtering and destroying bacteria from the lymph, the lymph nodes help prevent the spread of infection. When bacteria are present, lymph nodes may increase in size and become tender. You may have experienced the swollen cervical lymph nodes that often accompany a sore throat. An infection in almost any part of the body may result in swelling

and tenderness of the lymph nodes that drain that area.

TONSILS FILTER TISSUE FLUID

Tonsils are masses of lymph tissue located under the epithelial lining of the oral cavity and pharynx. Tonsils produce lymphocytes and filter tissue fluid. The **lingual** (ling'-gwal) **tonsils** are located at the base of the tongue. The **pharyngeal tonsil** is located in the posterior wall of the nasal portion of the pharynx above the soft palate. When enlarged (usually owing to infection or allergy), the pharyngeal tonsil is called the adenoids.

Most prominent are the paired **palatine tonsils** on each side of the throat. These oval masses of lymphatic tissue are thickenings in the mucous membrane of the throat. The stratified epithelium of the throat that overlies the tonsils dips down to form 10 to 20 pits, or crypts, in each tonsil. Bacteria often accumulate in these crypts and may invade the lymphatic tissue of the tonsil. This may cause an increase in the mass of the tonsil. Sometimes bacterial invasion of the tonsils becomes a chronic problem, and the tonsils are surgically removed by the well-known procedure called tonsillectomy. After about age 7, the lymphatic tissue of the tonsils begins to shrink in size.

THE SPLEEN IS THE LARGEST LYMPHATIC ORGAN

The spleen is the largest organ of the lymphatic system (Fig. 12–10). It lies in the abdominal cavity protected by the ribs, posterior and lateral to the stomach. Because it holds a great deal of blood, the spleen has a distinctive rich purple color.

One of the main functions of the spleen is to bring blood into contact with lymphocytes. As blood flows slowly through the spleen, any disease organisms within it activate lymphocytes in the spleen tissue. The activated lymphocytes then attack the foreign invaders. As blood flows through the spleen, macrophages remove worn-out red and white blood cells and platelets. The spleen stores platelets, and a large percentage of the body's platelets are normally found there.

Although the spleen performs these important functions, it is not vital to life. Fortunately so, for of

---

FIGURE **12–10** The lymphatic system. Lymphatic vessels extend into most tissues of the body, but lymph nodes are clustered in certain regions. The right lymphatic duct drains lymph from the upper right quadrant of the body. The thoracic duct drains lymph from other regions of the body.

all the abdominal organs, the spleen is the one most easily and most frequently injured. A severe blow or crushing injury to the upper abdomen or lower left chest may fracture the ribs that protect the spleen and cause rupture of the spleen itself. When the spleen is ruptured, extensive, sometimes massive, hemorrhage occurs. This condition is usually treated by prompt surgical removal of the spleen (splenectomy) to prevent death due to loss of blood and shock. When the spleen is surgically removed, some of its functions are taken over by the bone marrow and liver; other functions are simply absent, and the body does without them.

THE THYMUS GLAND PLAYS A ROLE IN IMMUNE FUNCTION

The thymus gland is a pinkish gray lymphatic organ located in the upper thorax anterior to the great vessels as they emerge from the heart and posterior to the sternum (Fig. 12–10). During fetal life and childhood, it is quite large. It reaches its largest size at puberty and then begins to become smaller with age. The thymus gland plays a key role in the body's immune processes. It produces several hormones and also prepares one type of lymphocyte for action.

SUMMARY

I. Blood is conducted through two circulatory circuits by a system of blood vessels. In each circuit blood leaving the heart flows through arteries, arterioles, capillaries, and veins.
   A. An artery conducts blood away from the heart and toward some organ.
   B. An arteriole is a small artery that can constrict or dilate, thereby changing the flow of blood into a tissue and affecting blood pressure.
   C. Capillaries are microscopic blood vessels with very thin walls through which oxygen, nutrients, and other materials diffuse.
   D. A vein conducts blood away from an organ and back toward the heart.
II. The blood vessel wall consists of three layers: the innermost layer is endothelium that lines the blood vessel; a middle layer consists of connective tissue and smooth muscle; and an outer connective tissue layer.
III. Blood is pumped by the left ventricle into the systemic circulation, which brings oxygen rich blood to all the tissues of the body.
   A. Blood is returned to the heart by veins.
   B. Blood passes through the right atrium and right ventricle, which pumps it into the pulmonary circulation. In the lungs, carbon dioxide wastes diffuse out from the blood, and oxygen diffuses into the blood.
   C. Blood recharged with oxygen returns to the left atrium of the heart and is pumped by the left ventricle back into the systemic circulation.
IV. The aorta is the largest artery in the body.
   A. The aorta receives blood from the left ventricle and gives off branches that deliver blood to all parts of the body.
   B. The main divisions of the aorta are: ascending aorta, aortic arch, thoracic aorta, and abdominal aorta.
   C. The main branches of each division of the aorta are listed in Table 12–1.
V. Blood is conducted into the brain by the internal carotid arteries and the vertebral arteries. Branches of these arteries join to form the circle of Willis. From the brain capillaries, blood passes into venous sinuses and then into the internal jugular veins (Table 12–2).
VI. Blood from the digestive system drains into the hepatic portal vein, which conducts it to the liver.
   A. Within the liver, blood flows into an extensive network of sinusoids from which the liver removes excess nutrients.
   B. Blood from the hepatic sinusoids passes into hepatic veins, which empty into the inferior vena cava. Note that there is an extra set of exchange vessels (sinusoids); instead of conducting blood into another vein, the hepatic portal vein empties into a set of sinusoids.
VII. Pulse is caused by the elastic expansion and recoil of arteries as they fill with blood; it is measured with a sphygmomanometer and a stethoscope.

VIII. Blood pressure is the force exerted by the blood against the inner walls of the blood vessels.
   A. Blood pressure is affected by the degree of constriction or dilation of the arterioles.
   B. Blood pressure is greatest in the arteries, decreases in the arterioles, and continues to decrease as blood flows through capillaries, and finally veins.
   C. Blood pressure is regulated by baroreceptors that provide feedback to the cardiac centers in the medulla.
IX. The lymphatic system collects and returns tissue fluid to the blood, defends the body against disease, and absorbs lipids from the intestine.
   A. The lymph is formed from tissue fluid.
   B. The lymph circulates through a system of lymph capillaries and lymphatics; as it passes through lymph nodes it is filtered.
   C. The lymphatic system includes the tonsils, spleen, and thymus gland.

POST TEST

1. Blood vessels that transport blood away from the heart and toward some organ or tissue are called _____ .

2. Materials are exchanged between blood and tissues through the thin walls of

   _____ .

3. By constricting and dilating, arterioles help regulate blood

   _____ .

4. The left ventricle pumps blood into the _____ circulation.

5. Blood from the right ventricle is pumped into the

   _____ artery.

6. The pulmonary vein carries _____ (oxygen-rich or oxygen-poor) blood.

7. The _____ aorta is the region of the aorta that descends from the aortic arch.

8. Blood returning to the heart from the tissues, above the level of the diaphragm, drains into a large vein, the _____

   _____   _____ .

9. An important arterial circuit at the base of the brain is the

   _____ of _____ .

10. Blood is delivered to the brain by the _____ and the
   _____ arteries.

11. Blood from the digestive tract passes from the superior mesenteric vein into the _____   _____ vein, which takes it to the

   _____ .

12. The alternate expansion and recoil of an artery is called

   _____ .

13. The force exerted by the blood against the inner walls of the blood vessels is called _____   _____ .

14. The _____ system returns tissue fluid to the blood.

15. Tonsils are masses of _____ tissue.

16. Two main functions of lymph nodes are to _____ and to

   _____ .

17. Vessels that conduct lymph into a lymph node are called

   _____ .

18. The spleen filters _____ .
19. Label the diagram.

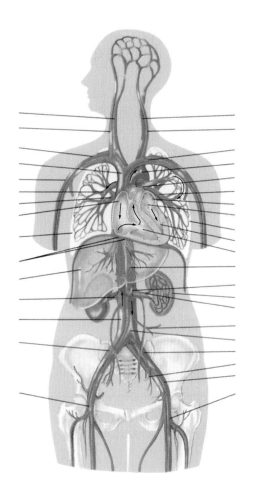

REVIEW QUESTIONS

1. Compare the wall of an artery with that of a capillary.

2. Why is the ability of arterioles to dilate and constrict important?

3. Why do some veins have valves?

4. Why are capillaries referred to as the exchange vessels of the circulatory system?

5. Name the divisions of the aorta and list the main arteries that branch from each division.

6. Trace a drop of blood from the inferior vena cava to the thoracic aorta by listing (in order) each blood vessel and each part of the heart through which it must pass.

7. What blood vessels bring blood to the brain? What is the significance of the circle of Willis?

8. Trace a drop of blood from the: (a) subclavian vein to the left ventricle; (b) right atrium to the renal vein; (c) inferior vena cava to the superior vena cava; (d) hepatic portal vein to the right common carotid artery.

9. Trace a drop of blood from the: (a) coronary vein to a pulmonary capillary; (b) iliac vein to the brain; (c) kidney to the liver; (d) inferior vena cava to the arm.

10. How does blood manage to travel against gravity through veins in the legs on its way back to the heart?

POST TEST ANSWERS

1. arteries
2. capillaries
3. pressure
4. systemic
5. pulmonary
6. oxygen-rich
7. thoracic
8. superior vena cava
9. circle; Willis
10. carotid; vertebral

11. hepatic portal; liver
12. pulse
13. blood pressure
14. lymphatic
15. lymph
16. filter lymph; produce lymphocytes
17. lymphatics
18. blood
19. see Figure 12–4

Thirteen

THE BODY'S DEFENSE MECHANISMS

CHAPTER OUTLINE

    I. The body distinguishes self from nonself
   II. Nonspecific defense mechanisms operate rapidly
  III. Specific defense mechanisms include cell- and antibody-mediated immunity
      A. T cells are responsible for cell-mediated immunity
      B. B cells are responsible for antibody-mediated immunity
      C. There are five classes of antibodies
      D. Antibodies combine with antigens
      E. The thymus is important in immune function
      F. Active immunity develops after exposure to antigens
      G. Passive immunity is borrowed immunity

LEARNING OBJECTIVES

After you have studied this chapter, you should be able to:

1. Identify several nonspecific defense mechanisms.
2. Define the terms antigen and antibody.
3. Describe cell-mediated immunity, including development of memory cells.
4. Describe antibody-mediated immunity, including the effects of antigen-antibody combination upon pathogens both directly and through the complement system.
5. Describe the role of the thymus in immune mechanisms.
6. Contrast active and passive immunity and give examples of each.

The body has remarkable defense mechanisms that protect against **pathogens** (**path′**-o-jens), organisms that cause disease. Defense mechanisms can be nonspecific or specific (Fig. 13–1). Nonspecific defense mechanisms are directed against foreign agents in general. Specific defense mechanisms are directed against particular pathogens.

Specific defense mechanisms are collectively referred to as **immune responses.** The term immune is derived from a Latin word meaning safe. Immunology is the study of the body's specific defense mechanisms.

THE BODY DISTINGUISHES SELF FROM NONSELF

Defense mechanisms depend upon the body's ability to distinguish between itself and pathogens that infect it. The body can recognize the difference because each of us is biochemically unique. Many cell types have large surface proteins that are different in different types of organisms and slightly different in each individual human. The body "knows" its own molecules and "recognizes" those of other organisms as foreign.

189

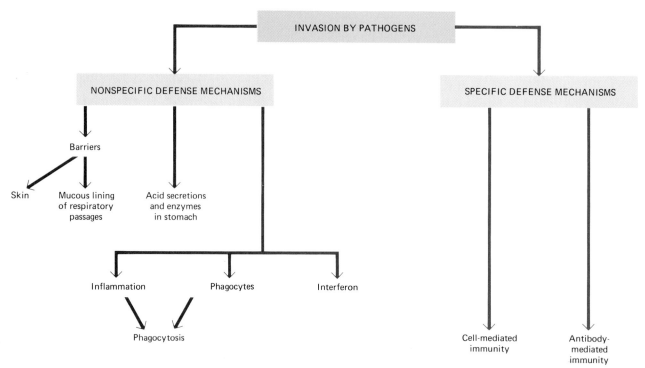

FIGURE 13–1 Summary of nonspecific and specific defense mechanisms. Nonspecific mechanisms prevent entrance of a great many pathogens and act rapidly to destroy those that do manage to cross the barriers. Specific defense mechanisms take longer to mobilize but are highly effective in destroying invaders.

A single bacterium may have 10 to more than 1000 distinct proteins on its surface. When a bacterium invades the body, these surface proteins are recognized as foreign and stimulate the body to defend itself. A substance capable of stimulating the body's defense mechanisms is called an **antigen.**

NONSPECIFIC DEFENSE MECHANISMS OPERATE RAPIDLY

Nonspecific defense mechanisms prevent pathogens from entering the body. When pathogens do succeed in penetrating the body's barriers, nonspecific defense mechanisms destroy them quickly. Some important nonspecific defense mechanisms are as follows:

1. The **skin** is the body's first line of defense against pathogens and other harmful substances. The skin is a mechanical barrier that blocks the entry of pathogens. However, the skin is more than just a mechanical barrier. It is populated by large numbers of harmless bacteria that inhibit the multiplication of harmful bacteria that happen to land on it. Sweat and sebum, found on the surface of the skin, also contain chemicals that destroy certain types of bacteria.

2. Pathogens that enter the body with inhaled air may be filtered out by hairs in the **nose** or trapped in the sticky mucous lining of the **respiratory passageway.** Once trapped, pathogens may be destroyed by phagocytes.

3. Bacteria that enter with food are usually destroyed by the acid and enzymes of the **stomach.**

4. When pathogens invade tissues, **inflammation** occurs (Fig. 13–2). Blood vessels in the affected area dilate, increasing blood flow to the area. This makes the skin look red and feel warm. Capillaries in the inflamed area become more permeable, and more plasma leaves the circulation and enters the tissues. As the amount of tissue fluid increases, **edema** (swelling) occurs. The clinical characteristics of inflammation are redness, edema, heat, and pain. The increased blood flow that occurs during inflammation brings phagocytic cells to the infected area. Increased permeability of the blood vessels permits gamma globulins (plasma proteins that serve as antibodies) to leave the circulation and enter the tissues.

5. Although inflammation often occurs in an injured or infected tissue, sometimes the entire body reacts. **Fever** is a common clinical symptom of widespread inflammation. Fever interferes with the activity of viruses and decreases the amount of iron circulating in the blood. Many pathogens require iron and cannot grow and multiply without it.

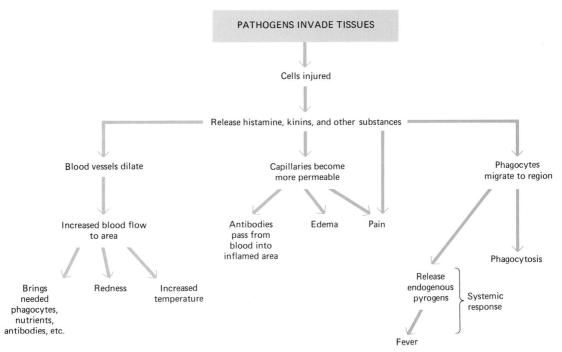

PATHOGENS INVADE TISSUES

Cells injured

Release histamine, kinins, and other substances

Blood vessels dilate

Capillaries become more permeable

Phagocytes migrate to region

Increased blood flow to area

Antibodies pass from blood into inflamed area

Edema

Pain

Phagocytosis

Brings needed phagocytes, nutrients, antibodies, etc.

Redness

Increased temperature

Release endogenous pyrogens } Systemic response

Fever

FIGURE 13–2 Inflammation is a defense mechanism that allows phagocytic cells, antibodies, and other needed compounds to enter infected tissues.

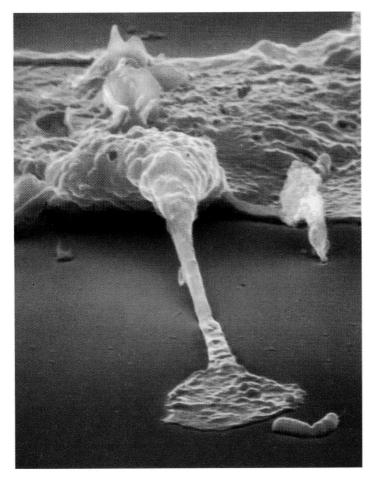

FIGURE 13–3 The macrophage is an incredibly efficient warrior. A macrophage (gray) extends a pseudopod toward an invading E. coli bacterium (green) that is already multiplying. The macrophage will trap the bacterium and take it into the macrophage cell. The macrophage's plasma membrane will seal over the bacterium, and powerful lysosomal enzymes will destroy it. *(From Nilsson, L.: The Incredible Machine. Boehringer Ingelheim International GmbH, p. 171.)*

6. One of the main functions of inflammation appears to be increased **phagocytosis.** Recall that a phagocyte, such as a macrophage, ingests bacteria by flowing around them and engulfing them (Fig. 13–3). As a bacterium is ingested, it is packaged within a vesicle formed by membrane pinched off from the plasma membrane. Lysosomes adhere to the vesicle and release enzymes into it that kill the bacterium.

7. When infected by viruses, or some types of bacteria or fungi, certain types of cells respond by secreting proteins called **interferons** (in-ter-**feer'**-ons). These proteins trigger other cells to produce antiviral proteins. Viruses produced in cells exposed to interferon are less effective at infecting new cells.

SPECIFIC DEFENSE MECHANISMS INCLUDE CELL- AND ANTIBODY-MEDIATED IMMUNITY

While nonspecific defense mechanisms rapidly destroy pathogens and prevent the spread of infection, specific defense mechanisms are being mobilized. Specific defense is the job of the lymphatic system. This system can mobilize armies of highly specialized cellular soldiers and can wage sophisticated chemical warfare. The principal warriors in specific immune responses are the trillion or so lymphocytes stationed strategically in the lymph tissue

TABLE 13–1

Some cells important in immune responses

TYPE OF CELL	FUNCTION
Macrophages	Phagocytize bacteria; process antigens, display them on their cell surface, and present them to lymphocytes; secrete a variety of substances that regulate immune responses
T cells	When stimulated by antigens, divide giving rise to clone of identical cells; some become killer T cells, others become helper T cells, or memory T cells
Killer T cells	Recognize cells bearing antigens and destroy these foreign cells; secrete a variety of substances that attract and activate macrophages and activate other lymphocytes
Memory T cells	Remain in lymph nodes for many years after an infection; should the same pathogen enter the body again, these cells produce new clones of T cells, permitting a rapid response
B cells	When stimulated by antigen, divide to form a clone of identical cells; some differentiate into plasma cells while others become memory B cells
Plasma cells	Secrete antibodies
Memory B cells	Continue to produce small amounts of antibody for years after an infection; should the same pathogen enter the body again, these cells multiply producing new clones of plasma cells; this results in a rapid, antibody response
Natural killer cells (NK cells)	Important in destroying cells infected by virus and cancer cells

throughout the body. Two main types of lymphocytes are **T cells** and **B cells.** Other cells important in internal defense are macrophages and natural killer cells. Some of the types of cells important in immunity are described in Table 13–1.

T CELLS ARE RESPONSIBLE FOR CELL-MEDIATED IMMUNITY

In cell-mediated immunity, T cells attack invading pathogens directly. Cell-mediated immunity is

the responsibility of T cells and macrophages. There are thousands of different varieties of T cells, each capable of responding to a specific type of antigen.

When an antigen enters the body, the types of T cells able to react to that antigen, that is, the competent T cells, become activated, or sensitized. It is thought that this activation process occurs when macrophages take up the antigens and present them to the lymphocytes.

Once stimulated, T cells multiply by mitosis, each giving rise to a sizable clone (family) of cells

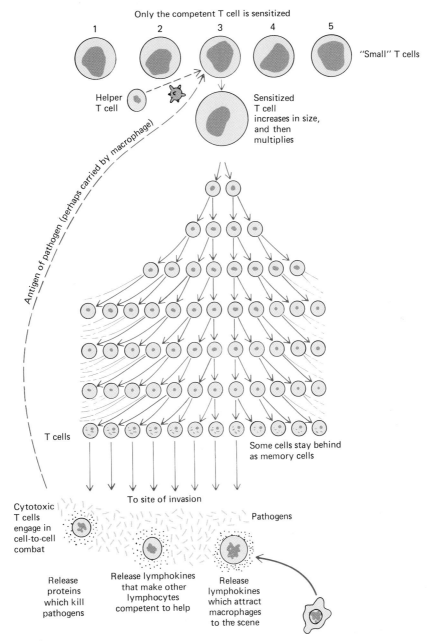

FIGURE 13–4 Cell-mediated immunity. When activated by an antigen, a competent T cell gives rise to a large clone of cells. Many of these differentiate to become killer T cells, which migrate to the site of infection. There they release proteins that destroy invading pathogens. They also release substances that stimulate macrophages and other lymphocytes. Some of the T cells remain in the lymph nodes as memory cells.

identical to itself (Fig. 13–4). T cells then differentiate (develop and specialize) to perform specific functions, and the specialized cells make their way to the site of infection.

One type of specialized T cell, the killer T cell, combines with antigens on the surface of an invading cell. Killer T cells release a powerful group of substances that kill the foreign cell directly and increase inflammation.

> Pathogen infects body → antigens on pathogen activate certain T cells → activated T cells multiply → clones of activated T cells → killer T cells migrate to infected area → release proteins that destroy the pathogens

When T cells in the lymph nodes are sensitized and multiply, not all of them leave the lymph tissue and travel to the scene of battle. Some remain behind as **memory cells.** If the same type of pathogen ever attacks again, the memory cells quickly go into action, destroying the invaders so rapidly that they usually do not have time to cause symptoms of the disease. This explains why we do not usually become ill from the same type of infection more than once.

You may wonder, then, how someone can get a cold or influenza (the "flu") more than once. The answer is that these infections have many varieties, each caused by a slightly different virus. Furthermore, viruses frequently mutate (that is, their gene structure changes), and develop slightly different surface antigens. Even a slight change in an antigen can prevent memory cells from recognizing the pathogen; the body must treat each different antigen as a new immunologic challenge.

B CELLS ARE RESPONSIBLE FOR ANTIBODY-MEDIATED IMMUNITY

As with T cells, thousands of different kinds of B cells exist, each specialized to respond to a specific type of antigen. However, B cells respond differently. Instead of going out to meet the invader, like T cells, B cells produce specific antibodies and send them out to do the job. As already defined antibodies are highly specific proteins (also known as immunoglobulins) that are manufactured in response to specific antigens. They are among the body's most powerful chemical weapons.

When bacteria invade the body, some of their antigens find their way to the lymph tissue. Some of the antigens come into contact with the type of B cell

that can produce antibodies against them. This activates the B cells. Certain T cells, called **helper T cells,** play a role in the stimulation of B cells.

The activated B cells multiply. Within a few days they produce a large clone of identical B cells (Fig. 13–5). Most of these cells become **plasma cells,** the mature B cells that secrete antibodies. The antibodies are carried by the lymph to the blood and are then transported to the infected region.

> Pathogen infects body → antigens on pathogen activate certain B cells → activated B cells multiply → clones of activated B cells → develop into plasma cells → plasma cells secrete antibodies → antibodies are transported to infected area

Some of the activated B cells become memory cells and continue for years to produce small amounts of antibody. Should the pathogen ever enter the body again, this circulating antibody (part of the gamma globulin fraction of the plasma) will immediately bind with it. At the same time, the memory cells will respond by quickly multiplying to produce new clones of the needed type of plasma cells.

THERE ARE FIVE CLASSES OF ANTIBODIES

Antibodies are grouped into five classes according to their structure. Using the abbreviation "Ig" (for immunoglobulin), the classes are designated IgG, IgM, IgA, IgD, and IgE. Each class has different functions. Normally about 75% of the antibodies in the body belong in the IgG group (part of the gamma globulin fraction of the blood).

ANTIBODIES COMBINE WITH ANTIGENS

The principal job of an antibody is to identify a pathogen as foreign. It does this by combining with one or more antigens on the surface of the pathogen. An antibody usually combines with several antigens, creating a mass of clumped antigen-antibody complex. The antigen-antibody complex activates several defense mechanisms:

1. The antigen-antibody complex may inactivate the pathogen or its toxin. For example, once an antibody has attached to the surface of a virus, the virus loses its ability to infect a new cell.

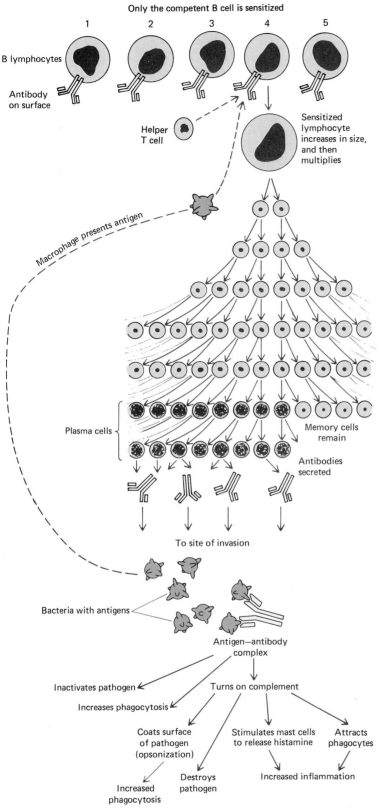

Only the competent B cell is sensitized

B lymphocytes

Antibody on surface

Helper T cell

Macrophage presents antigen

Sensitized lymphocyte increases in size, and then multiplies

Plasma cells

Memory cells remain

Antibodies secreted

To site of invasion

Bacteria with antigens

Antigen—antibody complex

Inactivates pathogen

Turns on complement

Increases phagocytosis

Coats surface of pathogen (opsonization)

Stimulates mast cells to release histamine

Attracts phagocytes

Increased phagocytosis

Destroys pathogen

Increased inflammation

FIGURE 13–5 Antibody-mediated immunity. When a macrophage presents an antigen to a competent B cell, the B cell becomes activated. Once activated in this way, the competent B lymphocyte multiplies, producing a large clone of cells. Some of these differentiate and become plasma cells, which secrete antibodies. The plasma cells remain in the lymph tissues, but the antibodies are transported to the site of infection by the circulatory system. Antigen-antibody complexes form, directly inactivating some pathogens and also turning on the complement system. Some of the B lymphocytes become memory cells that persist and continue to secrete small amounts of antibody for years after the infection is over.

2. The combination of antibody with antigen on the surface of a pathogen stimulates phagocytes to destroy it.

3. Antibodies of the IgG and IgM groups work by activating the **complement system.** This is a group of about 11 proteins found in plasma and other body fluids. Normally the proteins are inactive, but an antigen-antibody complex stimulates a series of reactions that activate the complement system. The antibody is said to "fix" complement. Proteins of the complement system then destroy pathogens. The complement system also increases inflammation.

THE THYMUS IS IMPORTANT IN IMMUNE FUNCTION

In some way, the thymus helps T cells develop the ability to specialize. Apparently, the thymus "instructs" the T cells just before birth and during the first few months of infancy. The thymus gives T cells the ability to be immunologically competent, that is, to develop into cells that can carry out certain specific immune reactions to specific antigens.

The thymus secretes several hormones, including **thymosin (thy′-mow-sin).** Thymosin is thought to stimulate immature T cells to become immunologically active. Thymosin has been successfully administered to patients who have poorly developed thymus glands and, thus, low immunity. Investigators are currently testing thymosin in patients with certain types of cancer. By stimulating cellular immunity, thymosin may help prevent the spread of the disease.

ACTIVE IMMUNITY DEVELOPS AFTER EXPOSURE TO ANTIGENS

Active immunity develops from exposure to antigens. If you had chickenpox as a young child, for example, you developed immunity that prevents you from contracting chickenpox again. Active immunity

can also be developed by **immunization,** that is, by injection of a vaccine. For example, if you are immunized against measles, your body reacts just as though it had been exposed to someone with measles. The body launches an immune response against the antigens in the measles vaccine and develops memory cells.

Effective vaccines can be prepared in a number of ways. Some vaccines (for example, typhoid fever vaccine) are made from killed pathogens. Measles and smallpox vaccine are made from viruses that have been weakened so that they can no longer cause disease.

PASSIVE IMMUNITY IS BORROWED IMMUNITY

In passive immunity, an individual is given antibodies actively produced by other humans or by animals. Passive immunity is borrowed immunity, so its effects do not last. It is used to boost one's defenses temporarily against a particular disease. For example, during the Vietnam war, viral hepatitis was widespread in some areas. Soldiers were injected with gamma globulin (containing antibody to hepatitis virus) to help protect them from the disease. Unfortunately, such injected antibodies last only a few months. Do you know why? It is because the body has not actively launched an immune response. No memory cells have been developed, and the body cannot produce antibodies to the pathogen. Once the injected antibodies wear out, the immunity disappears.

Pregnant women confer passive immunity upon their developing babies by producing antibodies for them. Babies who are breast fed receive antibodies in their milk. These antibodies provide immunity to the pathogens responsible for gastrointestinal infection, and perhaps to other pathogens as well.

SUMMARY

I. Defense mechanisms depend on the body's ability to distinguish between itself and pathogens that infect it.
II. Nonspecific defense mechanisms include the skin, acid secretions in the stomach, the mucous lining of the respiratory passageways, inflammation, fever, phagocytosis, and interferons.
III. Specific defense mechanisms include cell-mediated immunity and antibody-mediated immunity.
  A. In cell-mediated immunity, specific T cells are activated when they come into contact with specific antigens. Activated T lymphocytes multiply, giving rise to a clone of identical cells.
    1. Some T cells differentiate to become killer T cells, migrate to the site of infection, and kill pathogens.
    2. Some activated T cells remain in the lymph nodes as memory cells.

B. In antibody-mediated immunity, specific B cells are activated by the presence of specific antigens. Activated B cells multiply and give rise to plasma cells that secrete specific antibodies.
1. Antibodies are transported by the circulatory system to the site of infection.
2. Antibodies combine with specific antigens to form antigen-antibody complex. This may activate several defense mechanisms, including the complement system.
C. Active immunity, whether natural or by vaccine, involves exposure to an antigen and an active immune response. Memory cells are produced and provide long-term protection.
D. In passive immunity, antibodies are borrowed from another person or animal that has produced them. Passive immunity is temporary.

POST TEST

1. Disease-causing organisms such as bacteria and viruses are called

   _____ .

2. The body's first line of defense against pathogens is the

   _____ .

3. The increased blood flow characteristic of inflammation brings _____ cells to the infected area.

4. When certain types of cells are infected by viruses, they release proteins called

   _____ .

5. Proteins that stimulate immune responses are called _____ .

6. Plasma cells produce proteins called _____ , which help destroy antigens.

7. B lymphocytes are responsible for _____ -mediated immunity.

8. T lymphocytes are responsible for _____ -mediated immunity.

9. Activated B or T cells that remain in the lymph nodes for many years after an infection are called _____ cells.

10. The main job of an antibody is to identify a pathogen as foreign by combining with _____ on its surface.

11. The _____ system is a group of proteins found in plasma and other body fluids.

12. The temporary immunity gained when one is injected with gamma globulin is called _____ immunity.

13. Vaccines can stimulate _____ immunity.

REVIEW QUESTIONS

1. Contrast nonspecific and specific types of defense mechanisms. Which type acts immediately?

2. How does the inflammatory response help to restore homeostasis?

3. What is fever? Why is it considered a defense mechanism?

4. How does interferon work?

5. Define: (a) antigen; (b) antibody.

6. Contrast the actions of T and B cells.

7. Contrast cell-mediated immunity with antibody-mediated immunity, giving their principal differences.

8. Compare the immune response that occurs when someone with measles sneezes on you with the response stimulated when you are immunized against measles.

9. Why is passive immunity temporary?

POST TEST ANSWERS

1. pathogens
2. skin
3. phagocytic (white blood cells)
4. interferons
5. antigens
6. antibodies
7. antibody
8. cell
9. memory
10. antigen
11. complement
12. passive
13. active

Fourteen

THE RESPIRATORY SYSTEM

CHAPTER OUTLINE

I. The nasal cavities are lined with a mucous membrane
II. The pharynx is divided into three regions
III. The larynx is the voice box
IV. The trachea is the windpipe
V. The bronchi enter the lungs
VI. The air sacs are called alveoli
VII. The lungs provide a large surface area
VIII. Ventilation moves air into and out of the lungs
IX. Gas exchange occurs by diffusion
X. Gases are transported by the circulatory system
XI. Respiration is regulated by the brain
XII. The respiratory system defends itself against dirty air

LEARNING OBJECTIVES

After you have studied this chapter, you should be able to:
1. Trace a breath of air through the respiratory system from nose to alveoli.
2. Describe the structure of the lungs.
3. Define ventilation and summarize how breathing takes place.
4. Summarize the process of oxygen and carbon dioxide exchange in the lungs and in the tissues.
5. Outline how oxygen and carbon dioxide are transported in the blood.
6. Describe how respiration is regulated.

Respiration means to "breathe again." Respiration supplies the cells of the body with oxygen and rids them of carbon dioxide. The process of respiration includes breathing, gas exchange between the lungs and the blood, transport of gases through the body by the blood, gas exchange between the blood and the cells, and cellular respiration (use of oxygen by the cells and production of carbon dioxide by the cells).

The respiratory system consists of the lungs and the tubes through which air reaches them (Fig. 14–

1). A breath of air enters the body through the **nose,** flows through the **nasal cavities** to the **pharynx** (**far'**-inks), through the **larynx** (**lar'**-inks) (voice box), and into the **trachea** (**tray'**-kee-ah) (windpipe). Air then enters the **bronchi** (**brong'**-kie). One bronchus enters each **lung.** Air then passes into the many **bronchioles** (**brong'**-kee-oles) of the lungs. These divide again and again until the air reaches the microscopic **air sacs,** called **alveoli** (**al-vee'**-o-lee). Oxygen diffuses from the air sacs into the blood.

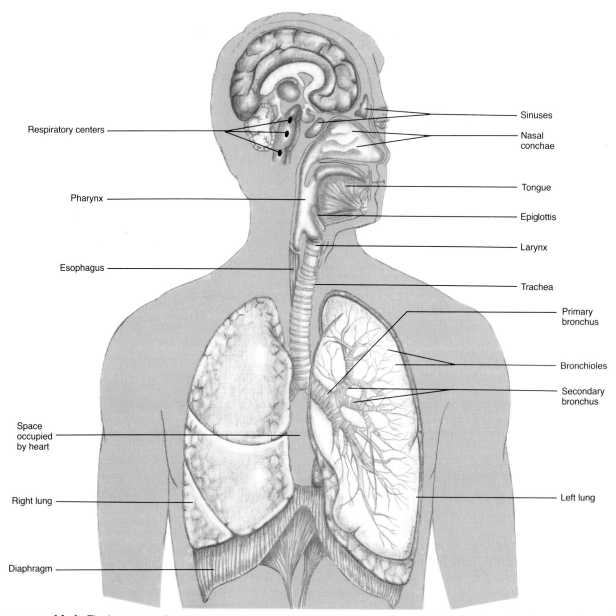

Respiratory centers

Sinuses

Nasal conchae

Pharynx

Tongue

Epiglottis

Larynx

Esophagus

Trachea

Primary bronchus

Bronchioles

Secondary bronchus

Space occupied by heart

Right lung

Left lung

Diaphragm

FIGURE 14–1   The human respiratory system includes a series of air passageways and the paired lungs. The lungs are located in the thoracic cavity. The muscular diaphragm forms the floor of the thoracic cavity, separating it from the abdominal cavity below. An internal view of one lung illustrates its extensive system of air passageways. The microscopic air sacs (alveoli) are shown in Figure 14–2.

Nasal cavities → pharynx → larynx → trachea → bronchus (enters lung) → bronchioles (in lung) → air sacs (in lung)

THE NASAL CAVITIES ARE LINED WITH A MUCOUS MEMBRANE

Whether you breathe through your nose or your mouth, air finds its way into the pharynx. Nose breathing has advantages. The nose "air conditions" air. It filters and moistens the air and brings it to body temperature. The nose also contains the receptors for the sense of smell.

Air passes into the nose through its two openings, the **nares (nay′**-reez), or nostrils. Coarse hairs in the nostrils prevent large particles from entering the nose. The nostrils open into the two nasal cavities, which are separated by a partition, the **nasal septum.** The septum and walls of the nose consist of bone covered with a mucous membrane. Three bony projections, the conchae, project from the lateral walls of the nose. The conchae increase the surface area over which air must pass as it moves through the nose. The mucous membrane lining the nose has a rich blood supply that heats and moistens the lining and the air that comes into contact with it.

Mucous cells within the lining produce more than a pint of mucus a day, more in the event of allergy or infection. Inhaled dirt and other foreign particles are trapped in the layer of mucus that forms along the surface of the mucous membrane. Ciliated epithelial cells of the membrane push a steady stream of mucus along with its trapped particles toward the throat. The mucus is swallowed with the saliva. In this way foreign particles are delivered to the digestive system, which is far more capable of disposing of them than are the delicate lungs.

Several sinuses (small cavities) in the bones of the skull communicate with the nasal cavities by small channels. They are lined with mucous membrane that sometimes becomes inflamed and infected (sinusitis).

THE PHARYNX IS DIVIDED INTO THREE REGIONS

Posteriorly, the nasal cavities are continuous with the pharynx, or throat. Air enters the **nasopharynx** (nay″-zo-**far**′-inks), the superior part of the pharynx. Air then moves down into the **oropharynx** (oh″-row-**far**′-inks) behind the mouth. The oropharynx also receives food from the mouth. Finally, air passes through the **laryngopharynx** (lah-ring″-oh-**far**′-inks) and enters the larynx. Behind the opening into the larynx is a second opening into the esophagus (part of the digestive tract).

THE LARYNX IS THE VOICE BOX

The larynx, or voice box, contains the vocal cords. The vocal cords are muscular folds of tissue that project from the lateral walls of the larynx. They vibrate as air from the lungs rushes past them during expiration (breathing out). The opening into the larynx is the **glottis.**

During swallowing, a flap of tissue, the **epiglottis** (ep″-ih-**glot**′-is), automatically closes off the larynx so food cannot enter the lower airway. When this mechanism fails, foreign matter comes into contact with the sensitive larynx. A cough reflex is stimulated to expel the material from the respiratory system.

The wall of the larynx is supported by cartilage that protrudes from the midline of the neck and is sometimes referred to as the Adam's apple. The

Adam's apple is more prominent in males than females. Inflammation of the larynx, or laryngitis, is most often caused by a respiratory infection or by irritating substances such as cigarette smoke.

THE TRACHEA IS THE WINDPIPE

The trachea, or windpipe, is located anterior to the esophagus. It extends from the larynx to the middle of the chest. Like the larynx, the trachea is kept from collapsing by rings of cartilage in its wall. The open parts of these C-shaped rings of cartilage face posteriorly, toward the esophagus.

The larynx, trachea, and bronchi are lined by a mucous membrane that traps dirt and other foreign matter. Ciliated cells in this lining continuously beat a stream of mucus upward to the pharynx, where the mucus is swallowed. This cilia-propelled mucus elevator keeps foreign material out of the lungs.

THE BRONCHI ENTER THE LUNGS

The trachea divides into right and left bronchi. One bronchus enters each lung. The structure of these main bronchi is similar to that of the trachea. Each bronchus branches again and again like the branches of a tree. The branches give rise to smaller and smaller bronchi and finally to very small bronchioles. Each lung has more than a million bronchioles. The network of branching air passageways within the lungs is referred to as the bronchial tree.

THE AIR SACS ARE CALLED ALVEOLI

Each bronchiole leads into a cluster of microscopic air sacs, the alveoli (Fig. 14–2). The wall of an alveolus consists of a single layer of epithelial cells and elastic fibers that permit it to stretch and contract during breathing. Each alveolus is surrounded by a network of capillaries so that gases diffuse easily between the alveolus and blood. Alveoli are coated by a thin film of surfactant, a substance that prevents the alveoli from collapsing.

THE LUNGS PROVIDE A LARGE SURFACE AREA

The lungs are large, paired, spongy organs that occupy the thoracic cavity. They are separated medi-

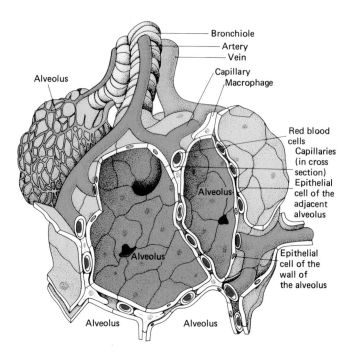

F I G U R E **14–2** Structure of an alveolus. Note that the wall of the alveolus consists of extremely thin epithelium that permits gas exchange. Capillary networks surround each alveolus. *(From Kessell, R.G., and Kardon, R.H.: Tissues and organs.* In *A Text-Atlas of Scanning Electron Microscopy. San Francisco, W.H. Freeman, 1979.)*

ally by the mediastinum (which contains the heart, esophagus, thymus gland, and parts of other organs). The right lung is divided into three lobes, the left lung into two lobes (see Fig. 14–1). Each bronchus enters its lung at a depression called the **hilus** (hi′-lus). Blood vessels and nerves also enter and leave the lung at the hilus.

Inside, each lung consists mainly of bronchi, bronchioles, alveoli, blood vessels, and elastic tissue. Lymph tissue and nerves are also present. Because there are millions of tiny air passageways, the surface area of the lung through which gases can be exchanged is very large. Its surface area is about the size of a tennis court!

Each lung is covered with a **pleural membrane** (**ploor′**-al), which forms a sac enclosing the lung and continues as the lining of the thoracic cavity. The part of the pleural membrane that covers the lung is the **visceral pleura;** the portion that lines the thoracic cavity is the **parietal pleura.** The pleural membrane is a serous membrane. Recall from Chapter 2 that a serous membrane lines a body cavity that does not open to the outside of the body.

Between the visceral and parietal pleura is a potential space, the **pleural cavity.** A film of fluid secreted by the pleural membranes fills the pleural cavity. This fluid lubricates and reduces the friction between the two pleural membranes during breathing. Inflammation of the pleural membrane, called pleurisy, may be caused by infection or injury. A

symptom of pleurisy is pain during breathing, when the swollen membranes contact each other.

The thoracic cavity is completely enclosed. It is bounded on the front and sides by the chest wall, which contains the ribs. Its floor is a strong, dome-shaped muscle, the **diaphragm.**

VENTILATION MOVES AIR INTO AND OUT OF THE LUNGS

Pulmonary ventilation is the movement of air into and out of the lungs. We generally accomplish pulmonary ventilation by breathing. Breathing in is called **inspiration** (or inhalation); breathing out is **expiration** (exhalation).

During inspiration the diaphragm contracts and flattens and the intercostal muscles contract (Fig. 14–3). The size of the chest cavity increases. The chest cavity is closed, so when it expands, the film of fluid on the pleural membranes holds the lung surfaces against the chest wall. This causes the lungs to move outward along with the chest walls. As a result, the space within each lung increases.

The air in the lungs at first tends to spread out to fill the larger space. However, the pressure of the air in the lungs falls below the pressure of the air outside the body (that is, a partial vacuum results). As a result, air from the outside rushes in through the respi-

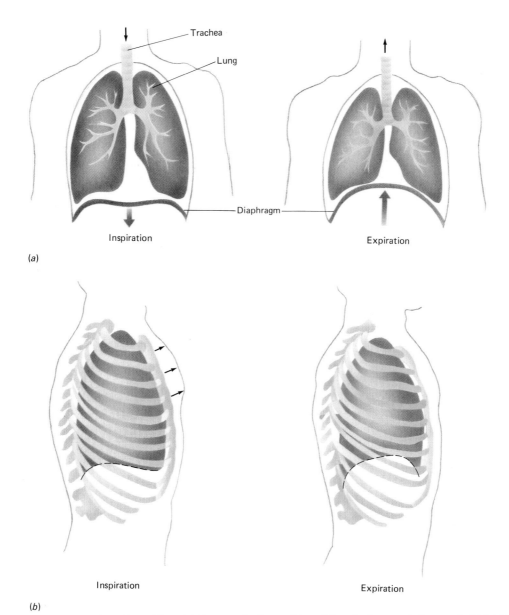

Trachea

Lung

Diaphragm

Inspiration

Expiration

(a)

Inspiration

Expiration

(b)

FIGURE 14–3 The mechanics of breathing. *(a)* Changes in the position of the diaphragm during inspiration and expiration result in changes in volume of the chest cavity. *(b)* Changes in position of the rib cage in expiration and inspiration. During inspiration the chest muscles pull the front ends of the ribs upward. The resulting increase in the volume of the chest cavity causes air to move into the lungs.

ratory passageways and fills the lungs until the two pressures are again equal.

> Diaphragm and intercostal muscles contract → volume of chest cavity increases → lungs expand → volume of lungs increases → air pressure in lungs decreases → air moves into lungs

Expiration occurs when the diaphragm and intercostal muscles relax, permitting the elastic tissues of the lung to recoil. The size of the thoracic cavity decreases. Pressure increases inside the lung and its elastic fibers push against the air, forcing it to rush out of the lung. The millions of alveoli deflate and the lung is ready for another inspiration. During forced expiration several sets of muscles, including the abdominal muscles, contract.

Diaphragm and intercostal muscles relax → volume of thoracic cavity decreases → lungs recoil → lung volume decreases → pressure in air sacs increases → air rushes out of lungs

Pressure in the space between the visceral and the parietal pleura is lower than atmospheric pressure. This pressure difference prevents the air sacs from completely deflating at the end of each expiration. If the chest wall is punctured, air enters this space and the pressure there becomes equal to atmospheric pressure. When this happens, the air sacs collapse like so many deflated balloons. This condition, referred to as a collapsed lung, blocks the movement of air.

GAS EXCHANGE OCCURS BY DIFFUSION

Breathing delivers oxygen to the alveoli of the lungs, However, if oxygen merely remained in the lungs, all the other body cells would die. The vital link between the alveoli and the body cells is the circulatory system. Each alveolus serves as a depot from which oxygen is loaded into the blood of the pulmonary capillaries.

Because the alveoli contain a greater concentration of oxygen than the blood entering the pulmonary capillaries, oxygen molecules diffuse from the alveoli into the blood (Fig. 14–4). Carbon dioxide moves from the blood, where it is more concentrated, to the alveoli, where it is less concentrated. Each gas diffuses through the thin lining of the capillary and the thin lining of the alveolus.

Table 14–1 shows the percentages of oxygen and carbon dioxide present in expired air compared with inspired air. Expired air has more than 100 times more carbon dioxide than air inspired from the environment. This is because carbon dioxide is produced by the cells of the body during cellular respiration (the chemical breakdown of fuel molecules).

As blood circulates through the tissues, oxygen moves from the blood, where it is more concentrated, into the cells, where it is less concentrated. On the other hand, carbon dioxide is more concentrated in the cells than in the blood. As a result, carbon dioxide diffuses from the cells into the blood and is transported to the lungs.

GASES ARE TRANSPORTED BY THE CIRCULATORY SYSTEM

When oxygen diffuses into the blood, it enters the red blood cells and forms a weak chemical bond with hemoglobin, forming oxyhemoglobin.

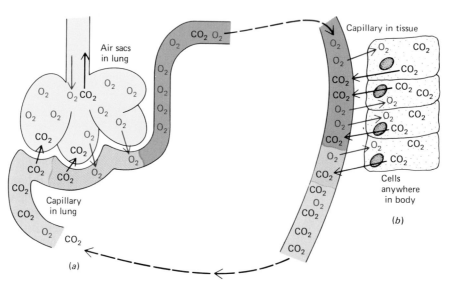

FIGURE 14–4 Gas exchange. (a) Exchange of gases between air sacs and capillaries in the lung. The concentration of oxygen is greater in the air sacs than in the capillary, so oxygen moves from the air sacs into the blood. Carbon dioxide is more concentrated in the blood, so it moves out of the capillary and into the air sacs. (b) Exchange of gases between capillary and body cells. Here oxygen is more concentrated in the blood, so it moves out of the capillary and into the cells. Carbon dioxide is more concentrated in the cells, and so it diffuses out of the cells and into the blood.

TABLE 14–1

Composition of inhaled air compared with that of exhaled air

	% OXYGEN (O_2)	% CARBON DIOXIDE (CO_2)	% NITROGEN (N_2)
Inhaled air (atmospheric air)	20.9	0.04	79
Exhaled air (alveolar air)	14.0	5.60	79

As indicated, the body uses up about one-third of the inhaled oxygen. The amount of CO_2 increases more than 100-fold because it is produced during cellular respiration.

$$\text{Hemoglobin} + \text{oxygen} \longrightarrow \text{oxyhemoglobin}$$

Because the chemical bond linking the oxygen with the hemoglobin is weak, this reaction is readily reversible. In tissues that are low in oxygen, oxyhemoglobin dissociates, releasing oxygen. The oxygen then diffuses out of the capillaries and into the cells.

$$\text{Oxyhemoglobin} \longrightarrow \text{oxygen} + \text{hemoglobin}$$

Carbon dioxide is transported in the blood in three ways. Most is transported as a compound called bicarbonate. Bicarbonate is produced when carbon dioxide chemically combines with water. Some carbon dioxide is transported attached to hemoglobin. A small amount of carbon dioxide is simply dissolved in plasma.

RESPIRATION IS REGULATED BY THE BRAIN

The normal adult breathing rate is about 12 to 20 times per minute. When you are engaged in a strenuous game of racketball, you require more oxygen than when you are quietly watching television. The rate, depth, and rhythm of breathing are regulated by **respiratory centers** in the medulla and pons (see Fig. 14–1).

During exercise, body tissues produce greater amounts of carbon dioxide. The carbon dioxide (after combining with water to form carbonic acid) causes the blood to be more acidic. Within the medulla is an area that is very sensitive to increased concentrations of carbon dioxide, or sharp decreases in oxygen concentration. Similar receptors are located in certain blood vessels (the carotid artery and aorta). When these receptors are stimulated, the medulla sends impulses that increase the rate and depth of breathing. Impulses from the medulla reach the diaphragm by way of the **phrenic (fren´-ik) nerves.**

Breathing is an involuntary process, but the action of the respiratory centers can be consciously stimulated or inhibited. For example, you can inhibit breathing by holding your breath. You could not kill yourself by holding your breath, however, because when carbon dioxide builds up to a certain level you do breathe, want to or not.

Underwater swimmers and divers not using scuba gear may voluntarily hyperventilate before going under water. Taking a series of deep breaths does not increase the oxygen in the blood, but it does reduce the carbon dioxide content. This permits them to remain under water for a few extra moments before the urge to breathe becomes irresistible. Hyperventilation can result in dizziness and even unconsciousness. This is because a certain concentration of carbon dioxide in the blood is necessary to maintain normal blood pressure.

When an individual has stopped breathing because of drowning, electric shock, cardiac arrest, or other crisis, the victim can often be kept alive by mouth-to-mouth resuscitation until his or her breathing reflexes can take over again. Cardiopulmonary resuscitation (CPR) is a method for helping victims who have suffered respiratory and cardiac arrest.

THE RESPIRATORY SYSTEM DEFENDS ITSELF AGAINST DIRTY AIR

We breathe about 20,000 times each day, inhaling about 35 pounds of air—6 times more than the food and drink we take in. Most of us breathe dirty urban air containing carbon monoxide, particles of dirt, and other harmful substances. The respiratory system has a number of defense mechanisms that help protect the delicate lungs from damage.

The hair in the nose and the mucous lining of the respiratory passageways help trap foreign particles in inspired air. When we breathe dirty air the bronchial tubes narrow. This constriction increases the chances that inhaled particles land on the sticky mucous lining.

The smallest bronchioles and the alveoli are not equipped with cells with cilia or with mucus. Foreign particles that slip through the respiratory defenses and find their way into the alveoli may remain there indefinitely or may be engulfed by macrophages. The macrophages may then accumulate in the lymph tissue of the lungs. Lung tissue of chronic smokers and of those who work in dirty industries contains large, blackened areas where carbon particles have been deposited.

Continued insult to the respiratory system results in disease. Chronic bronchitis and emphysema are chronic pulmonary diseases that have been linked to smoking and breathing polluted air. Cigarette smoking is also the main cause of lung cancer.

SUMMARY

I. The nose filters and moistens inspired air and brings it to body temperature.

II. From the nasal cavities, air passes through the pharynx and into the larynx. The larynx protects the lungs by initiating a cough reflex when it is touched by foreign matter.

III. From the larynx, inhaled air passes into the trachea and then into the right or left bronchus.

IV. Within the lungs, the bronchi branch and rebranch, giving rise to an extensive system of bronchioles.

V. Each bronchiole gives rise to a cluster of alveoli through which gas exchange takes place with the blood.

VI. The lungs are large, spongy organs covered with pleural membranes.

VII. Pulmonary ventilation is the process of moving air into and out of the lungs. We ventilate the lungs by breathing.

   A. When the diaphragm and intercostal muscles contract, the thoracic cavity expands. The lungs expand and pressure in the lungs decreases. Air rushes into the lungs.

   B. When the diaphragm and intercostal muscles relax, pressure in the lung increases and air rushes out of the lungs.

VIII. Oxygen diffuses from the alveoli into the blood and is transported to the body cells in the form of oxyhemoglobin. As oxygen is needed by the cells, oxyhemoglobin dissociates, and oxygen diffuses from the blood into the cells.

IX. Carbon dioxide is transported mainly in the form of bicarbonate ions. In the lungs, carbon dioxide diffuses from the blood in the pulmonary capillaries into the alveoli and then is expired.

X. Breathing is normally regulated by respiratory centers in the medulla and pons that are sensitive to the concentration of carbon dioxide in the blood.

XI. Among the defense mechanisms of the respiratory system are its cilia-mucus lining, bronchial constriction, and the action of macrophages. Continued insult to the respiratory system may result in chronic bronchitis, emphysema, or lung cancer.

POST TEST

1. Inhaled air passing through the pharynx would next enter the _____ and then pass through the _____ .

2. Gas exchange takes place through the thin walls of the _____ .

3. The floor of the thoracic cavity is formed by the _____ .

4. The _____ seals off the larynx during swallowing.

5. When foreign matter contacts the larynx it may initiate a _____ reflex.

6. The part of the pleural membrane that encloses the lung is the
   _____ pleura.

7. Pulmonary _____ is the process of moving air into and out of
   the lungs.

8. Breathing in is called _____ ; breathing out is called
   _____ .

9. Oxygen is transported in the blood chemically bound to
   _____ .

10. Impulses from the medulla reach the diaphragm by way of the
    _____ nerves.

11. Label the diagram.

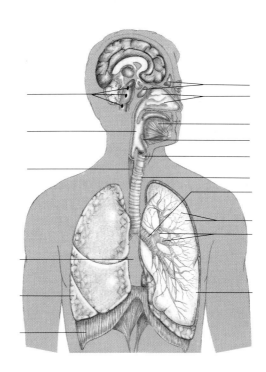

REVIEW QUESTIONS

1. Trace a breath of inspired air from nose to alveoli. List each structure in sequence through which the air must pass.

2. What are the advantages of having millions of alveoli rather than a pair of simple, balloon-like lungs?

3. Compare inspiration with expiration.

4. The larynx is sometimes referred to as the watchdog of the lungs. Why do you
   think this is appropriate?

5. What are the advantages of breathing through the nose?

6. How is the structure of the respiratory system especially designed to permit gas
   exchange? (Hint: consider the thickness of alveolar and capillary walls as part of
   your answer.)

7. How is breathing regulated?

8. How does the respiratory system protect itself from harmful pollutants in the air we breathe? Describe several defense mechanisms.

POST TEST ANSWERS

1. larynx; trachea
2. alveoli
3. diaphragm
4. epiglottis
5. cough
6. visceral
7. ventilation
8. inspiration; expiration
9. hemoglobin
10. phrenic
11. see Figure 14–1

Fifteen

THE DIGESTIVE SYSTEM

CHAPTER OUTLINE

    I. The digestive system consists of the digestive tract and accessory organs
    II. The digestive system processes food
    III. The wall of the digestive tract has four layers
    IV. Folds of the peritoneum support the digestive organs
    V. The mouth ingests food
        A. The teeth break down food
        B. The salivary glands produce saliva
    VI. The pharynx is important in swallowing
    VII. The esophagus conducts food to the stomach
    VIII. The stomach digests food
    IX. Most digestion takes place in the small intestine
    X. The pancreas secretes enzymes
    XI. The liver secretes bile
    XII. Digestion occurs as food moves through the digestive tract
        A. Glucose is the main product of carbohydrate digestion
        B. Bile digests fat
        C. Proteins are digested to amino acids
    XIII. The intestinal villi absorb nutrients
    XIV. The large intestine eliminates waste
    XV. A balanced diet is necessary to maintain health

LEARNING OBJECTIVES

After you have studied this chapter, you should be able to:

1. List in sequence each structure through which a bite of food passes on its way through the digestive tract; label a diagram of the digestive system.
2. Describe in general terms the following steps in processing food: ingestion, digestion, absorption, and elimination.
3. Describe the wall of the digestive tract, distinguish between the visceral and parietal peritoneums, and describe their major folds.
4. Describe the structures of the mouth, including the teeth, and give their functions.
5. Describe the structure and function of the pharynx and esophagus.
6. Describe the structure of the stomach and its role in processing food.
7. Identify the three main regions of the small intestine, and give the function of the small intestine.
8. Summarize the functions of the pancreas and liver.
9. Summarize carbohydrate, lipid, and protein digestion.
10. Describe the structure of an intestinal villus, and explain the role of villi in absorption of nutrients.
11. Describe the structure and functions of the large intestine.
12. List the nutrients that make up a balanced diet and summarize the functions of each.

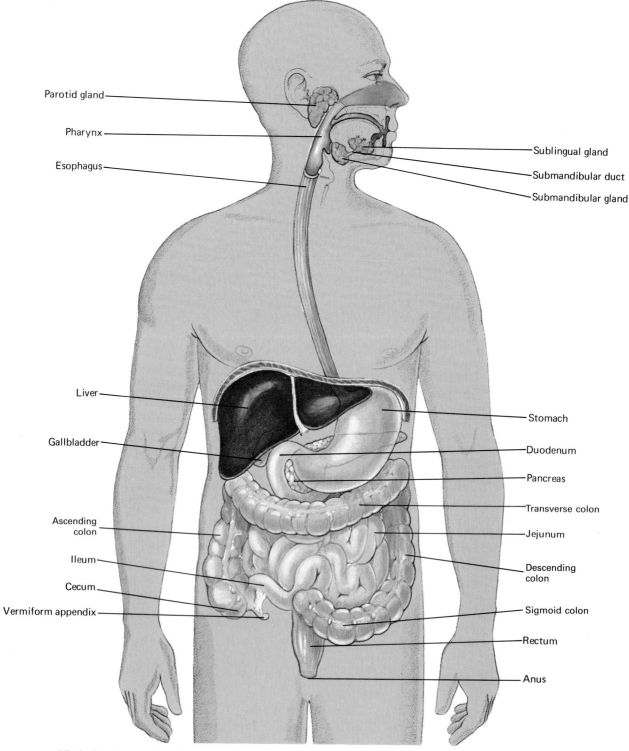

Parotid gland

Pharynx

Esophagus

Sublingual gland

Submandibular duct

Submandibular gland

Liver

Gallbladder

Ascending colon

Ileum

Cecum

Vermiform appendix

Stomach

Duodenum

Pancreas

Transverse colon

Jejunum

Descending colon

Sigmoid colon

Rectum

Anus

F I G U R E 15–1 The human digestive system. Note that the digestive tract is a long, coiled tube extending from mouth to anus. Locate the three types of accessory glands.

Nutrients are the substances in food that are used as an energy source to run the machinery of the body. The body also uses nutrients as building blocks to make new cells and as ingredients to make the chemical compounds needed for metabolism. The food we eat consists of large pieces and large molecules. It is not in a form that can reach the cells of the body or that can be used for nourishment. The digestive system processes the food and breaks it down into a form that can be delivered to the cells, and then used by the cells. This chapter focuses on the long and eventful journey that food takes through the digestive tract.

THE DIGESTIVE SYSTEM CONSISTS OF THE DIGESTIVE TRACT AND ACCESSORY ORGANS

The **digestive tract,** also called the alimentary canal, is a long tube about 8 meters (m) (23 feet) long. It extends from the mouth, where food is taken in, to the anus, through which unused food is eliminated (Fig. 15–1). Below the diaphragm, the digestive tract is often referred to as the GI (gastrointestinal) tract. The digestive tube is like a long, coiled hose. Some sections of the tube are narrow; others are wide.

The parts of the digestive tract through which food passes in sequence are the mouth, pharynx (throat), esophagus, stomach, small intestine (subdivided into duodenum, jejunum, and ileum), and large intestine (subdivided into cecum, colon, and rectum).

Mouth → pharynx → esophagus → stomach → small intestine → large intestine

Three types of **accessory digestive glands**—salivary glands, liver, and pancreas—are not part of the digestive tract but secrete digestive juices into it.

THE DIGESTIVE SYSTEM PROCESSES FOOD

The digestive system is responsible for four major processes:

1. **Ingestion** involves taking food into the mouth, chewing it, and swallowing it.

2. **Digestion** is the breakdown of food into smaller molecules. The food we eat consists mainly of big pieces and large molecules—far too large to pass through the wall of the digestive tract or into the cells of the body. During digestion, food is broken down into small molecules. Each reaction is regulated by a specific enzyme.

3. **Absorption** is the transfer of digested food through the wall of the intestine and into the circulatory system. The circulatory system transports the food molecules, or nutrients, to the liver, where many are removed and stored. Those remaining in the blood are transported to the cells of the body. Each cell uses nutrients for its metabolic activities.

4. **Elimination** removes undigested and unabsorbed food from the body.

THE WALL OF THE DIGESTIVE TRACT HAS FOUR LAYERS

From esophagus to anus, the wall of the digestive tract consists of four layers (Fig. 15–2):

1. The **mucosa** (mew-koe'-sah) is the lining of the digestive tract. It consists of epithelial tissue resting upon a layer of loose connective tissue. In the esophagus and anal canal the epithelium is specialized for protection of underlying tissues. The epithelium in other regions of the digestive tract is specialized for secretion of mucus or digestive juices or for absorption of nutrients. In the stomach and small intestine the mucosa is thrown into folds, which greatly increase its surface for digestion and absorption.

2. Beneath the mucosa lies a layer of connective tissue (**submucosa**) rich in blood vessels and nerves.

3. The third layer consists of muscle. This muscle contracts in a wavelike motion called **peristalsis** (per"-ih-**stal**'-sis) that pushes food along through the digestive tract.

4. The outer coat of the wall of the digestive tract consists of connective tissue. Below the level of the diaphragm this layer is called the **visceral peritoneum** (per"-ih-toe-**nee**'-um). By various folds it connects to the **parietal peritoneum,** the sheet of connective tissue that lines the walls of the abdominal and pelvic cavities. Between the visceral and the parietal peritoneum is a potential space, the **peritoneal cavity.** Inflammation of the peritoneum, called peritonitis, can have very serious consequences, be-

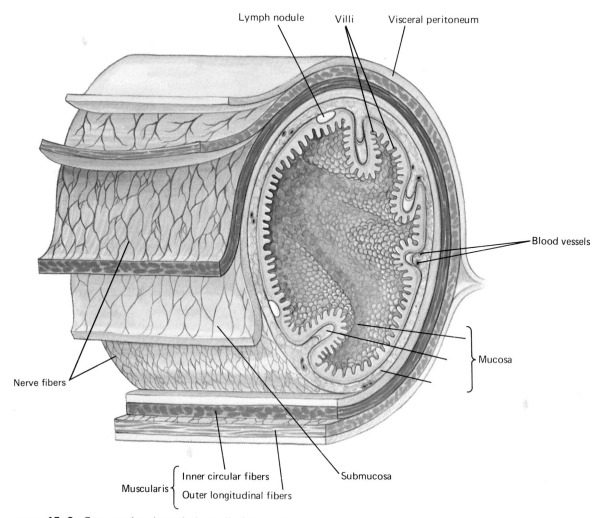

Lymph nodule   Villi   Visceral peritoneum

Blood vessels

Mucosa

Nerve fibers

Muscularis { Inner circular fibers / Outer longitudinal fibers }

Submucosa

FIGURE 15–2 Cross section through the wall of the small intestine illustrating the four layers: mucosa, submucosa, muscle layers, and visceral peritoneum.

cause infection can easily spread to all the adjoining organs.

FOLDS OF THE PERITONEUM SUPPORT THE DIGESTIVE ORGANS

A large double fold of peritoneal tissue, the **mesentery** (**mes′**-en-ter-ee), extends from the parietal peritoneum and attaches to the small intestine (Figs. 15–2 and 15–3). The mesentery is shaped somewhat like a fan. The handle part of the fan anchors the intestine to the posterior abdominal wall. Blood and lymph vessels, and nerves that supply the intestine, are present between the folds of the mesentery.

Other important folds of peritoneum are the greater omentum, the lesser omentum, and the meso-

colon (Fig. 15–3). The **greater omentum** (o-**men′**-tum), also known as the "fatty apron," is a large double fold of peritoneum attached to the stomach and intestine. It hangs down over the intestine like an apron. The greater omentum contains large deposits of fat. It also contains lymph nodes that help prevent spread of infection to the peritoneum. The **lesser omentum** suspends the stomach and duodenum from the liver. The **mesocolon** is a fold of peritoneum that attaches the colon to the posterior abdominal wall.

THE MOUTH INGESTS FOOD

The mouth, or **oral cavity**, ingests food and prepares it for digestion. The flexible, muscular tongue on the floor of the mouth pushes the food about to

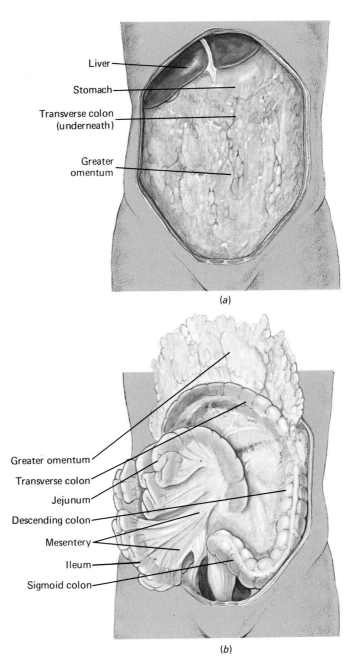

Liver
Stomach
Transverse colon (underneath)
Greater omentum

(a)

Greater omentum
Transverse colon
Jejunum
Descending colon
Mesentery
Ileum
Sigmoid colon

(b)

FIGURE **15–3** Folds of the peritoneum anchor the digestive organs to the abdominal wall and to one another. *(a)* Frontal view of abdomen. The greater omentum hangs down over the intestine like an apron. *(b)* Frontal view of abdomen. The greater omentum and transverse colon have been lifted to show the mesentery.

aid in chewing and swallowing. Taste buds on the tongue enable us to taste foods as sweet, sour, salty, or bitter (see Chap. 8). The tongue is also important in speech.

THE TEETH BREAK DOWN FOOD

The teeth are rooted in sockets (alveoli) of the alveolar processes, bony ridges that project from the mandible and maxilla. Each tooth consists of a **crown,** the part above the gum, and one or more **roots,** the portion beneath the gum line (Fig. 15–4). A section through a tooth, or an x-ray film of it, shows

that each tooth is composed mainly of **dentin,** a calcified connective tissue that imparts shape and rigidity to the tooth. In the crown region the dentin is protected by a tough covering of **enamel.** The bone-like enamel is the hardest substance in the body, comparable in hardness to quartz. Enamel helps protect the tooth against the wear and tear of chewing and against chemical substances that might dissolve the dentin.

The dentin encloses a **pulp cavity** filled with pulp, an extremely sensitive connective tissue containing blood vessels and nerves. Narrow extensions of the pulp cavity, called **root canals,** pass through the roots of the tooth. Each root canal has an opening

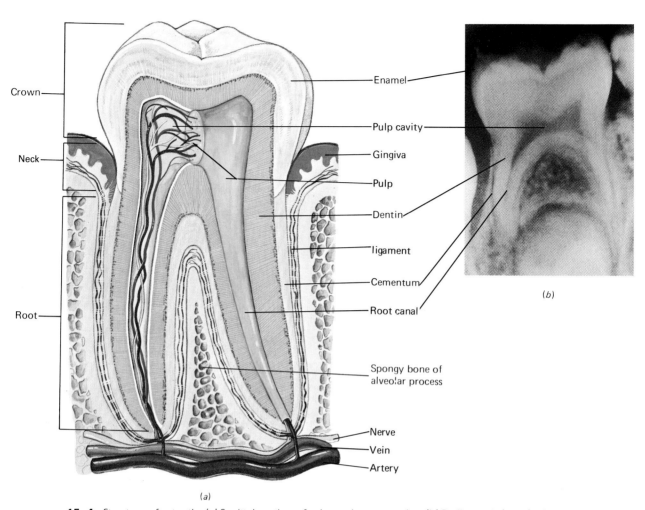

Crown

Neck

Root

Enamel

Pulp cavity

Gingiva

Pulp

Dentin

ligament

Cementum

Root canal

Spongy bone of
alveolar process

Nerve

Vein

Artery

(a)

(b)

FIGURE 15—4 *Structure of a tooth. (a) Sagittal section of a lower human molar. (b) Radiograph (x-ray) of a healthy tooth.*

at its base through which nerves and blood and lymph vessels enter the tooth.

By about 6 months of age, the first of the temporary **deciduous** (dee-**sid'**-u-us) **teeth,** also called baby teeth, show their crowns above the gums. After that, new teeth erupt every few weeks, so that a full set of 20 deciduous teeth is present by the time a child is about 2 years old (Fig. 15—5). These teeth are fairly small, and between the ages of 6 and 13 years they are slowly shed and replaced by larger, permanent teeth.

The adult set of teeth consists of a maximum of 32 teeth (Fig. 15—5). We can describe the number of each type of tooth in one quadrant of the mouth. Closest to the midline are 2 **incisors** (a total of 8, 4 on top and 4 on the bottom). The incisors are specialized for biting and cutting. Lateral to them are the **canines,** one in each quadrant. In humans the canines assist the incisors in biting, but in many mammals they are enlarged and are adapted for stabbing and tearing prey. The more posterior teeth are modified for grinding and crushing. Each quadrant has 2

premolars and 3 **molars.** The third molars are the wisdom teeth, which often appear after age 18. In many persons, the jaw is too small to accommodate the wisdom teeth. They may remain embedded (impacted). Sometimes they cause pain and must be surgically removed.

THE SALIVARY GLANDS PRODUCE SALIVA

The three main pairs of salivary glands are as follows:

1. The **parotid** (pah-**rot'**-id) **glands** are the largest salivary glands. They are located in the tissue inferior and anterior to the ears. When one has mumps, the parotid glands become infected and swell.

2. The **submandibular** (sub-man-**dib'**-u-lar) **glands** lie below the jaw.

3. The **sublingual** (sub-**ling'**-gwal) **glands** are under the tongue.

Saliva consists of two main components: (1) a

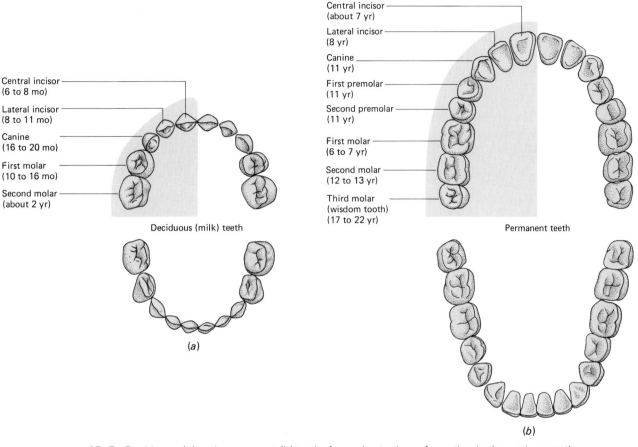

Central incisor
(about 7 yr)

Lateral incisor
(8 yr)

Canine
(11 yr)

First premolar
(11 yr)

Second premolar
(11 yr)

First molar
(6 to 7 yr)

Second molar
(12 to 13 yr)

Third molar
(wisdom tooth)
(17 to 22 yr)

Central incisor
(6 to 8 mo)

Lateral incisor
(8 to 11 mo)

Canine
(16 to 20 mo)

First molar
(10 to 16 mo)

Second molar
(about 2 yr)

Deciduous (milk) teeth

Permanent teeth

(a)

(b)

FIGURE 15–5 Deciduous (a) and permanent (b) teeth. Approximate time of eruption is shown in parentheses.

thin, watery secretion containing the digestive enzyme **salivary amylase;** and (2) a mucous secretion that lubricates the mouth. Salts, antibodies, and other substances that kill bacteria are also found in the saliva.

Saliva lubricates the tissues of the mouth and pharynx, making it easier to talk as well as chew. By moistening food, saliva helps the tongue convert the mouthful of food to a semisolid mass called a **bolus** (**bow′**-lus) that can be swallowed easily.

THE PHARYNX IS IMPORTANT IN SWALLOWING

After a bite of food has been chewed, moistened, tasted, and formed into a bolus, it must be swallowed. Swallowing moves the bolus from the mouth through the pharynx and down the esophagus. The **pharynx,** or throat, is a muscular tube about 12 centimeters (cm) (4.8 inches) long that serves as the hallway of both the respiratory and digestive systems. As noted in Chapter 14, the three regions of the pharynx are the oropharynx, posterior to the mouth; the naso-

pharynx, posterior to the nose; and the laryngopharynx, which opens into the larynx and esophagus.

The oropharynx and nasopharynx are partitioned by the **soft palate,** which hangs down like a curtain between them. The muscular soft palate is a posterior extension of the bony **hard palate,** which serves as the roof of the mouth. A small mass of tissue, the **uvula,** hangs from the lower border of the soft palate. During swallowing, the bolus is forced into the oropharynx by the tongue. Reflex contractions of muscles in the wall of the pharynx propel the food into the esophagus. During swallowing, the opening to the larynx is closed by a small flap of tissue, the **epiglottis.** This flap prevents food from straying into the respiratory passageways.

THE ESOPHAGUS CONDUCTS FOOD TO THE STOMACH

The esophagus extends from the pharynx through the thoracic cavity. It passes through the diaphragm and empties into the stomach. The bolus is swept through the pharynx and into the esophagus by a wave of muscle contraction—a peristaltic contraction. As the bolus enters the esophagus, the peristaltic wave continues pushing the food down toward the stomach. Two layers of muscle in the wall of the esophagus work together in pushing the bolus downward.

At the lower end of the esophagus is a sphincter muscle (cardiac sphincter), a circular muscle that constricts the tube so that the entrance to the stomach is generally closed. This prevents the highly acidic gastric juice from splashing up into the esophagus. Occasionally, gastric juice does spurt up into the esophagus, and the wall of the esophagus becomes irritated. The resulting spasms cause "heartburn" (probably so named because the pain seems to occur in the general region of the heart).

THE STOMACH DIGESTS FOOD

When a peristaltic wave passes down the esophagus, the cardiac sphincter relaxes, permitting the bolus to enter the **stomach.** The stomach is a large, muscular organ that, when empty, is shaped like the letter J (Fig. 15–6). When the stomach is empty, its lining has many folds, called **rugae** (**roo'**-jee). As food fills the stomach, the rugae gradually smooth out, increasing the stomach's capacity to more than a quart. As it fills, the stomach begins to look like a football.

Contractions of the stomach mix the food thoroughly. The stomach mashes and churns food and also moves it along by peristalsis. The stomach is lined with simple epithelium that secretes large amounts of mucus. Millions of gastric glands in the wall of the stomach secrete hydrochloric acid and enzymes. The hydrochloric acid kills bacteria and breaks down the connective tissues in meat. Even after mixing with mucus and food, the stomach is very acidic. The main enzyme secreted in the gastric juice is pepsin, which begins the digestion of proteins. Small amounts of water, salts, and fat-soluble substances such as alcohol are absorbed through the stomach mucosa.

As food is digested over a 3- to 4-hour period, it is converted into a soupy mixture called **chyme** (**kime**). The exit of the stomach is guarded by the **pyloric sphincter** (pie-**lor'**-ik), a strong ring of muscle. When this sphincter relaxes, chyme passes into the small intestine.

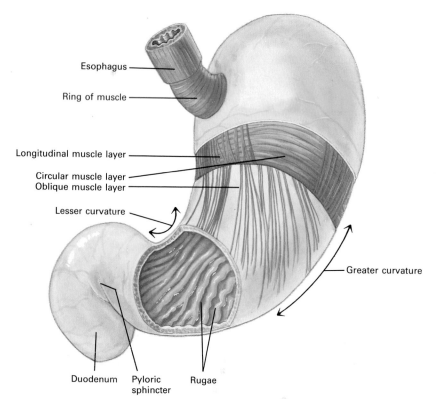

Esophagus

Ring of muscle

Longitudinal muscle layer

Circular muscle layer
Oblique muscle layer

Lesser curvature

Greater curvature

Duodenum   Pyloric   Rugae
            sphincter

FIGURE 15–6 Structure of the stomach. From the esophagus, food enters the stomach, where it is broken down mechanically. Protein digestion begins in the stomach.

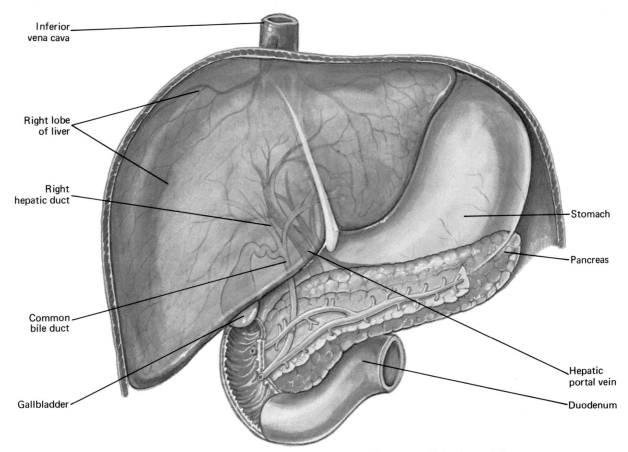

Inferior vena cava

Right lobe of liver

Right hepatic duct

Common bile duct

Gallbladder

Stomach

Pancreas

Hepatic portal vein

Duodenum

FIGURE 15–7 *Structure of the liver and pancreas. Note the gallbladder and ducts.*

MOST DIGESTION TAKES PLACE IN THE SMALL INTESTINE

The small intestine is a long, coiled tube more than 5 to 6 m (about 17 feet) long by 4 cm (1.5 inches) in diameter. The first 22 cm or so of the small intestine make up the **duodenum** (do″-o-**dee′**-num), which is curved like the letter C. As the tube turns downward, it is called the **jejunum** (je-**joo′**-num), which extends for about 2 m (6 feet) before becoming the **ileum** (**il′**-e-um) (Fig. 15–1).

The lining of the small intestine has millions of tiny fingerlike projections, called **villi** (**vill′**-ee) (Fig. 15–6). The villi increase the surface area of the small intestine, providing a greater surface for digestion and absorption of nutrients. If the lining of the intestine could be completely unfolded and spread out, its surface would approximate the size of a tennis court!

Most digestion takes place in the duodenum rather than in the stomach. The liver and pancreas release digestive juices into the duodenum that act upon the chyme. Then enzymes produced by the epithelial cells lining the duodenum complete the job of breaking down food molecules so they can be absorbed.

THE PANCREAS SECRETES ENZYMES

The pancreas is a large, long gland that lies in the abdomen posterior to the stomach (Fig. 15–7). The pancreas is both an exocrine and an endocrine gland. Its exocrine portion secretes pancreatic juice, which contains a number of digestive enzymes. The pancreatic duct from the pancreas joins the duct coming from the liver, forming a single duct that passes into the duodenum. An accessory pancreatic duct is often present as well.

If the pancreas becomes damaged, its ducts may become blocked. When this happens, the pancreas may be digested by its own enzymes. This condition, called acute pancreatitis, is frequently associated with alcoholism.

THE LIVER SECRETES BILE

The liver is the largest and one of the most complex organs in the body (Fig. 15–7). A single liver cell can carry on more than 500 separate metabolic activities. The right lobe of the liver is larger than the left lobe and has three main parts.

Oxygen-rich blood is brought to the liver by the hepatic arteries. However, the liver also receives blood from the hepatic portal vein. Recall that the hepatic portal vein delivers nutrients just absorbed from the intestine.

The liver:

1. Secretes **bile,** which is important in the digestion of fats. **Bilirubin** (bil″-ee-**roo**′-bin), a pigment released when red blood cells are broken down, is excreted in the bile.

2. Removes nutrients from the blood.

3. Converts glucose to glycogen and stores it; then when glucose is needed, it breaks down the glycogen and releases glucose into the blood.

4. Stores iron and certain vitamins.

5. Converts excess amino acids to fatty acids and urea.

6. Performs many important functions in the metabolism of proteins, fats, and carbohydrates.

7. Manufactures many of the plasma proteins found in the blood.

8. Detoxifies many drugs and poisons that enter the body.

9. Phagocytizes bacteria and worn-out red blood cells.

Bile is stored and concentrated in the pear-shaped **gallbladder** (see Fig. 15–5). A hormone (cholecystokinin, or CCK) is secreted by the intestinal mucosa, mainly when fat is present in the duodenum. This hormone stimulates the gallbladder to contract, releasing bile into the cystic duct. The cystic duct from the gallbladder joins the hepatic duct from the liver to form the **common bile duct,** which (together with the duct from the pancreas) opens into the duodenum.

DIGESTION OCCURS AS FOOD MOVES THROUGH THE DIGESTIVE TRACT

Secretion of digestive juices is stimulated by hormones and by chyme. For example, the hormone gastrin, which is released by the stomach mucosa, stimulates the gastric glands to secrete. The intestinal glands are stimulated to release their fluid mainly by local reflexes that occur when the small intestine is stretched by chyme.

GLUCOSE IS THE MAIN PRODUCT OF CARBOHYDRATE DIGESTION

Large carbohydrates such as starch and glycogen consist of long chains of glucose molecules. Starch digestion begins in the mouth. There the enzyme salivary amylase begins breaking down some of the long starch molecules to smaller compounds and then to the sugar maltose.

$$\text{Starch} \xrightarrow{\text{salivary amylase}} \begin{array}{l}\text{smaller}\\\text{carbohydrates}\\\text{and maltose}\end{array}$$

In the duodenum, pancreatic amylase (in the pancreatic juice) splits the remaining starch molecules to maltose.

$$\text{Carbohydrates} \xrightarrow{\text{pancreatic amylase}} \text{maltose}$$

Then the enzyme maltase (released by the epithelial cells lining the duodenum) breaks down each maltose molecule to two molecules of glucose. Sucrose, the sugar we use in our coffee, and lactose (milk sugar) are also broken down to simple sugars in the duodenum.

$$\text{Maltose} \xrightarrow{\text{maltase}} \text{glucose} + \text{glucose}$$

Many plant foods are rich in starch. However, this starch is not readily available to us because it is encased within the tough cellulose cell walls of plant cells. We do not have enzymes that digest cellulose, so much of this starch passes through the digestive tract without being digested. Cooking destroys the cellulose walls so that the starch can be more easily reached by amylase and other enzymes.

Glucose is the major product of carbohydrate digestion. Carbohydrate digestion is summarized in Table 15–1.

BILE DIGESTS FAT

Digestion of fat takes place mainly in the duodenum. Bile emulsifies (mechanically breaks down) fat by a detergent action that breaks large fat droplets down into smaller droplets.

$$\text{Large fat droplets} \xrightarrow{\text{bile}} \begin{array}{l}\text{small fat droplets}\\\text{containing}\\\text{triglycerides}\end{array}$$

These droplets are acted on by an enzyme in the pancreatic juice called **lipase.** Pancreatic lipase breaks

TABLE 15–1

Summary of carbohydrate digestion

PLACE OF ACTION	SOURCE OF ENZYME	DIGESTIVE PROCESS
Mouth	Salivary glands	Starch $\xrightarrow{\text{salivary amylase}}$ smaller carbohydrates + maltose
Small intestine	Pancreas	Starch and smaller carbohydrates $\xrightarrow{\text{pancreatic amylase}}$ maltose
	Intestine	Maltose $\xrightarrow{\text{maltase}}$ glucose + glucose
		Sucrose (table sugar) $\xrightarrow{\text{sucrase}}$ glucose + fructose
		Lactose (milk sugar) $\xrightarrow{\text{lactase}}$ glucose + galactose

TABLE 15–2

Summary of lipid digestion

PLACE OF ACTION	SOURCE OF DIGESTIVE SUBSTANCE	DIGESTIVE PROCESS
Small intestine	Liver	Drop of fat $\xrightarrow{\text{bile}}$ small fat droplets containing triglycerides 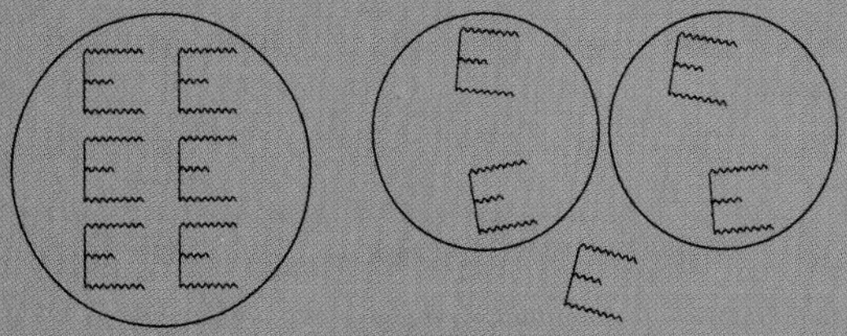
	Pancreas	Fat (triglycerides) $\xrightarrow{\text{lipase}}$ fatty acids + glycerol 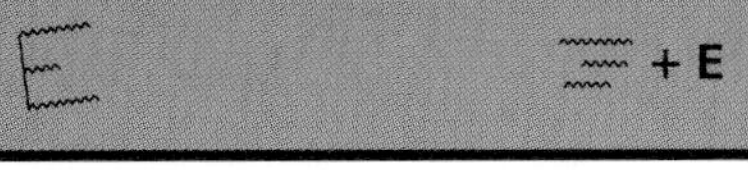

⌐ = triglyceride;   **E** = glycerol;   ⌀⌀⌀ = fatty acid.

down the fat molecules (triglycerides) to free fatty acids and glycerol.

$$\text{Triglycerides} \xrightarrow{\text{lipase}} \text{fatty acids and glycerol}$$

Fat digestion is summarized in Table 15–2.

PROTEINS ARE DIGESTED TO AMINO ACIDS

Proteins consist of smaller molecules called amino acids. These amino acid subunits are linked together by chemical bonds called peptide bonds. The goal of protein digestion is to break the peptide bonds and release free amino acids.

Protein digestion begins in the stomach with the enzyme pepsin. Pepsin breaks down most proteins to smaller molecules (called polypeptides). In the duodenum, the enzyme **trypsin** in the pancreatic juice further breaks down these molecules.

$$\text{Proteins} \xrightarrow{\text{pepsin, trypsin}} \text{polypeptides}$$

Then the protein fragments are digested by enzymes called **peptidases,** secreted by epithelial cells lining the intestine. Peptidases split some of these peptides into free amino acids.

$$\text{Polypeptides} \xrightarrow{\text{peptidases}} \text{free amino acids}$$

The products of protein digestion are free amino acids. Protein digestion is summarized in Table 15–3.

THE INTESTINAL VILLI ABSORB NUTRIENTS

After food has been digested, the nutrients are absorbed by the intestinal villi. The structure of a villus is illustrated in Figure 15–8. Within each villus is a network of capillaries that branches from an arteriole and empties into a venule. A central lymph vessel, called a **lacteal** (lak′-tee-al), is also present.

To reach the blood or lymph, a nutrient must pass through the single layer of epithelial cells lining the villus and through the single layer of cells forming the wall of the capillary or the lacteal. Amino

---

TABLE 15–3
Summary of protein digestion

PLACE OF ACTION	SOURCE OF ENZYME	DIGESTIVE PROCESS	
Stomach	Stomach (gastric glands)	Protein $\xrightarrow{\text{pepsin}}$ polypeptides	
		A–A–A–A–A–A	A–A–A–A–A–A
		A–A–A–A–A–A	A–A–A–A–A–A
		A–A–A–A–A–A	A–A–A–A–A–A
Small intestine	Pancreas	Protein, polypeptides $\xrightarrow{\text{trypsin}}$ polypeptides and smaller protein fragments	
		A–A–A–A–A–A	A–A–A–A–A–A
		A–A–A–A–A–A	A–A–A A–A–A
		A–A–A–A–A–A	A–A A–A A–A
	Small intestine	Polypeptides and smaller protein fragments $\xrightarrow{\text{peptidases}}$ free amino acids	
		A–A–A–A–A–A	A A A
		A–A–A	A A A A
		A–A A–A	A
			A A A

A represents amino acids.

Villi

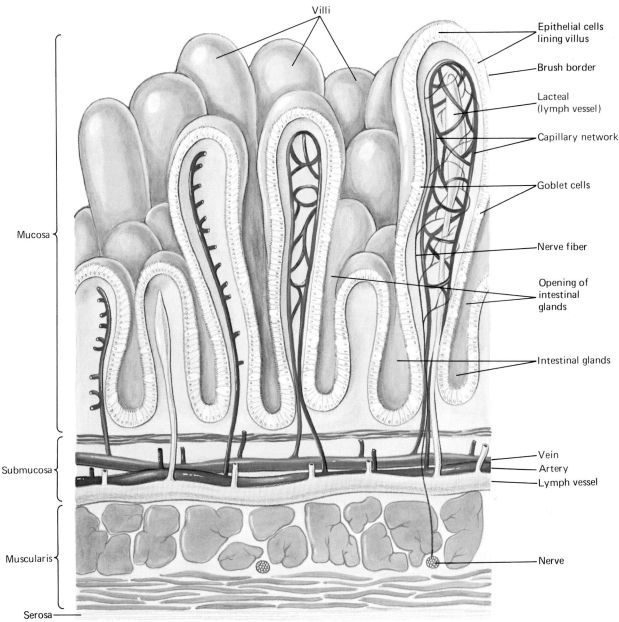

Epithelial cells lining villus

Brush border

Lacteal (lymph vessel)

Capillary network

Goblet cells

Nerve fiber

Opening of intestinal glands

Intestinal glands

Mucosa

Submucosa

Vein

Artery

Lymph vessel

Muscularis

Nerve

Serosa

FIGURE 15–8 *The surface of the small intestine is studded with villi and tiny openings into the intestinal glands. Here some of the villi have been opened to show the blood and lymph vessels within.*

acids and simple sugars are absorbed into the blood. They are transported directly to the liver by the hepatic portal vein. Fatty acids are absorbed into the lacteals. They circulate through the lymph system before entering the blood.

THE LARGE INTESTINE ELIMINATES WASTES

After the chyme has moved through the stomach and small intestine, it consists mainly of water and indigestible wastes such as cellulose. The small intestine is normally shut off from the large intestine by a sphincter called the **ileocecal** (il″-ee-o-**see′**-kal) **valve.** When a peristaltic contraction brings chyme toward it, the ileocecal valve opens, allowing the chyme to enter the large intestine.

One to 3 days or even longer may be required for the slow journey through the large intestine. Bacteria that live in the large intestine nourish themselves on the last remnants of the meal. In exchange, these bacteria produce certain vitamins that we can absorb and use. As the chyme slowly passes through the large intestine, water and sodium are absorbed from it, and what remains becomes feces.

Although only about a little more than 1.5 m (about 5 feet) long, the large intestine is called "large" because its diameter is much greater than the diameter of the small intestine. The small intestine joins the large intestine about 7 cm above the end of the large intestine. This creates a pouch called the **cecum (see′-kum)** (Fig. 15–1). The **vermiform appendix,** a worm-shaped blind tube, hangs down from the end of the cecum. The function of the appendix is unknown, but it is rich in lymph tissue. Inflammation of the appendix, known as appendicitis, can lead to peritonitis and other complications if not diagnosed and treated promptly.

From the cecum to the rectum the large intestine is known as the **colon (koe′-lon)**. The **ascending colon** extends from the cecum straight up to the lower border of the liver. As it turns horizontally, it becomes the **transverse colon.** The transverse colon extends across the abdomen below the liver and stomach. On the left side of the abdomen the descending colon turns downward. It forms the S-shaped **sigmoid colon,** which empties into the short **rectum.** The rectum is the last 12 cm or so of the digestive tract. It ends in the anus, the opening for elimination of feces. The last 4 cm of the rectum are called the **anal canal.**

The mucosa of the large intestine lacks villi and produces no digestive enzymes. Its surface epithelium consists of cells specialized for absorption and goblet cells that secrete mucus. The functions of the large intestine may be summarized as follows:

1. Absorption of sodium and water.

2. Incubation of bacteria. Because the movements of the large intestine are quite sluggish, bacteria have time to grow and reproduce there. These bacteria produce vitamin K and some of the B-complex vitamins.

3. Elimination of wastes. Undigested and unabsorbed food as well as bile pigments are eliminated from the body by the large intestine in the form of feces. The bile pigments give feces their characteristic brown color.

After meals, contractions of the large intestine increase. This stimulates the desire to **defecate** (expel feces). Two sphincters, an internal anal sphincter and an external anal sphincter in the wall of the anal canal, guard the anal opening. When the rectum fills with feces, the internal sphincter relaxes, but the external sphincter remains contracted until relaxed voluntarily. Thus, defecation is a reflex action that can be voluntarily inhibited by keeping the external sphincter contracted.

Cancer of the colon is one of the most common causes of cancer death in the United States. Research indicates that this type of cancer may be related to diet, because the disease is more common in those whose diets are very low in fiber.

A BALANCED DIET IS NECESSARY TO MAINTAIN HEALTH

Nutrients required for good health are provided by a balanced diet consisting of water, minerals, vitamins, carbohydrates, lipids, and proteins. Carbohydrates, lipids, and proteins can all be used as energy sources.

1. **Water**—An average adult requires a daily intake of about 2.4 liters (2.5 quarts) of water. About two thirds of this amount is ingested in the form of water or other fluids. The rest comes from solid foods, which actually contain quite a bit of water. For example, a raw apple is actually about 85% water by weight. Water is one of the main components of the body and is used by the body to transport materials. All the chemical reactions in the body take place in a watery medium.

2. **Minerals** are inorganic nutrients ingested in the form of salts dissolved in food and water. Some required minerals and their functions are listed in Table 15–4.

3. **Vitamins** are organic compounds required for certain reactions to take place. Many vitamins serve as coenzymes, compounds that work with enzymes to regulate chemical reactions. Table 15–5 lists essential vitamins and their functions.

4. **Carbohydrates** are ingested mainly as starch or cellulose. Sugars account for about 25% of the carbohydrates we ingest. Carbohydrates are digested to glucose or other simple sugars that can be absorbed into the blood. The cells use glucose as an energy source. Excess glucose can be stored in the liver and muscles as glycogen.

5. **Lipids**—Most of the lipids we ingest are fats (mainly triglycerides). Another important lipid is cholesterol. Lipids are used as fuel and also to make cell membranes. Diets high in triglycerides and cholesterol have been associated with heart disease.

6. **Proteins** are digested into their component amino acids. These smaller molecules are then assembled to make the types of proteins the body needs. Proteins are essential building blocks of cells and many serve as enzymes. Other proteins are used to make hemoglobin and muscle proteins.

TABLE 15–4

Some important minerals and their functions

MINERAL	FUNCTIONS	SOURCES
Calcium	Component of bones and teeth; essential for normal blood clotting; needed for normal muscle and nerve functions	Dairy products, green leafy vegetables
Phosphorus	As calcium phosphate, an important structural component of bone; essential in energy transfer and storage (component of ATP) and in many other metabolic processes; component of DNA and RNA; performs more functions than any other mineral; antacids can impair absorption	Beef, dairy products
Sulfur	Component of many proteins (e.g., insulin)	High-protein foods, such as meat, fish, legumes, nuts
Potassium	Influences muscle contraction and nerve excitability	Present in fruits and many other foods
Sodium	Important in fluid balance; essential for conduction of nerve impulses	Present in most foods; sodium chloride (table salt) added as seasoning; too much is ingested in average American diet; excessive amounts may lead to high blood pressure
Chlorine	Important in fluid balance and acid-base balance	Most foods; ingested as sodium chloride
Copper	Component of many enzymes; essential for hemoglobin synthesis	Liver, eggs, fish, whole wheat flour, beans
Iodine	Component of thyroid hormones (hormones that stimulate metabolic rate)	Seafoods, iodized salt, vegetables grown in iodine-rich soil; deficiency results in goiter (abnormal enlargement of thyroid gland)
Cobalt	As component of vitamin B_{12}, essential for red blood cell production	Meat, dairy products; strict vegetarians may become deficient in this mineral
Manganese	Necessary to activate an enzyme essential for urea formation; activates many other enzymes	Whole-grain cereals, egg yolks, green vegetables; poorly absorbed from intestine
Magnesium	Appropriate balance between magnesium and calcium ions needed for normal muscle and nerve function; component of many coenzymes	Present in many foods
Iron	Component of hemoglobin, important respiratory enzymes, and other enzymes essential to oxygen transport and cellular respiration	Meat (especially liver), nuts, egg yolk, legumes; mineral most likely to be deficient in diet; deficiency results in anemia
Fluorine	Component of bones and teeth; makes teeth resistant to decay	Where it does not occur naturally, fluorine may be added to municipal water supplies (fluoridation); excess causes tooth mottling
Zinc	Component of at least 70 enzymes; component of some peptidases, and thus important in protein digestion; may be important in wound healing	Present in many foods

TABLE 15–5

The vitamins

VITAMINS (U.S. RDA*)	ACTIONS	EFFECT OF DEFICIENCY	SOURCES
Fat-Soluble			
A (5000 IU†)	Essential for normal vision; essential for normal growth and health of epithelial tissue; promotes normal growth of bones and teeth; excessive amounts harmful	Failure of growth; night blindness; epithelium subject to infection; scaly skin	Liver, fish-liver oils, eggs, yellow and green vegetables
D (400 IU)	Promotes calcium absorption from digestive tract; essential to normal growth and maintenance of bone; excessive amounts harmful	Bone deformities; rickets in children; osteomalacia in adults	Liver, fish-liver oils, egg yolk, fortified milk, butter, margarine
E (30 IU)	Inhibits oxidation of unsaturated fatty acids that help form cell membranes; precise biochemical role not known	Increased catabolism of unsaturated fatty acids, so not enough are available for maintenance of cell membranes and other membranous organelles; prevents normal growth	Oils made from cereals, seeds, liver, eggs, fish
K (probably about 1 mg)	Essential for blood clotting	Prolonged blood-clotting time	Normally supplied by intestinal bacteria; green leafy vegetables
Water-Soluble			
C (ascorbic acid) (60 mg)	Needed for synthesis of collagen and other intercellular substances; aids formation of bone matrix and tooth dentin; may help body withstand injury from burns and bacterial toxins	Scurvy (wounds heal slowly and scars become weak and split open; capillaries become fragile; bone does not grow or heal properly)	Citrus fruits, strawberries, tomatoes
B complex vitamins			
Thiamine (B₁) (1.5 mg)	Required as coenzyme in many enzyme systems; important in carbohydrate and amino acid metabolism	Beriberi (weakened heart muscle, enlarged right side of heart, nervous system and digestive tract disorders)	Liver, yeast, cereals, meat, green leafy vegetables
Riboflavin (B₂) (1.7 mg)	Used to make coenzymes essential in cellular respiration	Dermatitis, inflammation of mouth and cracking at corners; mental depression	Liver, cheese, milk, eggs, green leafy vegetables
Niacin (nicotinic acid) (20 mg)	Component of important coenzymes essential to cellular respiration	Pellagra (dermatitis, diarrhea, mental symptoms, muscular weakness, fatigue)	Liver, meat, fish, cereals, legumes, whole-grain and enriched breads
Pyridoxine (B₆) (2 mg)	Needed for amino acid synthesis and protein metabolism	Dermatitis, digestive tract disturbances, convulsions	Liver, meat, cereals, legumes
Pantothenic acid (10 mg)	Important in cellular metabolism	Deficiency extremely rare	Widespread in foods
Folic acid (0.4 mg)	Required for nucleic acid synthesis and for maturation of red blood cells	A type of anemia	Produced by intestinal bacteria; liver, cereals, dark-green leafy vegetables

Table continued on opposite page

TABLE 15–5 *Continued*

The vitamins

VITAMINS (U.S. RDA*)	ACTIONS	EFFECT OF DEFICIENCY	SOURCES
Water-Soluble			
Biotin (0.3 mg)	Needed for fat metabolism	Deficiency unknown	Produced by intestinal bacteria; liver, chocolate, egg yolk
B₁₂ (6 mg)	Important in nucleic acid metabolism	Pernicious anemia	Liver, meat, fish

* RDA, the recommended dietary allowance, established by the Food and Nutrition Board of the National Research Council, to maintain good nutrition for healthy persons.

† International Unit, the amount that produces a specific biological effect and is internationally accepted as a measure of the activity of the substance.

SUMMARY

I. In sequence, a bite of food passes through the mouth, pharynx, esophagus, stomach, small intestine (duodenum, jejunum, ileum), large intestine (cecum, colon, rectum), and unabsorbed food passes out through the anus.

II. The digestive system functions in the ingestion, digestion, and absorption of nutrients. Food that is not absorbed is eliminated as feces by the process of defecation.

III. The lining of the digestive tract is its mucosa; beneath that is a layer of connective tissue (submucosa); then comes a layer of muscle; the outer coat of the wall is connective tissue. Below the diaphragm, the outer layer is called the visceral peritoneum.
   A. The parietal peritoneum lines the walls of the abdominal and pelvic cavities.
   B. The two peritoneums are connected by various folds including the greater omentum, the lesser omentum, and the mesocolon.

IV. Digestion begins in the mouth.
   A. The teeth grind and crush the food.
      1. The crown of a tooth is covered by tough enamel.
      2. Beneath the enamel is the dentin that makes up most of the tooth.
   B. Saliva contains salivary amylase, which begins the digestion of carbohydrates.

V. In swallowing, reflex movements propel the bolus through the pharynx and into the esophagus. Peristaltic contractions push the food through the esophagus to the stomach.

VI. Food is further processed in the large muscular stomach.
   A. The stomach churns the food, reducing it to chyme.
   B. Gastric glands in the stomach wall secrete gastric juice containing enzymes and hydrochloric acid.

VII. Most chemical digestion takes place within the duodenum.
   A. Bile from the liver and pancreatic juice from the pancreas are released into the duodenum.
   B. Cells of the small intestine produce enzymes needed for the final digestion of proteins, fats, and carbohydrates.

VIII. The pancreas releases enzymes that digest proteins, lipids, and carbohydrates.

IX. The liver performs many functions including secretion of bile.
   A. As blood circulates through the liver, nutrients are removed from it and stored.
   B. Bile produced in the liver is stored in the gallbladder.

X. Secretion of digestive juices is stimulated by the presence of chyme and by hormones. Food is slowly digested as it moves along through the digestive tract.
   A. Carbohydrate digestion begins in the mouth, where salivary amylase breaks down starches to smaller carbohydrates and maltose. In the duodenum pancreatic amylase continues the digestion of carbohydrates to maltose. Then specific enzymes in the duodenum break down maltose and other sugars to simple sugars, mainly glucose.

B. Lipid digestion begins in the duodenum when bile emulsifies large fat droplets. Then lipase from the pancreas digests the fat to fatty acids and glycerol.

C. Digestion of proteins begins in the stomach with the action of pepsin. In the duodenum enzymes from the pancreas continue to reduce proteins to polypeptides and then smaller protein fragments. Finally, peptidases produced by the epithelial cells lining the duodenum break down the peptides to free amino acids.

XI. Absorption takes place through the villi of the small intestine.

A. Glucose and amino acids are absorbed through the villi, enter the blood, and are transported to the liver.

B. Fatty acids are absorbed through the villi, pass into the lymph system, and eventually enter the blood.

XII. Indigestible material such as cellulose and unabsorbed nutrients pass into the large intestine.

A. Excess water and sodium are absorbed from the chyme as it passes through the large intestine.

B. Undigestible material, unabsorbed food, and bile pigments that have been excreted by the liver are eliminated by the large intestine in the form of feces.

XIII. A balanced diet includes water, minerals, vitamins, carbohydrates, lipids, and proteins.

POST TEST

1. The process of taking food into the mouth, chewing it, and swallowing it is called _____ .

2. _____ consists of breaking down food into molecules small enough to be absorbed.

3. The inner lining of the wall of the digestive tract is the _____ .

4. Inferior to the diaphragm, the outer layer of the wall of the digestive tract is called the _____ _____ .

5. Waves of contraction that push food along through the digestive tract are referred to as _____ .

6. The double fold of peritoneum that hangs down over the intestine like an apron is called the _____ _____ .

7. The normal maximum number of teeth in the adult mouth is _____ .

8. The portion of a tooth above the gum is the _____ ; the part below the gum is the _____ .

9. Each tooth is composed mainly of _____ , which in the crown region is covered by _____ .

10. The largest salivary glands are the _____ .

11. Salivary amylase begins the digestion of _____ .

12. The folds in the mucosa of the stomach are called _____ .

13. Two substances produced by the gastric glands are _____ and _____ .

14. The three divisions of the small intestine are the _____ , _____ , and _____ .

15. The _____ increase the surface area of the small intestine.

16. Bile is stored in the _____ .

17. The end products of protein digestion are _____
_____ .

18. Nutrients are absorbed by the intestinal _____ .

19. Chyme passing through the transverse colon would next enter the
_____ colon.

20. _____ are ingested mainly in the form of salts.

21. Label the diagram.

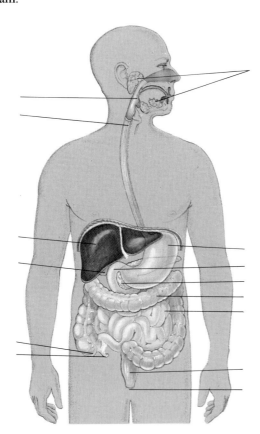

REVIEW QUESTIONS

1. Trace the journey of a bite of food containing mainly carbohydrate through the digestive tract, listing each structure through which it must pass and describing what happens to the carbohydrate in each place.

2. Trace the journey of a protein food through the digestive tract, describing how it changes along the way. Do the same for a lipid.

3. Describe (or label on a diagram) the structure of a tooth.

4. Why is it important to increase the surface area of the small intestine?

5. Draw a diagram of a villus and label its parts.

6. List the three types of accessory glands that release secretions into the digestive tract, and give the composition and functions of each type of secretion.

7. Describe four functions of the liver.

8. What are the functions of the large intestine?

9. What are the components of a balanced diet?

POST TEST ANSWERS

1. ingestion
2. Digestion
3. mucosa
4. visceral peritoneum
5. peristalsis
6. greater omentum
7. 32
8. crown; root
9. dentin; enamel
10. parotid
11. carbohydrates
12. rugae
13. hydrochloric acid; enzymes
14. duodenum; jejunum; ileum
15. villi
16. gallbladder
17. amino acids
18. villi
19. descending
20. Minerals
21. see Figure 15–1

Sixteen

THE URINARY SYSTEM

CHAPTER OUTLINE

I. The urinary system consists of the kidneys, urinary bladder, and ducts
II. The kidneys consist of a cortex and medulla
    A. The nephrons produce urine
    B. Urine is produced by filtration, reabsorption, and secretion
        1. Glomerular filtration is not a selective process
        2. Tubular reabsorption and secretion are selective processes
    C. Urine consists mainly of water
    D. Urine volume is regulated by ADH
    E. The kidneys help maintain homeostasis
III. Urine is transported by ducts and stored in the bladder
IV. Urination empties the bladder

LEARNING OBJECTIVES

After you have studied this chapter, you should be able to:
1. Identify the principal metabolic waste products and the organs that excrete them.
2. Label a diagram of the urinary system and give the function of each structure.
3. Describe a nephron and give the functions of the following structures: Bowman's capsule, glomerulus, renal tubule, collecting duct, afferent arteriole, efferent arteriole. (Be able to label a diagram of a nephron.)
4. Trace a drop of filtrate from glomerulus to urethra, listing in sequence each structure through which it passes.
5. Describe the process of urine formation and give the composition of urine.
6. Summarize the regulation of urine volume including the role of ADH.
7. Summarize the functions of the kidney in maintaining homeostasis.
8. Describe the process of urination.

As cells carry on metabolic activities, they produce waste products. If permitted to accumulate, these metabolic wastes could reach toxic concentrations and threaten homeostasis. To prevent this threat, metabolic wastes must be excreted. **Excretion** is the removal of metabolic wastes. Excretion is different from **elimination,** the discharge of undigested or unabsorbed food from the digestive tract.

The principal metabolic waste products are water, carbon dioxide, and wastes that contain nitrogen. Amino acids and nucleic acids contain nitrogen. When excess amino acids are broken down in the liver, the nitrogen-containing amino group is removed. The amino group is chemically converted to ammonia, which is then converted to urea. Somewhat similarly, uric acid is formed from the breakdown of nucleic acids. Urea and uric acid are trans-

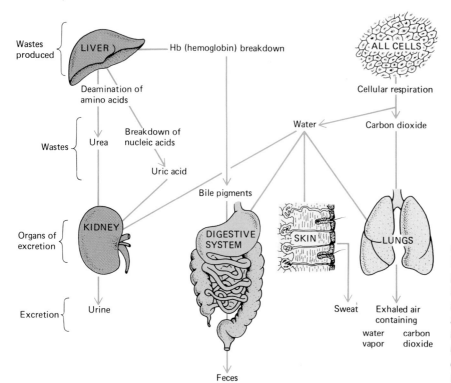

Deamination of
amino acids

Wastes
produced

LIVER

Hb (hemoglobin) breakdown

ALL CELLS

Cellular respiration

Water

Carbon dioxide

Wastes

Urea

Breakdown of
nucleic acids

Uric acid

Bile pigments

Organs of
excretion

KIDNEY

DIGESTIVE
SYSTEM

SKIN

LUNGS

Excretion

Urine

Sweat

Exhaled air
containing

water
vapor

carbon
dioxide

Feces

FIGURE 16–1 *The kidneys, lungs, skin, and digestive system all participate in the disposal of metabolic wastes. Wastes containing nitrogen are produced by the liver and transported to the kidneys. The kidneys excrete these wastes in the urine. All cells produce carbon dioxide and some water during cellular respiration.*

ported from the liver to the kidneys by the circulatory system.

Although metabolic wastes are excreted mainly by the urinary system, the skin, lungs, and digestive system also function in waste disposal (Fig. 16–1). Sweat glands in the skin excrete 5 to 10% of all metabolic wastes. Sweat contains the same substances—water, salts, and nitrogen wastes—as urine, but is much more dilute.

The lungs excrete carbon dioxide and water (in the form of water vapor). The liver excretes bile pigments, which are breakdown products of hemoglobin. These pigments pass into the intestine as part of the bile and then leave the body with the feces.

THE URINARY SYSTEM CONSISTS OF THE KIDNEYS, URINARY BLADDER, AND DUCTS

The principal organs of the urinary system are the paired **kidneys,** which remove wastes from the blood and produce the urine (Fig. 16–2). From the kidneys, urine is conducted to the **urinary bladder** by the paired **ureters** (u-ree′-ters). The single urinary bladder collects and stores urine. Eventually, urine is discharged from the body through the single **urethra** (u-ree′-thruh).

Kidney → ureter → urinary bladder → urethra

THE KIDNEYS CONSIST OF A CORTEX AND MEDULLA

The kidneys are located behind the peritoneum lining the abdominal cavity and so are described as **retroperitoneal** (re″-trow-per″-i-tow-nee′-al). They are located near the posterior body wall just below the diaphragm. The lower ribs protect the kidneys. Each kidney receives blood from a renal artery and is drained by a renal vein.

Each kidney looks something like a large, dark-red lima bean about the size of a fist. The ureters and blood vessels connect with the kidney at its **hilus** (hi′-lus), the notch on its medial border. Covering the kidney is a strong capsule of connective tissue, the **renal capsule.**

The kidney consists of an outer renal **cortex** and an inner renal **medulla** (Fig. 16–3). The medulla contains between 5 and 18 triangular structures called the **renal pyramids.** The tip of each pyramid is called a **renal papilla.** Each renal papilla extends into a small tube called a **calyx** (kay′-liks). Each pa-

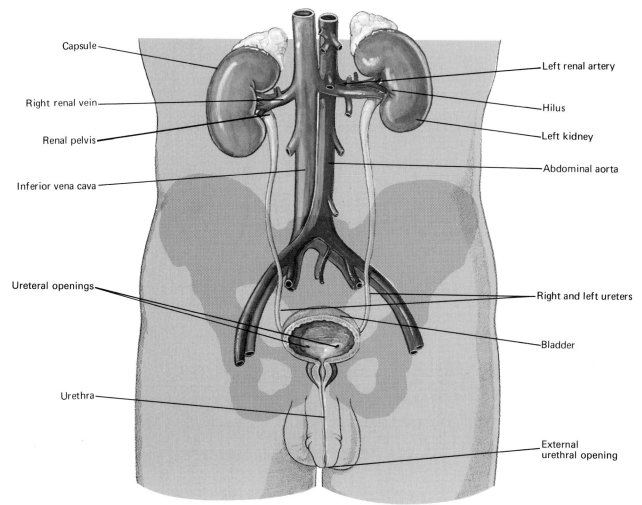

Capsule

Right renal vein

Renal pelvis

Inferior vena cava

Ureteral openings

Urethra

Left renal artery

Hilus

Left kidney

Abdominal aorta

Right and left ureters

Bladder

External urethral opening

FIGURE 16–2 The urinary system.

FIGURE 16–3 Structure of the kidney.

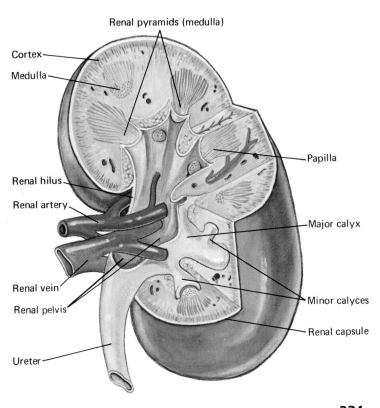

Renal pyramids (medulla)

Cortex

Medulla

Renal hilus

Renal artery

Renal vein

Renal pelvis

Ureter

Papilla

Major calyx

Minor calyces

Renal capsule

pilla has several pores, the openings of collecting ducts, through which urine passes into the calyx. The calyces join to form a large cavity, the **renal pelvis.** As urine is produced, it flows into the renal pelvis. From the renal pelvis, urine flows into the ureter. Urine flows through these structures in the following sequence:

> Collecting duct → renal papilla → calyx → renal pelvis → ureter

THE NEPHRONS PRODUCE URINE

Each kidney contains more than a million microscopic units called **nephrons** (**nef′**-rons). The neph-

rons filter the blood and produce urine. Each nephron consists of two main structures: (1) a **renal corpuscle;** and (2) a **renal tubule.** Blood is filtered in the renal corpuscle. Then the filtered fluid, called the **filtrate,** passes through the renal tubule. As the filtrate moves through the long tubule, substances needed by the body are returned to the blood. Waste products, excess water, and other substances not needed by the body pass into the collecting ducts as urine.

The renal corpuscle consists of a network of capillaries, the **glomerulus** (glow-**mare′**-you-lus), surrounded by a cuplike structure known as **Bowman's capsule** (Fig. 16–4). Blood flows into the glomerulus through a small **afferent arteriole** and leaves the glomerulus through an **efferent arteriole.** This arteriole conducts blood to a second set of capillaries,

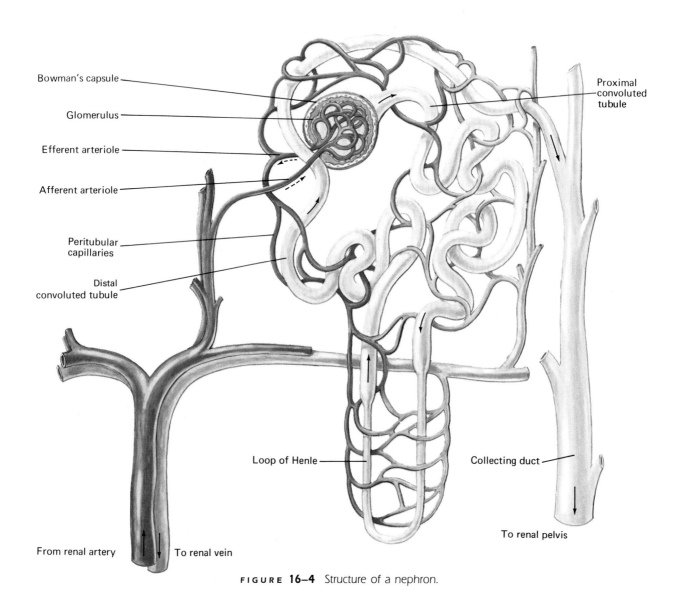

FIGURE 16–4 Structure of a nephron.

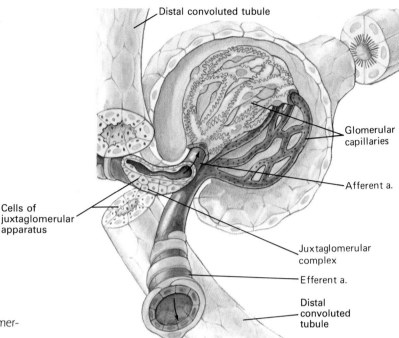

FIGURE **16–5** *Close-up view of the glomerulus and Bowman's capsule.*

the **peritubular capillaries** that surround the renal tubule.

> Afferent arteriole → capillaries of glomerulus → efferent arteriole → peritubular capillaries

Bowman's capsule has an opening in its bottom through which filtrate passes into the renal tubule. The first part of the renal tubule is the coiled **proximal convoluted tubule.** After passing through the proximal convoluted tubule, filtrate flows into the **loop of Henle (Hen′-lee)** and then into the **distal convoluted tubule.** Urine from the distal convoluted tubules of several nephrons drain into a **collecting duct.** Thus, the filtrate flows through the following structures:

> Bowman's capsule → proximal convoluted tubule → loop of Henle → distal convoluted tubule → collecting duct

Part of the distal convoluted tubule curves upward and contacts the afferent arteriole. The cells that make this contact form the **juxtaglomerular (jux-tah-glow-mer′-u-lar) apparatus** (Fig. 16–5). This structure secretes the enzyme renin. Renin acti-

vates a hormone (angiotensin) in the blood that helps regulate blood pressure.

The renal corpuscle, the proximal convoluted tubule, and the distal convoluted tubule of each nephron are located within the renal cortex. Loops of Henle dip down into the medulla.

URINE IS PRODUCED BY FILTRATION, REABSORPTION, AND SECRETION

Urine formation involves three processes: (1) glomerular filtration; (2) tubular reabsorption; and (3) tubular secretion (Fig. 16–6).

Glomerular Filtration Is Not a Selective Process

The first step in urine production is **glomerular filtration.** The afferent arteriole is larger in diameter than the efferent arteriole, so blood enters the glomerulus more rapidly than it can leave. This causes the blood pressure to be higher in the glomerular capillaries than in other capillaries. The high pressure forces plasma and substances dissolved in the plasma out of the capillaries and into Bowman's capsule.

The filtrate consists of blood plasma containing small, dissolved molecules. Glomerular filtration is not a selective process. Useful substances such as glucose, amino acids, and salts are present in the filtrate.

Blood cells and proteins are too large to pass through the walls of the capillary and capsule. When

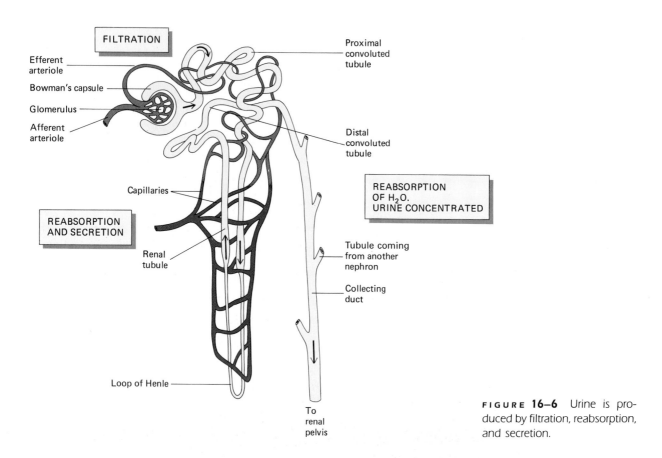

FILTRATION

Proximal
convoluted
tubule

Efferent
arteriole

Bowman's capsule

Glomerulus

Afferent
arteriole

Distal
convoluted
tubule

Capillaries

REABSORPTION
OF H₂O.
URINE CONCENTRATED

REABSORPTION
AND SECRETION

Renal
tubule

Tubule coming
from another
nephron

Collecting
duct

Loop of Henle

To
renal
pelvis

FIGURE **16–6** Urine is produced by filtration, reabsorption,
and secretion.

blood cells or proteins do appear in the urine, they are signs of a problem with glomerular filtration.

Almost 25% of the cardiac output is delivered to the kidneys each minute, so every 4 minutes the kidneys receive a volume of blood equal to the total volume of blood in the body. Every 24 hours about 180 liters (45 gallons) of filtrate are produced. Common sense suggests that we could not excrete urine at the rate of 45 gallons per day. If we were losing fluid that quickly, dehydration would become a life-threatening problem within a few moments.

Tubular Reabsorption and Secretion Are Selective Processes

Dehydration does not normally occur because about 99% of the filtrate is returned to the blood by **tubular reabsorption.** This leaves only about 1.5 liters to be excreted as urine during a 24-hour period. Tubular reabsorption is the job of the renal tubules and collecting ducts.

Unlike glomerular filtration, tubular reabsorption is highly selective. Wastes, surplus salts, and excess water are kept as part of the filtrate. Glucose, amino acids, and other needed substances are reabsorbed into the blood.

A few substances are actively **secreted** from the blood in the peritubular capillaries into the renal tu-

bules. Tubular secretion is important in regulating the potassium and hydrogen ion concentrations in the blood. Some toxic substances and certain drugs, such as penicillin, are removed from the body by tubular secretion.

URINE CONSISTS MAINLY OF WATER

By the time the filtrate reaches the ureter, its composition has been carefully adjusted. Useful materials have been returned to the blood while wastes and excess materials have been cleared from the blood. The adjusted filtrate is called **urine.** It is composed of about 96% water, 2.5% nitrogen wastes (mainly urea), 1.5% salts, and traces of other substances.

Healthy urine is sterile. However, urine rapidly decomposes when exposed to bacterial action, forming ammonia and other products. The ammonia causes diaper rash in infants.

URINE VOLUME IS REGULATED BY ADH

When you drink a large amount of water, your kidneys produce a large volume of urine. Water is absorbed from the digestive tract into the blood. Excess water is removed from the blood by the kidneys. When you drink too little water, only a small volume of urine is produced. By regulating urine volume, the body maintains a steady volume and composition of blood.

The kidney receives information about the state of the blood indirectly (Fig. 16–7). When fluid intake is low, the body begins to dehydrate. When the volume of the blood decreases, the concentration of dissolved salts is greater, causing an increase in the osmotic pressure of the blood. Specialized receptors in the brain, heart, and in certain large blood vessels are sensitive to such change. The posterior lobe of the pituitary gland responds by releasing antidiuretic hormone (ADH). This hormone serves as a chemical messenger carrying information from the brain to the distal convoluted tubules and collecting ducts of the

kidneys. It causes the walls of these ducts to become much more permeable to water, so more water is reabsorbed into the blood. Blood volume increases, and homeostasis of fluid volume is restored. Only a small amount of concentrated urine is produced.

On the other hand, when a great deal of fluid is consumed, the blood becomes diluted and its osmotic pressure falls. Release of ADH by the pituitary gland decreases. This reduces the amount of water reabsorbed from the distal tubules and collecting ducts. As a result, a large volume of dilute urine is produced.

When the pituitary gland does not produce enough ADH, water is not efficiently reabsorbed from the ducts. This results in the production of a large volume of urine. This condition is called diabetes insipidus (not to be confused with the more common disorder, diabetes mellitus). An individual with se-

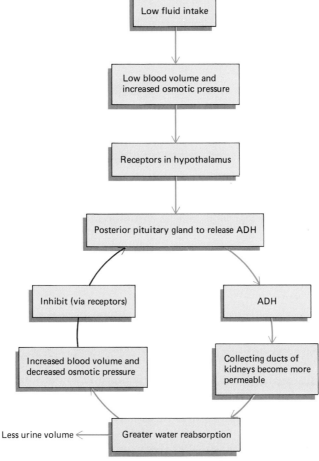

FIGURE **16–7** Regulation of urine volume reflects the blood volume and osmotic pressure. When the body is dehydrated, the hormone ADH increases the permeability of the collecting ducts to water. More water is reabsorbed, and only a small volume of concentrated urine is produced.

vere diabetes insipidus may excrete up to 25 quarts of urine each day and must drink almost continually to offset this fluid loss.

ADH regulates the excretion of water by the kidneys. Salt excretion is regulated by hormones, mainly aldosterone, secreted by the adrenal glands.

Coffee, tea, and alcoholic beverages contain chemicals called diuretics that increase urine volume. Diuretics inhibit reabsorption of water. Some diuretics inhibit secretion of ADH; others act directly on the tubules in the kidneys.

THE KIDNEYS HELP MAINTAIN HOMEOSTASIS

The kidneys are vital in maintaining homeostasis. Their functions include:

1. Excretion of metabolic wastes such as water, urea, and uric acid.

2. Disposal of excess water and salts.

3. Regulation of acid-base (pH) level of blood and body fluids. Acids and bases that are not needed are excreted in the urine.

4. Secretion of regulatory substances. The kidneys secrete the enzyme renin, which is important in regulating blood pressure. They also secrete a hormone (erythropoietin) that regulates production of red blood cells.

URINE IS TRANSPORTED BY DUCTS AND STORED IN THE BLADDER

Urine passes from the kidneys through the paired ureters, ducts about 25 centimeters (cm) (10 inches) long, which conduct it to the urinary bladder. Urine is forced along through the ureter by peristaltic contractions.

The urinary bladder is a temporary storage sac for urine. The bladder is lined with a mucous membrane that (like the stomach) has folds called rugae. This lining and smooth muscle in its wall permit the bladder to stretch so that it can hold up to 800 milliliters (ml) (about a pint and a half) of urine.

When urine leaves the bladder, it flows through the urethra, a duct leading to the outside of the body. In the male, the urethra is lengthy and passes through the prostate gland and the penis. Semen, as well as urine, is transported through the male urethra. In the female, the urethra is short and transports only urine. Its opening to the outside is just above the opening into the vagina. Bladder infections are more common in females than males because the long male urethra is a barrier to bacterial invasion.

URINATION EMPTIES THE BLADDER

The process of emptying the bladder and expelling urine is referred to as urination, or micturition (mik'-tyoo-**rish'**-un). When the volume of urine in the bladder reaches about 300 ml, special nerve endings in the bladder wall are stimulated. These receptors send neural messages to the spinal cord, initiating a urination reflex. This reflex contracts the bladder wall and also relaxes the internal urethral sphincter, a ring of smooth muscle at the upper end of the urethra. These actions stimulate a conscious desire to urinate.

If the time and place are appropriate, the external urethral sphincter, located a short distance below the internal sphincter, is voluntarily relaxed, allowing urination to occur. Voluntary control of urination cannot be exerted by an immature nervous system. That is why most babies under the age of 2 automatically urinate every time the bladder fills.

SUMMARY

 I. The principal waste products are water, carbon dioxide, and nitrogen wastes (urea, uric acid, creatinine).
 II. The kidneys produce urine, which passes through the ureters to the urinary bladder for storage. During urination, urine is discharged through the urethra to the outside of the body.
 III. Each kidney consists of an outer renal cortex and an inner renal medulla.
   A. The renal medulla consists of renal pyramids. Urine passes from the collecting ducts through the papilla of a pyramid and flows into a calyx.
   B. The calyx empties into the renal pelvis.
 IV. Each nephron consists of a renal corpuscle and a renal tubule.
   A. The renal corpuscle is composed of a glomerulus that fits into a Bowman's capsule.
   B. The renal tubule has three main regions: (1) proximal convoluted tubule; (2) loop of Henle; and (3) distal convoluted tubule.

V. Urine formation is accomplished by glomerular filtration, tubular reabsorption, and tubular secretion.
  A. Blood is delivered to the glomerular capillaries by the afferent arteriole under high pressure; some plasma containing dissolved substances is filtered out of the capillaries and into Bowman's capsule.
    1. A large volume of filtrate is produced.
    2. Glomerular filtration is not a selective process, so useful materials, as well as wastes, become part of the filtrate.
  B. About 99% of the filtrate is returned to the blood by tubular reabsorption.
    1. Tubular reabsorption is accomplished by the renal tubules and collecting ducts.
    2. Tubular reabsorption is highly selective; wastes, excess water, and surplus salts remain in the filtrate; glucose, amino acids, and other needed substances are reabsorbed (returned) into the blood.
  C. Tubular secretion is important in regulating potassium and hydrogen ion concentration in the blood.
VI. The adjusted filtrate is called urine; it consists of water, nitrogen wastes, salts, and traces of other substances.
VII. Urine volume is regulated by the hormone ADH released by the posterior lobe of the pituitary gland. ADH makes the distal convoluted tubules and collecting ducts more permeable to water so that more water is reabsorbed.
VIII. The kidneys help maintain homeostasis by excreting metabolic wastes, ridding the body of excess water and salts, and helping regulate the acid-base level of the blood (pH). The kidneys also secrete the enzyme renin; renin activates a hormone that helps regulate blood pressure.
IX. The reflex to urinate occurs when the volume of urine in the bladder reaches about 300 ml; if the external urethral sphincter is relaxed, urination occurs.

POST TEST

1. The process of disposing of metabolic wastes is called _____ .
2. Two nitrogen wastes excreted by the kidneys are _____ and _____ .
3. Urine is conducted from the renal pelvis to the urinary bladder by the _____ .
4. Urine in a calyx next passes into the renal _____ .
5. The outer portion of the kidney is the _____ and the inner portion is the _____ .
6. A nephron consists of two main structures: the renal _____ and the renal _____ .
7. The renal corpuscle consists of a tuft of capillaries, the _____ surrounded by _____ _____ .
8. Blood flows into the glomerulus through an _____ arteriole.
9. From the proximal convoluted tubule filtrate flows into the _____ of _____ .
10. In glomerular _____ , plasma leaves the glomerular capillaries and passes into _____ _____ .
11. The process of returning most of the filtrate to the blood is known as _____ .

12. The adjusted filtrate is called _____ .

13. The hormone _____ causes the walls of the collecting ducts to be more permeable to _____ .

14. The urinary _____ is a temporary storage sac for urine.

15. During urination, urine is discharged through the _____ .

16. Label the diagram.

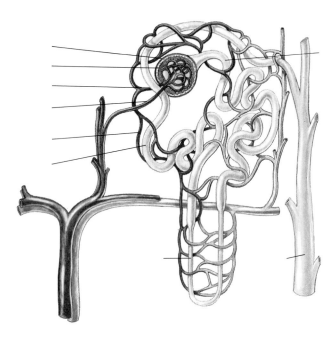

REVIEW QUESTIONS

1. What is the difference between excretion and elimination? Give specific examples.

2. What are the principal metabolic waste products? What organs excrete them?

3. In what ways do the kidneys help maintain homeostasis?

4. Trace a drop of filtrate from the glomerular capillaries to the renal pelvis.

5. Trace a drop of urine from the renal pelvis to the urethra.

6. What are the main steps in urine production? Where does each occur?

7. A large amount of protein is found in the urine of a patient. With what process would you suspect a problem?

8. The urination reflex can be consciously facilitated or inhibited. What does this mean?

POST TEST ANSWERS

1. excretion
2. urea; uric acid
3. ureter
4. pelvis
5. cortex; medulla
6. corpuscle; tubule
7. glomerulus; Bowman's capsule
8. afferent
9. loop; Henle
10. filtration; Bowman's capsule
11. (tubular) reabsorption
12. urine
13. ADH; water
14. bladder
15. urethra
16. see Figure 16–4

Seventeen

REGULATION OF FLUIDS AND ELECTROLYTES

CHAPTER OUTLINE

I. The body has two main fluid compartments
II. Fluid intake must equal fluid output
    A. The hypothalamus regulates fluid intake
    B. The hypothalamus also regulates fluid output
III. Electrolyte balance is affected by fluid balance
    A. Sodium is the major extracellular cation
    B. Potassium is the major intracellular cation
    C. Other major electrolytes include calcium, phosphate, chloride, and magnesium

LEARNING OBJECTIVES

After you have studied this chapter, you should be able to:
1. Identify the fluid compartments of the body.
2. Summarize the principal routes for fluid input and fluid output.
3. Describe how fluid input and output are regulated.
4. Define electrolyte balance and identify the functions of six major electrolytes.
5. Describe the mechanisms responsible for sodium and potassium homeostasis.

Fluid balance is critical to homeostasis. Whether you drink a pint of water or a gallon, whether you are on a salt-restricted diet or eat a bag of potato chips, the fluid and salt content of your body must be kept within strict limits. To keep the quantities of these substances steady, the body must replace water and salt losses and excrete excesses. Normal body function, and even survival, depend upon homeostasis of body fluids.

The term **body fluid** refers to the water in the body and the substances dissolved in it. Among the most important components of body fluid are **electrolytes** (ee-**lek′**-trow-lites), compounds such as salts that form ions (electrically charged particles) in solution. Most organic compounds dissolved in the body fluid are nonelectrolytes, compounds that do not form ions. Examples of nonelectrolytes in the body fluid are glucose and urea.

THE BODY HAS TWO MAIN FLUID COMPARTMENTS

The human body is about 60% water by weight. Water and electrolytes are distributed in certain regions, or compartments. The two principal compartments are the **intracellular compartment** and the **extracellular compartment.** About two thirds of the body fluid is found in the intracellular compartment, that is, within cells (Fig. 17–1). This fluid is referred to as intracellular fluid. The remaining third

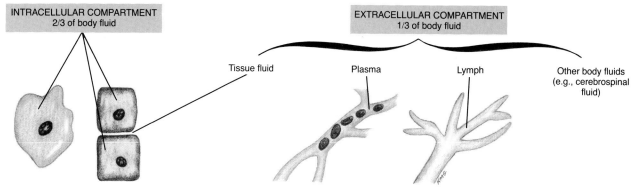

FIGURE 17–1 Fluid compartments.

is located outside the cells in the extracellular compartment. This extracellular fluid includes the tissue fluid, also called interstitial fluid, found in the tissue spaces between cells; the blood plasma and lymph; the cerebrospinal fluid; and all other fluids in the body.

Fluid constantly moves from one compartment to another. However, in a healthy person, the volume of fluid in each compartment remains about the same. The movement of fluid from one compartment to another depends upon blood pressure and osmotic concentration. Recall that blood pressure forces fluid out of the blood at the arterial ends of capillaries. When it leaves the blood, this fluid is called tissue fluid. Excess tissue fluid returns to the blood at the venous ends of capillaries because of osmotic pressure. (Plasma proteins in the plasma exert a pulling force on fluid.) Excess tissue fluid is also returned to the blood by way of the lymphatic system. Fluid movement between the intracellular and extracellular compartments occurs mainly as a result of changes in osmotic pressure.

Important differences in composition exist between the intracellular fluid and the extracellular fluid. For example, sodium ion concentration is much higher in the extracellular fluid than in the intracellular fluid. In contrast, potassium ion concentration is much higher within cells than in the extracellular fluid. To maintain these differences in ion distribution, cells must pump specific kinds of ions into or out of the cell. This is a form of cellular work known as active transport.

FLUID INTAKE MUST EQUAL FLUID OUTPUT

Normally, fluid input equals fluid output, so the total amount of fluid in the body remains constant (Fig. 17–2). We ingest about 2500 milliliters (ml) of water each day in the foods we eat and liquids we drink. This water is absorbed from the digestive tract into the blood. Water is also produced during catabolic processes. Most fluid (about 1500 ml per day) is discharged by the kidneys. Fluid is also lost through the skin, lungs, and the digestive tract.

When fluid output is greater than fluid input, dehydration occurs. Dehydration can result from not drinking enough fluid, from profuse sweating, or as a result of vomiting or diarrhea.

THE HYPOTHALAMUS REGULATES FLUID INTAKE

Fluid intake is regulated by the hypothalamus. Dehydration raises the osmotic pressure of the blood (when there is less fluid, the blood is saltier). The increased osmotic pressure stimulates the **thirst center** in the hypothalamus (Fig. 17–3). This results in the sensation of thirst and the desire to drink fluids. Dehydration also leads to a decrease in saliva secretion that results in dryness in the mouth and throat. This dryness also signals thirst. We feel thirsty when total body fluid is decreased more than 1 to 2%.

THE HYPOTHALAMUS ALSO REGULATES FLUID OUTPUT

The kidneys are primarily responsible for fluid output. This output is regulated by ADH (antidiuretic hormone). Recall that ADH, produced by the hypothalamus and secreted by the posterior lobe of the pituitary gland, regulates the volume of urine.

When the body begins to dehydrate, ADH secretion increases (see Fig. 16–7). This occurs because the plasma becomes saltier when the volume of water in the body decreases. Special receptors in the hypothalamus signal the posterior pituitary to release

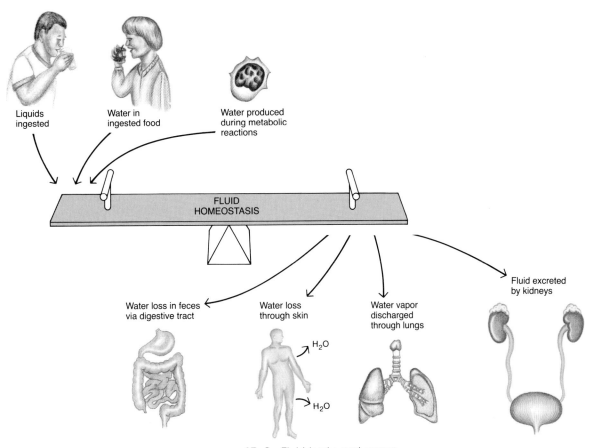

FIGURE 17–2 Fluid intake and output.

more ADH. The ADH makes the distal tubules and collecting ducts in the kidneys more permeable to water. More water is reabsorbed into the blood, and only a small volume of concentrated urine is excreted.

When blood volume increases, less ADH is secreted. Less water is reabsorbed, and a large volume of dilute urine is excreted. In this way, fluid homeostasis is restored.

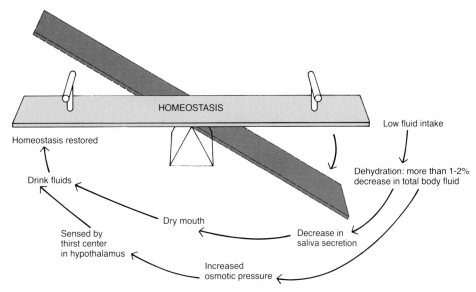

FIGURE 17–3 Regulation of fluid intake.

ELECTROLYTE BALANCE IS AFFECTED BY FLUID BALANCE

Normally, a person obtains adequate amounts of electrolytes in the food and fluid ingested. When the amounts of the various electrolytes taken into the body equal the amounts lost, the body is in **electrolyte balance.** Because electrolytes are dissolved in the body fluid, electrolyte balance and fluid balance are interdependent. When the fluid content decreases, the electrolytes become more concentrated; when fluid content increases, electrolytes are more diluted.

Electrolytes produce positively and negatively charged ions. Positively charged ions are referred to as cations; negatively charged ions are anions. Among the important cations in the body fluid are sodium, potassium, calcium, hydrogen, magnesium, and iron. Important anions include chloride and phosphate.

SODIUM IS THE MAJOR EXTRACELLULAR CATION

About 90% of the extracellular cations are **sodium** ions. Sodium is needed to transmit impulses in nervous and muscle tissue. Low sodium concentration can cause headache, mental confusion, rapid heart rate, low blood pressure, and even circulatory shock. Severe sodium depletion can result in coma.

Sodium concentration is adjusted mainly by regulating the amount of water in the body. When the sodium concentration is too high, we feel thirsty and drink water. In addition, sodium concentration is regulated by the hormone aldosterone secreted by the adrenal cortex. Aldosterone stimulates the distal convoluted tubules and collecting ducts to increase their reabsorption of sodium.

POTASSIUM IS THE MAJOR INTRACELLULAR CATION

Most of the cations in the intracellular fluid are **potassium** ions. These cations are important in nervous and muscle tissue function. Potassium ions are also important in maintaining the fluid volume within cells, and they help regulate acid-base levels (pH). An

abnormally low level of potassium may cause mental confusion, fatigue, and cramps, and it may affect the heart. When the potassium concentration is too high, nerve impulses are not effectively transmitted and the strength of muscle contraction decreases. In fact, a high potassium concentration can weaken the heart and lead to death from heart failure.

When the concentration of potassium ions is too high, potassium ions are secreted from the blood into the renal tubules, and the ions are excreted in the urine. This is due to a direct effect of the potassium ions on the tubules. A high potassium ion concentration also stimulates aldosterone secretion. The aldosterone further stimulates secretion of potassium. Loss of large numbers of potassium ions in the urine brings the potassium concentration in the body back to normal. When the potassium concentration becomes too low, aldosterone secretion decreases, and potassium secretion decreases almost to zero.

OTHER MAJOR ELECTROLYTES INCLUDE CALCIUM, PHOSPHATE, CHLORIDE, AND MAGNESIUM

Calcium is found mainly in the extracellular fluid. **Phosphate** is the most abundant intracellular anion. Calcium and phosphate are both important components of bone and teeth. Calcium is also important in blood clotting, transmission of neural impulses, and muscle contraction. Phosphate is needed to make ATP, DNA, and RNA. The concentrations of calcium and phosphate are regulated by parathyroid hormone and calcitonin.

Chloride ions are the most abundant extracellular anions. These ions can diffuse easily across plasma membranes. Their movement is closely linked to the movement of sodium ions. Chloride helps regulate differences in osmotic pressure between fluid compartments and is also important in pH balance. The hormone aldosterone indirectly regulates chloride concentration.

Magnesium ions are cations found mainly in the intracellular fluid and in bone. They are important in production of bone and teeth and play a role in neural transmission and muscle contraction. The hormone aldosterone increases reabsorption of magnesium ions by the kidneys.

SUMMARY

I. Body fluid is the water in the body and the substances dissolved in it.
II. Body fluid is distributed in the intracellular and extracellular compartments.

A. About two thirds of body fluid is located in the intracellular compartment.

B. The remaining third is located in the extracellular compartment; this includes the tissue fluid, the plasma and lymph, and the cerebrospinal fluid.

C. Fluid continuously moves from one compartment to another, but the volume in each compartment remains fairly constant.

D. Differences in composition exist between the intracellular fluid and the extracellular fluid.

III. Normally, fluid input equals fluid output. We ingest about 2500 ml each day, so about 2500 ml must be discharged from the body. Most fluid is excreted by the kidneys.

IV. When total body fluid is decreased by 1 to 2%, the hypothalamus is stimulated and we feel thirsty.

V. The kidneys are the organs mainly responsible for fluid output.

A. When the body begins to dehydrate, the posterior pituitary increases its secretion of ADH. This hormone stimulates the distal tubules and collecting ducts in the kidneys to reabsorb more water; fluid is conserved for the body.

B. When excess fluid is present, ADH secretion decreases and less water is reabsorbed; a large volume of dilute urine is excreted.

VI. When the amounts of the various electrolytes taken into the body equal the amounts lost, the body is in electrolyte balance.

A. Sodium ions account for about 90% of the extracellular cations. Sodium concentration is regulated by the amount of water in the body and by aldosterone, which stimulates reabsorption of sodium.

B. Potassium ions account for most intracellular cations. When the concentration of potassium ions rises above normal, potassium ions are secreted into the renal tubules and excreted in the urine. High potassium ion concentration also stimulates aldosterone secretion, which stimulates potassium excretion.

POST TEST

1. Compounds such as salts that form ions in solution are called

   _____ .

2. Most of the body fluid is located in the _____ compartment.

3. The movement of fluid from one compartment to another depends on blood
   _____ and _____ concentration.

4. Sodium ion concentration is much higher in the _____ fluid.

5. Fluid output is mainly the job of the _____ .

6. When total body fluid is decreased more than 2%, we feel

   _____ .

7. Excretion of water by the kidneys is regulated by the hormone

   _____ .

8. ADH causes the distal tubules and collecting ducts to reabsorb
   _____ (more, less) water; a _____ (small, large) volume of urine is excreted.

9. Aldosterone results in _____ (greater, less) excretion of sodium.

10. Aldosterone results in _____ (greater, less) excretion of potassium.

11. When fluid output is greater than fluid input, _____ occurs.

REVIEW QUESTIONS

1. What is body fluid? What are electrolytes?
2. What are the main compartments in the body where fluid is located? Describe each.
3. What is meant by fluid balance? How are fluid and electrolyte balance related?
4. What are some differences in composition between intracellular and extracellular fluid? How are these differences maintained?
5. How is fluid intake regulated?
6. What is the role of ADH in regulating fluid output? Explain.
7. How is sodium concentration regulated?
8. How is potassium concentration regulated?

POST TEST ANSWERS

1. electrolytes
2. intracellular
3. pressure; osmotic
4. extracellular
5. kidneys
6. thirsty
7. ADH
8. more; small
9. less
10. greater
11. dehydration

Eighteen

REPRODUCTION

CHAPTER OUTLINE

I. The male produces sperm and delivers them into the female
   A. The testes produce sperm
   B. The conducting tubes transport sperm
   C. The accessory glands produce semen
   D. The penis delivers sperm into the female reproductive tract
   E. Male hormones regulate male sexuality and reproduction
II. The female produces ova and incubates the embryo
   A. The ovaries produce ova and hormones
   B. The uterine tubes transport ova
   C. The uterus incubates the embryo
   D. The vagina functions in sexual intercourse, menstruation, and birth
   E. The external genital structures are the vulva
   F. The breasts contain the mammary glands
   G. Hormones regulate female reproduction
   H. The menstrual cycle prepares the body for pregnancy
   I. Menopause is marked by a decline in ovary function
III. Fertilization is the fusion of sperm and ovum
IV. The zygote gives rise to the new individual
   A. The embryo develops in the wall of the uterus
   B. Prenatal development requires about 266 days
   C. The birth process has three stages
   D. Multiple births may be fraternal or identical
V. The human life cycle extends from fertilization to death

LEARNING OBJECTIVES

After you have studied this chapter, you should be able to:

1. Label a diagram of the male reproductive system and describe the functions of each structure.
2. Trace the passage of sperm from the tubules in the testes through the conducting tubes, describing changes that may occur along the way.
3. Describe the actions of the male gonadotropic hormones and of testosterone.
4. Label diagrams of internal and external female reproductive organs and describe their structure and functions.
5. Trace the development of an ovum and its passage through the female reproductive system.
6. Describe the principal events of the menstrual cycle, and summarize the interactions of hormones that regulate the cycle.
7. Describe the process of fertilization and identify the time of the menstrual cycle at which sexual intercourse is most likely to result in pregnancy.
8. Summarize the course of development from fertilization to birth.
9. Describe the functions of the amnion and placenta.
10. Identify the three stages of the birth process.
11. List the stages of human development from fertilization to death.

247

Reproduction involves several processes including formation of specialized sex cells called gametes (**gam'**-eets) (eggs and sperm), preparation of the female body for pregnancy, sexual intercourse, fertilization (union of sperm and egg), pregnancy, and lactation (producing milk for nourishment of the infant). These events are regulated and coordinated by the interaction of hormones secreted by the anterior pituitary gland and the **gonads** (**go'**-nads), or sex glands.

THE MALE PRODUCES SPERM AND DELIVERS THEM INTO THE FEMALE

The male's function in reproduction is to produce sperm cells (spermatozoa) (sper''-mah-tow-**zow'**-ah) and to deliver them into the female reproductive tract. When a sperm combines with an egg, it contributes half the genes of the offspring and determines the sex of the baby. Male reproductive structures include the testes and scrotum, conducting tubes that lead from the testes to the outside of the body, accessory glands, and the penis (Fig. 18–1).

THE TESTES PRODUCE SPERM

In the adult male, millions of sperm cells are manufactured each day within the paired male gonads, the **testes** (**tes'**-teez). Each testis is a small, oval organ about 4 to 5 centimeters (cm) (1.6 to 2 inches) long and 2.5 cm (about an inch) wide and thick. Each testis is filled with about 1000 threadlike, coiled tubules (seminiferous tubules) (Fig. 18–2). These tubules are the sperm-cell factories. The mature sperm is a tiny, elongated cell with a tail that it uses for moving toward an egg.

The testes develop in the abdominal cavity of the male embryo. About 2 months before birth they *descend* into the **scrotum** (**skrow'**-tum), a skin-covered bag suspended from the groin. As the testes descend, they move through the inguinal canals, the passageways connecting the scrotal and abdominal cavities. The testes pull their arteries, veins, nerves, and conducting tubes after them. These structures, surrounded by muscle and by layers of connective tissue, make up the **spermatic cord.** The inguinal region remains a weak place in the abdominal wall. Straining the abdominal muscles by lifting a very heavy object may result in a tear, through which a loop of intestine can bulge into the scrotum; this is called an inguinal hernia.

Sperm cells are not able to develop at body temperature, and the scrotum serves as a cooling unit, maintaining them at about 2° C below body temperature. The wall of the scrotum is rich in sweat glands and blood vessels. These structures promote heat loss and so help maintain the cool temperature.

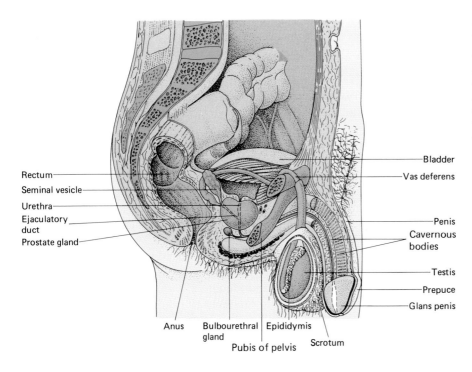

FIGURE **18–1** Anatomy of the human male reproductive system. The scrotum, penis, and pelvic region have been cut sagittally to show their internal structure. Identify the accessory glands and trace the conducting tubes from the testis to the urethra.

Rectum
Seminal vesicle
Urethra
Ejaculatory duct
Prostate gland
Bladder
Vas deferens
Penis
Cavernous bodies
Testis
Prepuce
Glans penis
Anus   Bulbourethral gland   Epididymis
Pubis of pelvis   Scrotum

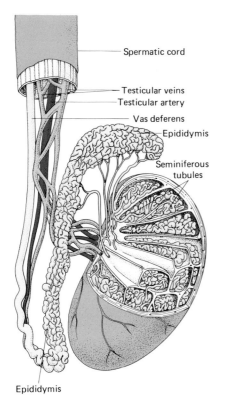

Spermatic cord

Testicular veins
Testicular artery
Vas deferens
Epididymis
Seminiferous tubules

Epididymis

FIGURE **18–2** *Structure of the testis and epididymis. The testis is shown in sagittal section to illustrate the arrangement of the tubules.*

THE CONDUCTING TUBES TRANSPORT SPERM

From the tubules inside the testis, sperm pass into a large, coiled tube, the **epididymis** (ep″-ih-**did′**-ih-mis) (Fig. 18–2). The epididymis of each testis is located within the scrotum. Sperm mature within the epididymis and are stored there. The epididymis empties into a straight tube, the **vas deferens** (**def′**-er-enz), or sperm duct. The vas deferens passes from the scrotum through the inguinal canal as part of the spermatic cord. After entering the pelvic cavity, the vas deferens loops over the side and then down the posterior surface of the urinary bladder.

The vas deferens is joined by the duct from the seminal vesicles (discussed in the next paragraph) to become the **ejaculatory duct.** This very short duct passes through the prostate gland (discussed in the next section) and then opens into the **urethra.** The single urethra, which conducts both urine and semen, passes through the penis to the outside of the body. Thus, sperm pass through the following path:

> Tubules in the testis → epididymis →
> vas deferens → ejaculatory duct →
> urethra

THE ACCESSORY GLANDS PRODUCE SEMEN

Semen (**see′**-mun) is a thick, whitish fluid consisting of sperm cells suspended in secretions of the accessory glands. The paired **seminal vesicles** are saclike glands. A seminal vesicle empties into each vas deferens. The mucuslike fluid secreted by the seminal vesicles contains the sugar fructose and other nutrients that nourish and provide fuel for the sperm cells. Secretions of the seminal vesicles account for about 60% of the semen volume.

The single **prostate** (**pros′**-tate) **gland** surrounds the urethra as the urethra emerges from the urinary bladder. The prostate gland produces a thick, milky, alkaline secretion that neutralizes the mildly acidic semen. This change in acidity level (pH) activates the sperm cells.

In older men, the prostate gland often enlarges and exerts pressure on the urethra, making urination difficult. When necessary, the prostate can be removed surgically. Cancer of the prostate is a common disorder in men over 50 years old.

The **bulbourethral** (bul″-bow-yoo-**ree′**-thrul) **glands** (also called Cowper's glands) are about the size and shape of two peas, one on each side of the urethra. When a male is sexually aroused, these glands release a few drops of clear, alkaline fluid into the urethra. This secretion neutralizes the acidity of the urethra and also lubricates the urethra and penis.

About 3 milliliters (ml) of semen is discharged from the penis during **ejaculation.** Semen consists of about 300 million sperm cells suspended in the secretions of the accessory glands. Sperm cells are so tiny that they account for very little (less than 1%) of the semen volume. Men with fewer than 20 million sperm/ml of semen usually are sterile. Fever or infection of the testes may cause temporary sterility.

THE PENIS DELIVERS SPERM INTO THE FEMALE REPRODUCTIVE TRACT

The penis is the male copulatory organ; it delivers sperm into the female reproductive tract during sexual intercourse. The penis consists of a long **shaft** that enlarges to form an expanded tip, the **glans** (see Fig. 18–1). Part of the loose-fitting skin of the penis folds down and covers the proximal portion of the glans, forming a cuff called the **prepuce** (**pree′**-pyous) or foreskin. This cuff of skin is removed during circumcision.

Under the skin, the penis consists of three cylinders of spongy tissue. This tissue contains large blood vessels (sinusoids). When the male is sexually stimulated, nerve impulses signal the arteries of the penis to dilate. Blood rushes into the blood vessels of the spongy tissue. As this tissue fills with blood, it swells and presses against the veins that conduct blood away from the penis. As a result, more blood enters the penis than can leave, and the spongy tissue becomes filled with blood. The penis becomes **erect,** that is, larger in circumference, and firm. The average penis is about 9 cm long when flaccid (relaxed) and 16 to 19 cm when erect.

When the level of sexual excitement reaches a peak, ejaculation occurs. Both erection and ejaculation are reflex actions.

MALE HORMONES REGULATE MALE SEXUALITY AND REPRODUCTION

Between the tubules in the testes are small islands of cells called interstitial cells (in-ter-**stish′**-al) that produce the male hormone **testosterone** (tes-**tos′**tur-own). Testosterone is responsible for the development of both primary and secondary sex characteristics in the male. **Primary sex characteristics** include the growth of the penis and scrotum, and the growth and activity of internal reproductive structures. **Secondary sex characteristics** include deepening of the voice, muscle development, and growth of pubic, facial, and underarm hair. Testosterone also stimulates the adolescent growth spurt and stimulates oil glands in the skin (sometimes causing acne).

Puberty, the period of sexual maturation, begins at about age 12 or 13 in the male. At puberty the hypothalamus begins to secrete releasing hormones that stimulate the anterior lobe of the pituitary gland to secrete gonadotropic hormones. These hormones are follicle-stimulating hormone (FSH) and luteinizing hormone (LH). FSH stimulates sperm production. LH stimulates the testes to secrete testosterone.

When a male is castrated (that is, his testes are removed) before puberty, he becomes a eunuch. His sex organs remain childlike, and he does not develop secondary sexual characteristics. If castration occurs after puberty, increased secretion of male hormone by the adrenal cortex helps to maintain masculinity.

THE FEMALE PRODUCES OVA AND INCUBATES THE EMBRYO

The female produces **ova** (eggs), receives the penis and the sperm released from it during sexual intercourse, houses and nourishes the embryo during its prenatal development, and nourishes the infant. Much of the activity of the female reproductive system centers about the **menstrual (mens′**-tru-al) **cycle,** the monthly preparation for possible pregnancy.

The organs of the female reproductive system include the ovaries (which produce ova and female hormones), the uterine tubes (where fertilization takes place), the uterus (incubator for the developing

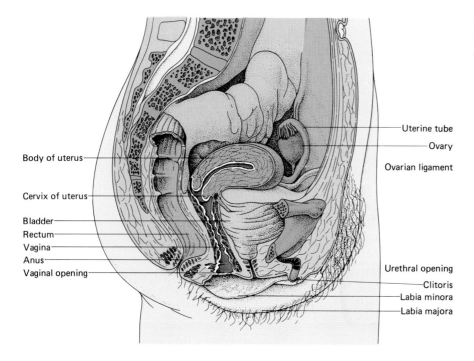

FIGURE **18–3** Midsagittal section of the female pelvis showing reproductive organs. Note the position of the uterus relative to the vagina.

Body of uterus

Cervix of uterus

Bladder
Rectum
Vagina
Anus
Vaginal opening

Uterine tube
Ovary
Ovarian ligament

Urethral opening
Clitoris
Labia minora
Labia majora

child), the vagina (which receives the penis and serves as a birth canal), the vulva (external genital structures), and the breasts.

THE OVARIES PRODUCE OVA AND HORMONES

The paired **ovaries** are the female gonads. The ovaries produce ova and the female sex hormones, estrogen and progesterone. About the size and shape of large almonds, the ovaries are located close to the lateral walls of the pelvic cavity (Figs. 18–3 and Fig. 18–4). The ovaries are held in position by several connective tissue ligaments. The ovarian ligament, for example, anchors the medial end of the ovary to the uterus.

Each ovary consists mainly of connective tissue through which developing ova (eggs) are scattered. All the ova are produced before birth. Each ovum matures within a little sac of cells and fluid. Together, the ovum and its surrounding sac make up a **follicle.**

With the onset of puberty, a few follicles develop each month. Their maturation is controlled by FSH secreted by the anterior lobe of the pituitary gland. Cells of the follicle secrete female hormones, called **estrogens.** As a follicle matures, it moves close to the wall of the ovary and can be seen as a

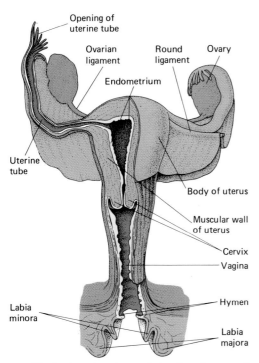

FIGURE 18–4 Anterior view of the female reproductive system. Some organs have been cut open to expose the internal structure. The ligaments help to hold the reproductive organs in place.

fluid-filled blister. Mature follicles are called graafian follicles. Usually, only one follicle matures each month. Several others may develop for about a week and then deteriorate.

In response to FSH and LH from the anterior pituitary gland, the mature follicle ruptures after about 2 weeks of development. During this process, called **ovulation,** the ovum is ejected through the wall of the ovary and into the pelvic cavity. The part of the follicle that remains behind in the ovary develops into an important endocrine structure, the **corpus luteum** ("yellow body"). LH stimulates the development of the corpus luteum. This temporary endocrine structure secretes progesterone and estrogens. These hormones stimulate the uterus to prepare for possible pregnancy.

THE UTERINE TUBES TRANSPORT OVA

Each **uterine tube** (also called the oviduct or fallopian tube) is about 12 cm long. Its free end is shaped like a funnel and has long, fingerlike projections called **fimbriae** (**fim′**-bree-ee). At ovulation, the mature ovum is released into the pelvic cavity. Movements of the fimbriae and the current created by the beating of cilia in the lining of the tube draw the ovum into the uterine tube.

Peristaltic contractions of the muscular wall and action of the cilia help move the ovum toward the uterus. Unlike sperm, the ovum is not capable of moving by itself. Normally, fertilization takes place in the upper third of the uterine tube. The fertilized egg, or **zygote** (**zye′**-goat), begins its development as it is moved along toward the uterus. If fertilization does not occur, the ovum degenerates in the uterine tube.

Because the uterine tubes open into the peritoneal cavity, bacteria that enter through the vagina can cause serious clinical problems. This route of infection has led to many deaths from abortions performed under nonsterile conditions.

THE UTERUS INCUBATES THE EMBRYO

Each month during a woman's reproductive life, the **uterus,** or womb, prepares for possible pregnancy. When pregnancy occurs, the uterus serves as the incubator for the developing embryo. The tiny embryo implants itself in the wall of the uterus and develops there until it is able to live independently. When that time comes, the uterine wall contracts powerfully and rhythmically (the process of labor), expelling the new baby from the mother's body. If pregnancy does not occur, the inner lining of the uterus sloughs off each month and is discarded. This process is called **menstruation** (men″-stroo-**ay′**-shun).

The uterus is a single, hollow organ shaped somewhat like a pear. In the nonpregnant condition, it is about the size of a small fist—about 7.5 cm (3 inches) in length and 5 cm (2 inches) in width at its widest region. The uterus lies in the bottom of the pelvic cavity, anterior to the rectum and posterior to the urinary bladder.

The main portion of the uterus is its **corpus,** or body. The rounded part of the uterus above the level of the entrance of the uterine tubes is the **fundus** (**fun′**-dus). The lower narrow portion is the **cervix** (**ser′**-viks). Part of the cervix projects into the vagina (see Fig. 18–3).

The uterus is lined by a mucous membrane, the **endometrium** (en-doe-**me′**-tree-um). Beneath the endometrium, the wall of the uterus consists of a thick layer of muscle. Just as the ovary develops a new ovum each month, the uterus also follows a cycle of activity. Each month, in response to estrogen and progesterone from the ovary, the endometrium prepares for possible pregnancy. The endometrium becomes thick and vascular and develops glands that secrete a nourishing fluid. If pregnancy does not occur, part of the endometrium sloughs off during menstruation.

Cancer of the cervix is one of the most common types of cancer in women. About 50% of cases of cervical cancer are now detected at very early stages, when cures are most likely. Detection is aided by the routine Papanicolaou test (Pap smear). A few cells are scraped from the cervix during a routine gynecological examination and are studied microscopically.

THE VAGINA FUNCTIONS IN SEXUAL INTERCOURSE, MENSTRUATION, AND BIRTH

The vagina functions as the sexual organ that receives the penis during sexual intercourse. It also serves as an exit through which the discarded endometrium is discharged during menstruation and as the lower part of the birth canal.

The vagina is located anterior to the rectum and posterior to the urethra and urinary bladder. The vagina is an elastic, muscular tube capable of considerable stretching. It extends from the cervix to its orifice (opening) to the outside of the body. The vagina surrounds the end of the cervix. The recesses formed between the vaginal wall and cervix are called **fornices** (**for′**-nee-seez).

The vagina is normally collapsed so that its walls touch each other. Two ridges run along anterior and posterior walls, and there are numerous **rugae** (folds). During sexual intercourse, when the penis is inserted into the vagina, or during childbirth, when the baby's head emerges into the vagina, the rugae straighten out, greatly enlarging the vagina. A thin ring of mucous membrane, the **hymen,** surrounds the entrance to the vagina.

THE EXTERNAL GENITAL STRUCTURES ARE THE VULVA

The term **vulva** (**vul′**-vah) refers to the external female genital structures. They include the mons pubis, labia, clitoris, and vestibule of the vagina (Fig. 18–5). The **mons pubis** is a mound of fatty tissue that covers the pubic symphysis. At puberty it becomes covered by coarse pubic hair.

The paired **labia** (**lay′**-be-ah) **majora** (meaning large lips) are folds of skin that pass from the mons pubis to the region behind the vaginal opening. Normally, the labia majora meet in the midline, providing protection for the genital structures beneath. After puberty the outer epidermis of the lips is pigmented and covered with coarse hair. Two thin folds of skin,

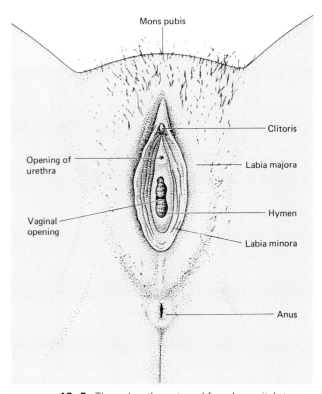

FIGURE 18–5 The vulva, the external female genital structures.

the **labia minora** (meaning small lips), are located just within the labia majora.

The **clitoris** (**klit′**-oh-ris) is a small structure that corresponds to the male glans penis. It projects from the anterior end of the vulva at the anterior junction of the labia minora. However, most of the clitoris is not visible because it is embedded in the tissues of the vulva. The clitoris is a main focus of sexual sensation in the female.

The space enclosed by the labia minora is the **vestibule.** Two openings can be seen in the vestibule—the opening of the urethra anteriorly, and the opening of the vagina posteriorly. Two small **Bartholin's glands** (greater vestibular glands) open on each side of the vaginal opening. A group of smaller glands (lesser vestibular) open into the vestibule near the opening of the urethra. All these glands secrete mucus. They help provide lubrication during sexual intercourse. These glands are vulnerable to infection, especially from the bacterium that causes gonorrhea. In both male and female the diamond-shaped region between the pubic arch and the anus is the **perineum** (peh-**rin′**-ee-um). In the female the region between the vagina and anus is referred to as the clinical perineum.

THE BREASTS CONTAIN THE MAMMARY GLANDS

The mammary glands are located within the breasts. The breasts overlie the pectoral muscles and are attached to them by connective tissue. Fibrous bands of tissue called ligaments of Cooper firmly connect the breasts to the skin. The function of the breasts is **lactation,** production of milk for nourishment of the baby.

Each breast is composed of 15 to 20 lobes of glandular tissue (Fig. 18–6). A duct drains milk from each lobe and opens onto the surface of the nipple. Thus, the surface of each nipple has 15 to 20 openings.

The amount of adipose tissue around the lobes of the glandular tissue determines the size of the breasts and accounts for their soft consistency. The size of the breasts does not affect their capacity to produce milk.

The nipple consists of smooth muscle that can contract to make the nipple erect in response to sexual stimuli. In the pinkish areola surrounding the nipple, several rudimentary milk glands may be found. In childhood, the breasts contain only rudimentary glands. At puberty, estrogen and progesterone stimulate development of the glands and ducts and the deposit of fatty tissue characteristic of the adult breast.

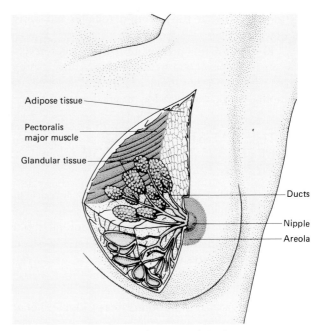

FIGURE **18–6** Structure of the breast.

During pregnancy, high concentrations of estrogen and progesterone stimulate the glands and ducts to develop, resulting in increased breast size. For the first few days after childbirth, the mammary glands produce a fluid called **colostrum** (koe-**los′**-trum), which contains protein and lactose but little fat. After birth, prolactin secreted by the anterior pituitary stimulates milk production. By the third day after delivery, milk is produced. When the infant suckles at the breast, a reflex action results in release of prolactin and oxytocin from the pituitary gland. Oxytocin permits actual release of milk from the glands and from the breasts.

The breasts are the most common site of cancer in women. Breast cancer now strikes 1 in every 10 women and is the leading cause of cancer deaths in women. Breast cancer often spreads to the lymphatic system, often to the axillary nodes or the nodes along the internal mammary artery. About two thirds of breast cancers have metastasized (i.e., spread) to the lymph nodes by the time the cancer is first diagnosed.

HORMONES REGULATE FEMALE REPRODUCTION

Like testosterone in the male, **estrogens** (**es′**-trow-jens) are responsible for the growth of sex organs at puberty and for the development of secondary sex characteristics. Female secondary sex characteristics include breast development, broadening of the pelvis, and distribution of fat and muscle that shape the female body. During the menstrual cycle, estrogens stimulate the growth of follicles and stimulate growth of the endometrium.

Progesterone (pro-**jes′**-ter-own) is secreted by the corpus luteum and by the placenta during pregnancy. This hormone stimulates the endometrium to complete its preparation for pregnancy.

THE MENSTRUAL CYCLE PREPARES THE BODY FOR PREGNANCY

As a female approaches puberty, the anterior pituitary gland secretes FSH and LH. These hormones signal the ovaries to begin functioning. Interaction of FSH and LH with estrogens and progesterone from the ovaries regulates the menstrual cycle. This cycle occurs every month from puberty until menopause, the end of a woman's reproductive life.

The menstrual cycle stimulates production of an ovum each month and prepares the uterus for pregnancy. Although there is wide variation, a "typical" menstrual cycle is 28 days long. The first day of menstruation marks the first day of the cycle. Menstruation lasts for about 5 days. Ovulation occurs about 14 days before the next cycle begins; in a 28-day cycle this would correspond to about the fourteenth day (Fig. 18–7).

During menstruation, the thickened endometrium of the uterus sloughs off. During this phase of the menstrual cycle, FSH is the principal hormone released by the pituitary gland. It stimulates a group of follicles to develop in the ovary.

During the first 2 weeks of the menstrual cycle, estrogens released from the developing follicles stimulate the growth of the endometrium once again. Its blood vessels and glands begin to develop anew. At midcycle, an increase in estrogen secretion from the follicles is followed by release of LH from the anterior pituitary. LH is necessary for final maturation of the follicle, for ovulation, and later for development of the corpus luteum.

After ovulation, the corpus luteum develops and releases progesterone as well as estrogens. These hormones stimulate continued thickening of the endometrium.

If pregnancy does not occur, the corpus luteum begins to degenerate. Progesterone and estrogen levels in the blood fall markedly. Small arteries in the uterine wall constrict, and the part of the endometrium they supply becomes deprived of oxygen. Menstruation begins once again as cells begin to die and damaged arteries rupture and bleed.

MENOPAUSE IS MARKED BY A DECLINE IN OVARY FUNCTION

At about age 50, a woman enters **menopause.** The ovaries become less responsive to gonadotropic hormones, and the amount of estrogens and progesterone secreted decreases. Perhaps not enough follicles are left to develop and secrete hormones. The ovaries then begin to degenerate, and the menstrual cycle becomes irregular and eventually halts. A sensation of heat ("hot flashes") sometimes occurs, probably because of the effect of decreased estrogen on the temperature-regulating center in the hypothalamus.

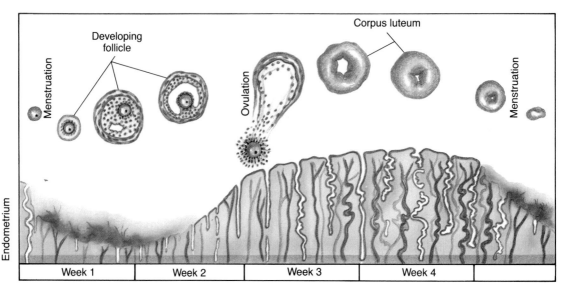

FIGURE 18–7 The menstrual cycle. The events that take place within the pituitary, ovary, and uterus are precisely synchronized. When fertilization does not occur, the cycle repeats itself about every 28 days.

Estrogen deficiency may also contribute to headaches and to feelings of depression experienced by some women. The vaginal lining thins, and the breasts and vulva begin to atrophy. Despite these physical changes, menopause does not usually affect a woman's interest in sex or her sexual performance. When missing hormones are replaced clinically, many of the symptoms of menopause cease.

FERTILIZATION IS THE FUSION OF SPERM AND OVUM

When sperm are released in the vagina, some find their way into the uterus and uterine tubes. Large numbers of sperm are necessary to penetrate the follicle cells surrounding the ovum (egg). As soon as one sperm penetrates the ovum, a series of reactions occurs in the membrane surrounding the ovum that prevents other sperm from entering the ovum. Sperm and ovum fuse to form a fertilized egg, or zygote.

After ejaculation, sperm remain viable for only about 48 hours. The ovum remains fertile for about 24 hours after ovulation. Thus there are only about 3 days each menstrual cycle (perhaps days 12 to 15 in a regular cycle) when sexual intercourse is likely to result in fertilization.

THE ZYGOTE GIVES RISE TO THE NEW INDIVIDUAL

The zygote contains all the genetic information (in its DNA) to produce a complete individual. The zygote divides to form an **embryo** composed of 2 cells. Each of these cells then divides to form 4 cells. As these first cell divisions take place, the embryo is pushed along the uterine tube toward the uterus (Fig. 18–8). By the time the embryo reaches the uterus on the fifth day of development, it is a tiny cluster of 16 cells.

THE EMBRYO DEVELOPS IN THE WALL OF THE UTERUS

On about the seventh day of development, the embryo begins to *implant* itself in the wall of the uterus. All further prenatal (before birth) development takes place within the uterine wall.

Several **fetal membranes** develop around the embryo. These membranes help protect, nourish, and support the developing embryo. They are discarded at birth. The **amnion** (am'-nee-ahn) is a membrane that forms a sac around the embryo. The fluid that fills the amnion keeps the embryo moist and cushions it (Fig. 18–9).

The **placenta** (plah-sen'-tah) is the organ of exchange between the mother and the embryo (Fig. 18–9). Nutrients and oxygen in the mother's blood move through the placenta and into the embryo. Wastes from the embryo move through the placenta and into the mother's blood.

The placenta produces a hormone called **human chorionic gonadotropin (hCG),** which signals the corpus luteum to increase in size and to release large amounts of estrogens and progesterone. These hormones stimulate the endometrium and the placenta to continue their development. Without hCG, the corpus luteum degenerates and the embryo is aborted. After about the eleventh week of preg-

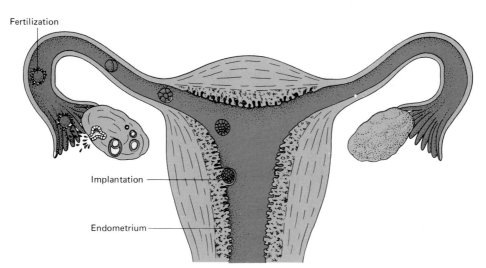

Fertilization

Implantation

Endometrium

FIGURE **18–8** Cell division takes place as the embryo is moved through the uterine tube to the uterus.

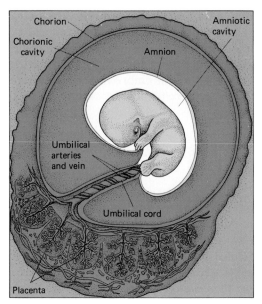

FIGURE **18–9** At about 45 days the embryo and its membranes together are about the size of a ping-pong ball, and the mother still may be unaware of her pregnancy. The amnion filled with amniotic fluid surrounds and cushions the embryo. Blood circulation has been established between the embryo and the maternal circulation through blood vessels that run through the umbilical cord to the placenta.

nancy, the placenta itself produces enough estrogens and progesterone to maintain pregnancy.

The stalk of tissue that connects the embryo with the placenta is the **umbilical cord** (Fig. 18–9). Two umbilical arteries deliver blood from the em-

bryo to the placenta, and an umbilical vein returns blood to the embryo.

PRENATAL DEVELOPMENT REQUIRES ABOUT 266 DAYS

From fertilization, about 266 days are required for the developing baby to complete its prenatal development (Figs. 18–10 to 18–12). By 4 weeks, many organs have begun to develop. The brain and spinal cord are among the first organs to develop, and by 4 weeks the eye and ear are visible. A simple circulatory system is working by this time. Small mounds of tissue called limb buds can be seen by the end of the first month and slowly lengthen and form the limbs.

After the second month, the embryo is referred to as a **fetus (fee'-tus)** (see Fig. 18–11). By the end of the third month, the fetus is almost 56 millimeters (mm) (2.2 inches) long and weighs about 14 grams (0.5 ounces). By 5 months of development, the fetus moves about in the amniotic fluid. At this time the mother usually becomes aware of fetal movements.

The last 3 months (last trimester) of development are a time of rapid growth and specialization of tissues and organs. If born prematurely before 7 months or weighing less than 1000 grams, the fetus is

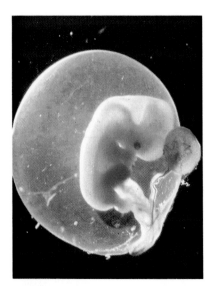

FIGURE **18–10** Human embryo at 5½ weeks, about 1 cm (0.4 inch) long. Note the developing limb buds. (Guigoz, Petit Format, Photo Researchers, Inc.)

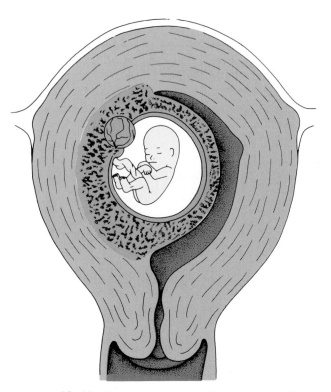

FIGURE **18–11** Human embryo at 10 weeks, 6 cm (2.4 inches) long.

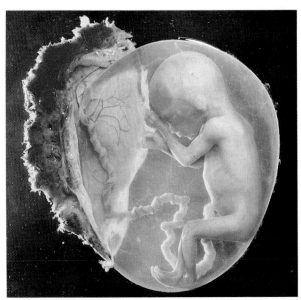

FIGURE 18-12 Human embryo at 16 weeks, about 16 cm (6.4 inches). *(From Nilsson, L.: A Child is Born. New York, Dell Publishing Co., Inc., 1977.)*

able to move about and cry but often dies because its brain is not developed enough to sustain such vital functions as breathing and regulation of body temperature.

During the seventh month, the cerebrum grows rapidly and develops convolutions. The grasp and sucking reflexes are present, and the fetus may suck its thumb. Most of the body is covered by downy hair (lanugo), which is usually shed before birth. At birth, the average full-term baby weights about 3000 grams (7 pounds) and measures about 52 cm (20 inches) in total length.

THE BIRTH PROCESS HAS THREE STAGES

Late in pregnancy the placenta begins to degenerate. The uterus is distended to its fullest capacity. Several days before birth, the fetus usually assumes an upside-down position preparing it to enter the birth canal head first. The factors that begin the birth process are not well understood.

Childbirth, or **parturition,** begins with a long series of involuntary contractions of the uterus, referred to as labor contractions. *Labor* may be divided into three stages.

During the **first stage,** regular uterine contractions occur. At first they may occur at about 30-minute intervals, but then they become more intense, rhythmical, and frequent, occurring as often as every minute (or even less) later in labor. As this

stage progresses, the cervix becomes *dilated* to about 10 cm (4 inches) and *effaced* (that is, continuous with the uterine wall, so it cannot be distinguished from the adjoining portion of the uterus), allowing passage of the fetal head. Rupture of the amnion with release of the amniotic fluid through the vagina may occur during this stage. The first stage of labor is the longest, often lasting 8 to 24 hours in a first pregnancy.

The **second stage** begins when the cervix is fully dilated and ends with the delivery of the baby. By contracting her abdominal muscles, the mother can help push the baby along through the vagina. When the **neonate** (newborn) emerges, it is still connected to the placenta by the umbilical cord. Most physicians clamp and cut the cord immediately after the infant has been delivered.

During the **third stage** of labor, the placenta separates from the uterus and is expelled. Generally, this occurs within 10 to 20 minutes after the birth of the baby. Now referred to as the afterbirth, the placenta is inspected for abnormalities and later discarded.

MULTIPLE BIRTHS MAY BE FRATERNAL OR IDENTICAL

In the United States, twins are born once in about 88 births, triplets once in 88 squared (7744), and quadruplets once in 88 cubed births. Twins (or other multiple births) can be either fraternal or identical. **Fraternal twins** develop when a woman ovulates 2 eggs and each is fertilized by a different sperm. Each fertilized egg has its own unique genetic endowment and the twins that develop are no more alike than any 2 siblings. Identical twins develop when the tiny mass of cells that makes up the early embryo divides to form 2 independent groups of cells, and each develops into a baby. Because the cells of each twin have developed from one fertilized egg, they have identical genes and are indeed **identical twins.** Rarely, the two masses of cells do not separate completely and develop into **conjoined** (Siamese) **twins.**

THE HUMAN LIFE CYCLE EXTENDS FROM FERTILIZATION TO DEATH

Development begins at fertilization and continues through the stages of the human life cycle until death. In this chapter we have briefly examined the development of the **embryo** and **fetus.** The **neonatal period** extends from birth to the end of the first month of postnatal life. **Infancy** follows the neonatal period and lasts until age 2 years; some consider infancy to end when the infant can assume an erect posture and walk, usually between the ages of 10 and 14 months. **Childhood,** also a period of rapid growth and development, continues from infancy until adolescence.

Adolescence is the time of development between puberty and adulthood. During adolescence, a young person experiences the physical and physiological changes that result in physical and reproductive maturity. This is also a time when young people make the psychological adjustments that prepare them to assume the responsibilities of adulthood. **Young adulthood** extends from adolescence until about age 40. **Middle age** is usually considered to be the period between ages 40 and 65. **Old age** begins after age 65.

SUMMARY

  I. The reproductive function of the male is to produce sperm and to deliver them into the female reproductive tract.
    A. Sperm are produced in tubules within the testes.
    B. From the tubules in the testes, sperm pass into an epididymis, where they complete maturation and may be stored. From the epididymis they enter the vas deferens. During ejaculation, sperm pass into the ejaculatory duct and then into the urethra, which extends through the penis.
    C. Most of the volume of the semen is produced by the seminal vesicles and the prostate gland. The bulbourethral glands produce a few drops of alkaline fluid prior to ejaculation.
    D. The penis consists of three columns of spongy tissue. When the large venous sinusoids of this tissue become engorged with blood, the penis becomes erect.
    E. The anterior lobe of the pituitary gland releases the gonadotropic hormones FSH and LH.
      1. FSH stimulates sperm production.
      2. LH stimulates the testes to secrete testosterone.
    F. Testosterone is responsible for the development of reproductive structures and the development and maintenance of secondary sex characteristics.
  II. The reproductive role of the female includes production of ova, receiving sperm, incubation and nourishment of the developing embryo, and lactation.
    A. Ova develop in the ovaries as part of follicles.
      1. After puberty, a few follicles begin to develop each month when stimulated by FSH.
      2. At ovulation, the ovum is ejected into the pelvic cavity. It then passes into the uterine tube, where it is either fertilized or deteriorates.
    B. If fertilized, the ovum begins to develop, and the embryo passes into the uterus, which serves as its incubator.
    C. The vagina is the lower part of the birth canal. It also receives the penis during sexual intercourse and serves as an outlet for menstrual discharge.
    D. The external female genital structures are collectively referred to as the vulva.
    E. The mammary glands within the breasts function in lactation.
    F. The first day of menstrual bleeding marks the first day of the menstrual cycle.
      1. In a "typical" 28-day cycle, ovulation occurs on about the fourteenth day.
      2. Events of the menstrual cycle are coordinated by the interaction of gonadotropic and ovarian hormones: (a) FSH stimulates follicle growth during the first 2 weeks of the cycle; (b) estrogens released from the developing follicles stimulate the endometrium to thicken; (c) LH released from the pituitary stimulates ovulation and the development of the corpus luteum; (d) the corpus luteum secretes progesterone and estrogens; (e) if fertilization does not occur, the corpus luteum begins to degenerate; (f) with the degeneration of the corpus luteum, estrogens and progesterone levels fall, and the endometrium begins to slough off again (menstruation).
    G. Estrogens are responsible for the development and maintenance of secondary sex characteristics; with progesterone, estrogens prepare the endometrium each month for possible pregnancy.

III. Millions of sperm are required for fertilization even though only one sperm actually fertilizes the ovum. The fertilized ovum is called a zygote.

IV. The zygote divides to form a two-celled embryo. Then each new cell divides again and again to form the new individual.
   A. On about the seventh day of development, the tiny embryo implants in the wall of the uterus.
   B. The amnion forms a protective sac of fluid around the embryo.
   C. The placenta is the organ of exchange between the mother and developing embryo.
   D. During the first stage of labor, the cervix dilates; during the second stage, the baby is delivered; during the third stage, the placenta is expelled.

V. The stages of the human life cycle include embryo, fetus, neonate, infant, child, adolescent, young adult, middle-aged adult, and old adult.

POST TEST

1. Sperm cells are produced in tubules within the _____ .

2. From the epididymis, sperm pass into the _____

   _____ .

3. Most of the semen is produced by the _____

   _____ .

4. Testosterone is produced by cells in the _____ .

5. The period of sexual maturation is called _____ .

6. Hormones produced by the ovary are _____ and

   _____ .

Match
Select the most appropriate answer in Column B for each question in Column A.

Column A
7. place where ova are produced
8. site of fertilization
9. part of uterus that projects into vagina
10. embryo implants here
11. external female genital structures

Column B
a. vulva
b. uterine tube
c. ovary
d. uterus
e. cervix

12. Ejection of the ovum from the follicle is called _____ .

13. In the female, FSH stimulates development of _____ .

14. The number of sperm that fertilize an ovum is _____ .

15. Lactation is the process of producing _____ .

16. A fertilized ovum is called a _____ .

17. The _____ is a fluid-filled sac around the embryo.

18. The _____ is the organ of exchange between mother and embryo.

19. The baby is delivered during the _____ stage of labor.

20. The hormone hCG (human chorionic gonadotropin) signals the

    _____ _____ that pregnancy has begun.

21. Label the diagrams on the following page.

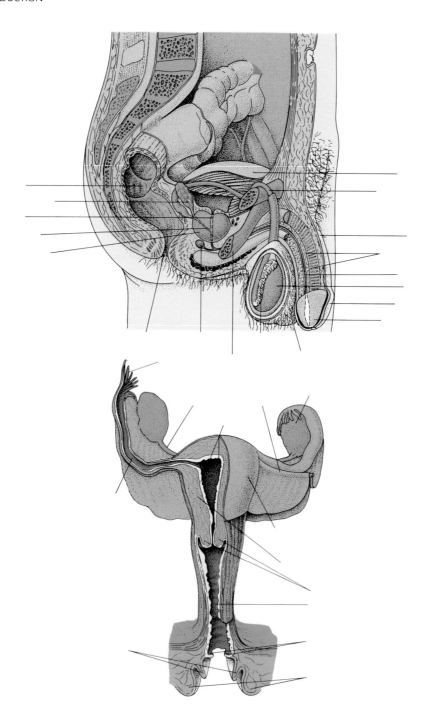

REVIEW QUESTIONS

1. The testes are located in the scrotum outside the pelvic cavity. Why?

2. What are the actions of testosterone?

3. Trace the path traveled by a sperm cell from the tubules of the testes until it is discharged from the body.

4. During sexual excitement the penis becomes erect. Relate this process to the internal structure of the penis.

5. What is the function of the corpus luteum? What hormone is necessary for its development?

6. In a typical 28-day menstrual cycle, when does ovulation occur? When does menstruation occur? When is a woman most likely to become pregnant?

7. What is puberty? What is menopause?

8. Trace the early development of the embryo.

POST TEST ANSWERS

1. testes
2. vas deferens
3. seminal vesicles
4. testes
5. puberty
6. estrogens; progesterone
7. c
8. b
9. e
10. d
11. a
12. ovulation
13. follicles
14. one
15. milk
16. zygote
17. amnion
18. placenta
19. second
20. corpus luteum
21. see Figures 18–1 and 18–4

APPENDICES

APPENDIX A   Dissecting Terms

APPENDIX B   The Metric System

APPENDIX A

Dissecting Terms
Common Prefixes, Suffixes, and Word Roots

Your task of mastering new terms will be greatly simplified if you learn to dissect each new word. Many terms can be divided into a prefix (the part of the word that precedes the main root), the word root itself, and often a suffix (a word ending that may add to or modify the meaning of the root). As you progress in your study of anatomy and physiology, you will learn to recognize the more common prefixes, word roots, and suffixes. Such recognition will help you analyze new terms so that you can determine their meaning and will also help you remember them.

PREFIXES

a-, ab- from, away, apart (*ab*duct, lead away, move away from the midline of the body)

a-, an- un-, -less, lack, not (*a*symmetrical, not symmetrical)

ad- (also **af-, ag-, an-, ap-**) to, toward (*ad*duct, move toward the midline of the body)

ambi- both sides (*ambi*dextrous, able to use either hand)

ante- forward, before (*ante*flexion, bending forward)

anti- against (*anti*coagulant, a substance that prevents coagulation of blood)

bi- two (*bi*ceps, a muscle with two heads of origin)

bio- life (*bio*logy, the study of life)

brady- slow (*brady*cardia, abnormally slow heart beat)

circum-, circ- around (*circum*cision, a cutting around)

co-, con- with, together (*con*genital, existing with or before birth)

contra- against (*contra*ception, against conception)

crypt- hidden (*crypt*orchidism, undescended or hidden testes)

cyt- cell (*cyt*ology, the study of cells)

di- two (*di*saccharide, a compound made of two sugar molecules chemically combined)

dis- (also **di-** or **dif-**) apart, un-, not (*dis*sect, cut apart)

dys- painful, difficult (*dys*pnea, difficult breathing)

end-, endo- within, inner (*endo*plasmic reticulum, a network of membranes found within the cytoplasm)

epi- on, upon (*epi*dermis, upon the dermis)

eu- good, well (*eu*phoria, a sense of well-being)

ex-, e-, ef- out from, out of (*ex*tension, a straightening out)

extra- outside, beyond (*extra*embryonic membrane, a membrane such as the amnion that protects the embryo)

hemi- half (cerebral *hemi*sphere, lateral half of the cerebrum)

hetero- other, different (*hetero*geneous, made of different substances)

homo-, hom- same (*homo*logous, corresponding in structure)

hyper- excessive, above normal (*hyper*secretion, excessive secretion)

265

hypo- under, below, deficient (*hypo*dermic, below the skin; *hypo*thyroidism, insufficiency of thyroid hormones)

in-, im- not (*im*balance, condition in which there is no balance)
inter- between, among (*inter*stitial, situated between parts)
intra- within (*intra*cellular, within the cell)
iso- equal, like (*iso*tonic, equal strength)

mal- bad, abnormal (*mal*nutrition, poor nutrition)
mega- large, great (*mega*karyocyte, giant cell of bone marrow)
meta- after, beyond (*meta*phase, the stage of mitosis after prophase)

neo- new (*neo*natal, newborn during the first 4 weeks after birth)

oo- egg (*oo*cyte, developing egg cell)
oligo- small, deficient (*oli*guria, abnormally small volume of urine)

para- near, beside, beyond (*para*central, near the center)
peri around (*peri*cardial membrane, membrane that surrounds the heart)
poly- multiple, complex (*poly*saccharide, a carbohydrate composed of many simple sugars)
post- after, behind (*post*natal, after birth)
pre- before (*pre*natal, before birth)

retro- backward (*retro*peritoneal, located behind the peritoneum)

semi- half (*semi*lunar, half-moon)
sub- under (*sub*cutaneous tissue, tissue immediately under the skin)
super-, supra- above (*supra*renal, above the kidney)
syn- with, together (*syn*drome, a group of symptoms that occur together and characterize a disease)

trans- across, beyond (*trans*port, carry across)

SUFFIXES

-able, -ible able (vi*able*, able to live)
-ac pertaining to (cardi*ac*, pertaining to the heart)
-ad used in anatomy to form adverbs of direction (cephal*ad*, toward the head)
-asis, -asia, -esis condition or state of (hemost*asis*, stopping of bleeding)

-cide kill, destroy (bio*cide*, substance that kills living things)

-ectomy surgical removal (append*ectomy*, surgical removal of the appendix)
-emia condition of blood (an*emia*, without enough blood)

-gen something produced or generated or something that produces or generates (patho*gen*, something that can cause disease)
-gram record, write (electrocardio*gram*, a record of the electrical activity of the heart)
-graph record, write (electrocardio*graph*, an instrument for recording the electrical activity of the heart)

-itis inflammation of (appendic*itis*, inflammation of the appendix)

-logy study or science of (physio*logy*, study of the function of the body)

-oid like, in the form of (thyr*oid*, in the form of a shield)
-oma tumor (carcin*oma*, a malignant tumor)
-osis indicates disease (psych*osis*, a mental disease)
-ous, -ose full of (poison*ous*, full of poison)

-scope instrument for viewing or observing (micro*scope*, instrument for viewing small objects)
-stomy refers to a surgical procedure in which an artificial opening is made (colo*stomy*, surgical formation of an artificial anus)

-tomy cutting or section (appende*ctomy*, cutting out the appendix)

-uria refers to urine (poly*uria*, excessive production of urine)

SOME COMMON WORD ROOTS

aden gland, glandular (*aden*osis, a glandular disease)
alg pain (neur*alg*ia, nerve pain)
arthr joint (*arthr*itis, inflammation of the joints)

bi, bio life (*bio*logy, study of life)
blast a formative cell, germ layer (osteo*blast,* cell that gives rise to bone cells)
brachi arm (*brachi*al artery, blood vessel that supplies the arm)
bronch branch of the trachea (*bronch*itis, inflammation of the bronchi)
bry grow, swell (em*bry*o, an organism in the early stages of development)

carcin cancer (*carcin*ogenic, cancer-producing)
cardi heart (*cardi*ac, pertaining to the heart)
cephal head (*cephal*ad, toward the head)
cerebr brain (*cerebr*al, pertaining to the brain)
cervic, cervix neck (*cervic*al, pertaining to the neck)
chol bile (*chol*ecystogram, an x-ray of the gallbladder)
chondr cartilage (*chondr*ocyte, a cartilage cell)
chrom color (*chrom*osome, deeply staining body in nucleus)
cran skull (*cran*ial, pertaining to the skull)
cyt cell (*cyt*ology, study of the cells)

derm skin (*derm*atology, study of the skin)
duct, duc lead (*duct,* passageway)

ecol dwelling, house (*ecol*ogy, the study of organisms in relation to their environment)
enter intestine (*enter*itis, inflammation of the intestine)
evol to unroll (*evol*ution, descent of complex organisms from simpler ancestors)

gastr stomach (*gastr*itis, inflammation of the stomach)
gen generate, produce (*gen*e, a hereditary factor)
glyc, glyco sweet, sugar (*glyco*gen, storage form of glucose)
gon semen, seed (*gon*ad, an organ producing gametes)

hem, em blood (*hem*atology, the study of blood)
hepat, hepar liver (*hepat*itis, inflammation of the liver)
hist tissue (*hist*ology, study of tissues)
hom, homeo same, unchanging, steady (*homeo*stasis, reaching a steady state)
hydr water (*hydr*olysis, a breakdown reaction involving water)

leuk white (*leuk*ocyte, white blood cell)

macro large (*macro*phage, large janitor cell)
mamm breast (*mamm*ary glands, the glands that produce milk to nourish the young)
micro small (*micro*scope, instrument for viewing small objects)
morph form (*morph*ogenesis, development of body form)
my, mys muscle (*my*ocardium, muscle layer of the heart)

nephr kidney (*nephr*on, microscopic unit of the kidney)
neur, nerv nerve (*neur*algia, pain associated with nerve)
neutr neither one nor the other (*neutr*on, a subatomic particle that is neither positively nor negatively charged)

occiput back part of the head (*occiput*al, back region of the head)
ost, oss bone (*ost*eology, study of bones)

path disease (*path*ologist, one who studies disease processes)
ped child (*ped*iatrics, branch of medicine specializing in children)
ped, pod foot (bi*ped,* organism with two feet)
phag eat (*phag*ocytosis, process by which certain cells ingest particles and foreign matter)
phil love (hydro*phil*ic, a substance that attracts water)
proct anus (*proct*oscope, instrument for examining rectum and anal canal)
psych mind (*psych*ology, study of the mind)

scler hard (arthero*scler*osis, hardening of the arterial wall)
som body (chromo*som*e, deeply staining body in the nucleus)
stas, stat stand (*stas*is, condition in which blood stands, as opposed to flowing)

thromb clot (*thromb*us, a clot within the body)

ur urea, urine (*ur*ologist, a physician specializing in the urinary tract)

visc pertaining to an internal organ or body cavity (*visc*era, internal organs)

APPENDIX B

The Metric System

Standard metric units		
METRIC UNITS		**ABBREVIATIONS**
Standard unit of mass	gram	g
Standard unit of length	meter	m
Standard unit of volume	liter	l

Some common prefixes		
PREFIXES		**EXAMPLES**
kilo	1,000	a kilogram is 1000 grams
centi	0.01	a centimeter is 0.01 meter
milli	0.001	a milliliter is 0.001 liter
micro (μ)	one-millionth	a micrometer is 0.000001 (one millionth) of a meter
nano (n)	one-billionth	a nanogram is 10^{-9} (one billionth) of a gram
pico (p)	one-trillionth	a picogram is 10^{-12} (one trillionth) of a gram

Some common units of length

UNIT	ABBREVIATION	EQUIVALENT
meter	m	approximately 39 in
centimeter	cm	10^{-2} m
millimeter	mm	10^{-3} m
micrometer	μm	10^{-6} m
nanometer	nm	10^{-9} m
angstrom	Å	10^{-10} m

LENGTH CONVERSIONS

1 in = 2.5 cm   1 mm = 0.039 in
1 ft = 30 cm   1 cm = 0.39 in
1 yd = 0.9 cm   1 m = 39 in
1 mi = 1.6 km   1 m = 1.094 yd
                 1 km = 0.6 mi

To convert	Multiply by	To obtain
inches	2.54	centimeters
feet	30	centimeters
centimeters	0.39	inches
millimeters	0.039	inches

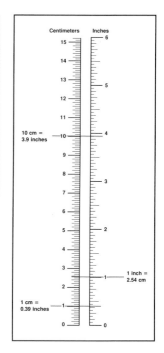

Temperature conversions

TEMPERATURE	SOME EQUIVALENTS
$^\circ C = \dfrac{(^\circ F - 32) \times 5}{9}$	$1^\circ C = 1.8^\circ F$
	$10^\circ C = 18^\circ F$
$^\circ F = \dfrac{^\circ C \times 9}{5} + 32$	$16^\circ C = 61^\circ F$

Think Celsius!

When room temperature is 20° C, you probably will not feel cold. That is the same as 68° F.

When the temperature reaches 100° C, water boils.

At 0° C, water freezes.

Normal human body temperature is about 37° C.

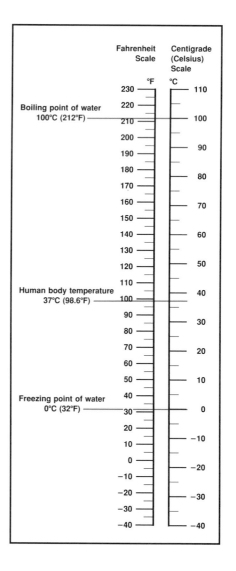

GLOSSARY

abdomen (**ab**-doe-men) The region of the body between the diaphragm and the pelvis.

abdominal cavity (ab-**dom**-ih-nal) The superior part of the abdominopelvic cavity containing the liver, gallbladder, spleen, stomach, pancreas, and small intestine and part of the large intestine.

abdominopelvic cavity (ab-*dom*-ih-no-**pel**-vic) The lower part of the ventral body cavity below the thoracic cavity.

abduction (ab-**duk**-shun) A movement whereby a body part is drawn away from the main body axis or the axis of a limb.

ABO blood types A system of categorizing blood, based on the presence or absence of specific surface antigens.

abortion (ah-**bor**-shun) Expulsion of an embryo or fetus before it is capable of surviving outside the uterus.

absorption (ab-**sorp**-shun) The passage of material into or through a cell or tissue, as in the movement of digested nutrients from the GI tract into the blood or lymph.

acetylcholine (*as*-ee-til-**koe**-leen) A neurotransmitter released by cholinergic nerves, such as those stimulating skeletal muscle contraction.

Achilles' tendon (ah-**kil**-eez) The tendon of the gastrocnemius and soleus muscle that inserts upon the calcaneus (heel bone).

acid (**as**-id) A proton donor or compound that dissociates in solution to produce hydrogen ions and some type of anion.

acquired immune deficiency syndrome (AIDS) A disease caused by the HIV virus in which a deficiency develops in helper T cells. Symptoms include fever, night sweats, sore throat, coughing, enlarged lymph nodes, body aches, fatigue, and weight loss. No cure is presently known.

acromegaly (*ak*-roe-**meg**-ah-lee) A condition resulting from a hypersecretion of growth hormone in the adult. It is characterized by enlarged bones in the extremities and face along with the enlargement of other tissues.

actin (**ak**-tin) A contractile protein of the thin filaments within a muscle cell.

action potential The electrical activity developed in a muscle or nerve cell during activity; also called a nerve or muscle impulse.

active immunity An acquired immunity resulting from the production of antibodies in response to exposure to antigens.

active transport The movement of substances through cell membranes against concentration gradients. Active transport requires energy expenditure.

acute (a-**kyout**) Having a short and relatively severe course; not chronic.

Adam's apple The thyroid cartilage of the larynx. In males, it is pronounced because of enlargement caused by testosterone.

adduction (ad-**duk**-shun) A movement whereby a body part is drawn toward the main body axis or the axis of a limb.

adenosine triphosphate (ATP) (a-**den**-oh-seen try-**fos**-fate) The energy currency of the cell; a chemical compound used to transfer energy from those biochemical reactions that yield energy to those that require it.

adipose tissue A type of connective tissue characterized by the presence of many fat cells.

adrenal cortex (ah-**dree**-nal **kore**-tekz) The outer part of the adrenal gland. It has three zones, each producing different hormones.

adrenal glands (ah-**dree**-nal) The two glands located superior to the kidneys. They are also known as the suprarenal glands.

adrenal medulla (ah-**dree**-nal meh-**dul**-ah) The inner part of the adrenal gland that secretes catecholamines (epinephrine and norepinephrine) in response to sympathetic stimulation.

adrenocorticotropic hormone (ACTH) (ad-*ree*-no-kore-ti-kow-**trope**-ik) A hormone produced and released by the anterior pituitary that causes the production and release of hormones of the adrenal cortex.

adventitia (*ad*-ven-**tish**-eah) The outermost layer or covering of an organ or structure.

aerobic (air-**oh**-bik) Requiring molecular oxygen.

afferent (**af**-er-ent) Indicates movement *toward* a structure.

afferent arteriole (**af**-er-ent ar-**tee**-ree-ole) The blood vessel within the kidney that carries blood to the glomerulus.

afferent neuron A nerve cell that carries information toward the central nervous system. It is also called a sensory neuron.

afterbirth The separated placenta and membranes expelled from the uterus after childbirth.

agglutination (a-*glue*-tin-**nay**-shun) The aggregation of particles into masses or clumps, especially in reference to microbes and blood cells.

albumin (al-**byou**-min) The smallest and most abundant of the plasma proteins.

aldosterone (al-**dos**-ter-own) The principal mineralocorticoid of the adrenal cortex. It increases sodium reabsorption in the kidneys. It also enhances water reabsorption and potassium excretion.

alimentary canal (*al*-ih-**men**-tah-ree) The digestive tract.

alkaline (**al**-kuh-line) A solution containing more hydroxyl ions than hydrogen ions resulting in a pH greater than 7.

allergen (**al**-er-jen) An antigen that produces an allergic reaction.

allergy (**al**-ur-jee) A state of altered immunological reactivity or hypersensitivity.

All-or-none law The phenomenon by which a stimulus produces maximal response or no response at all. If the stimulus is subthreshold, no response occurs. If the stimulus is threshold or greater, a maximal response occurs.

alpha cell (**al**-fah) Endocrine cells or the islets of Langerhans of the pancreas that produce the hormone glucagon.

alveolar gland (al-**vee**-oh-lar) A type of gland characterized by a small hollow sac.

alveolus (al-**vee**-oh-lus) A small hollow sac. 1. The air sacs of the lungs functioning in gas exchange with the blood. 2. The milk-secreting sacs of a mammary gland.

amino acid An organic acid possessing both an amine (NH_2) and a carboxyl group (COOH). Amino acids are the basic units of proteins.

amnion (**am**-nee-on) An extraembryonic membrane that forms a fluid-filled sac for the protection of the developing embryo.

amphiarthrosis (*am*-fee-ar-**throw**-sis) Joint showing slight movement; the joints between vertebrae.

anabolism (a-**nab**-o-*lizm*) The synthesizing or building-up part of metabolism in which small molecules combine to form larger ones.

anaerobic (*an*-air-**oh**-bik) Processes not requiring molecules of oxygen.

anal canal The terminal end of the rectum.

anaphase (**an**-ah-faze) Third stage of mitosis in which the chromatids of each chromosome separate at their centromeres and move to opposite poles.

anaphylaxis (*an*-ah-fih-**lak**-sis) An unusual or exaggerated allergic reaction.

anastomosis (ah-*nas*-toe-**moe**-sis) The union or communication of blood vessels, nerves, or lymphatics.

anatomical position (*an*-ah-**tom**-ih-kal) The positioning of the body for descriptive purposes in which the body stands erect, facing the viewer, with upper limbs at sides and palms facing anteriorly.

anatomy (a-**nat**-o-mee) The study of the structures of the body and their relationships.

androgen (**an**-drow-jen) A substance, such as testosterone, stimulating or producing male characteristics.

anemia (ah-**nee**-mee-ah) A deficiency of hemoglobin or number of red blood cells.

angiotensins (*an*-jee-o-**ten**-sins) A group of compounds found in blood that constrict blood vessels.

anion (**an**-eye-on) A negatively charged ion such as Cl^-.

antagonist (an-**tag**-o-nist) A muscle opposing the action of another muscle, its agonist.

anterior (an-**tee**-ree-or) Located in front of or nearer to the front of the body. Anterior is also ventral or at the belly side.

anterior root The ventral root of a spinal nerve; consists of motor fibers.

antibiotic (*an*-ti-bye-**ot**-ik) A chemical substance produced by a microbe that inhibits growth or kills other microorganisms.

antibody (**an**-ti-*bod*-ee) A protein compound that is produced by plasma cells in response to a specific antigen. The antibody renders the antigen harmless. It is also called an immunoglobulin.

antidiuretic (*an*-ti-die-you-**ret**-ik) A substance that decreases or inhibits the formation of urine.

antidiuretic hormone (ADH) A hormone produced in the hypothalamus and stored in the posterior pituitary. ADH increases water reabsorption in the kidneys.

antigen (**an**-tih-jen) A substance foreign to the body that causes the production of antibodies when introduced into the body.

antihistamine (*an*-ti-**his**-tah-min) A drug blocking the effects of histamine.

anus (**ay**-nus) The distal end and outlet of the digestive tract.

aorta (ay-**or**-tah) The largest and main systemic artery of the body. It arises from the left ventricle and branches to distribute blood to all parts of the body.

aqueous humor (**ak**-wee-us **hyou**-mor) A serous fluid within the anterior cavity of the eye.

arachnoid membrane (ah-**rak**-noyd) The middle meninx of the central nervous system located between the dura mater and the pia mater.

areola (ah-**ree**-o-lah) The dark pigmented area surrounding the nipple of the mammary gland.

arm The region of the upper limb between the shoulder and the elbow.

arrector pili (a-**rek**-tor **pi**-lee) The smooth muscle associated with hairs whose contraction causes the hair to assume a more vertical position. The contraction of the arrector pili results in "goose bumps."

arteriole (ar-**tee**-ree-ole) A small artery that carries blood to capillaries. Vasoconstriction and vasodilation of arterioles help regulate blood pressure and blood distribution to the tissues.

artery (**ar**-ter-ee) A thick-walled blood vessel that carries blood away from the heart.

arthritis (ar-**thrye**-tis) The inflammation of a joint.

ascending colon (**koe**-lon) The part of the large intestine that extends from the cecum upward to the lower border of the liver. The ascending colon is on the right side of the abdomen.

association area Cortical area of cerebrum having sensory and motor fibers connected to other cortical areas. The association area is involved with higher mental and emotional processes.

association neuron A nerve cell located entirely within the central nervous system that transmits information between sensory and motor neurons. It is also called an interneuron.

asthma (**az**-muh) A disease characterized by airway constriction, often leading to difficult breathing or dyspnea.

astigmatism (ah-**stig**-mah-tizm) A defect of vision resulting from irregularity in the curvature of the cornea or lens.

atherosclerosis (*ath*-er-o-skleh-**roe**-sis) A progressive disease in which smooth muscle cells and lipid deposits accumulate in the inner lining of arteries leading to decreased arterial diameters and impairment of circulation.

atom The smallest particle of an element with the chemical properties of that element.

ATP Abbreviation for adenosine triphosphate. The energy currency of the cell. A chemical compound used to transfer energy from those biochemical reactions that yield energy to those that require it.

atrioventricular node The part of the cardiac conduction system within the right atrium near the opening of the coronary sinus.

atrioventricular valve A valve between each atrium and its ventricle that prevents a backflow of blood.

atrium (**ay**-tree-um) A superior chamber of the heart that receives blood from veins.

auditory ossicle (**aw**-di-*toe*-ree **os**-sih-kul) One of the three bones of the middle ear.

auditory tube The tube connecting the middle ear cavity with the nasopharynx. It is also called the eustachian tube.

auricle (**or**-i-kul) 1. A small, muscular pouch of the atria of the heart. 2. The pinna or flap of the outer ear.

autoimmune disease A disease in which the body produces antibodies against its own cells or tissues.

autonomic ganglion (*aw*-toe-**nom**-ik **gang**-lee-on) A collection of cell bodies of either the sympathetic or parasympathetic nervous systems located outside of the central nervous system.

autonomic nervous system The portion of the peripheral nervous system that controls the visceral functions of the body by innervating smooth muscle, cardiac muscle, or glands.

axilla (ak-**sil**-ah) The armpit area of the shoulder region of the body.

axon (**ak**-son) The long, tubular extension of a neuron that transmits nerve impulses away from the cell body.

ball-and-socket joint The type of synovial joint in which the rounded head of one bone moves within a fossa or cup-shaped depression of another.

baroreceptor (*bar*-oh-re-**sep**-tor) Receptor found within certain blood vessels that is stimulated by changes in blood pressure.

basal ganglia (**bay**-sal **gang**-lee-ah) The cerebral nuclei located deep within the white matter of the cerebrum that play an important role in movement.

basal metabolic rate (BMR) The rate of metabolism measured under standard or basal conditions.

base A substance which when dissolved in water produces a pH greater than 7. Most bases yield hydroxyl ions (OH^-) when dissolved in water. A base is also referred to as an alkali.

basophil (**bay**-so-fil) A type of white blood cell (leukocyte), stained by basic dyes, that is involved in allergic and inflammatory reactions.

B cell A type of white blood cell responsible for antibody-mediated immunity. When stimulated, B cells differentiate to become plasma cells that produce antibodies. B cells are also called B lymphocytes.

belly 1. The bulge in the middle of spindle-shaped muscle. 2. The abdomen.

benign (be-**nine**) Refers to a tumor that is not malignant.

beta cell (**bay**-tah) A cell in the islets of Langerhans of the pancreas producing insulin.

beta receptor A receptor on visceral effectors innervated by postganglionic fibers of the sympathetic nervous system.

bicuspid valve (bye-**kus**-pid) The left atrioventricular valve separating the left atrium from the left ventricle. It is also known as the mitral valve.

bilateral (bye-**lat**-er-al) Referring to the two sides of the body.

bile (byl) The greenish fluid secreted by the liver containing bile salts and bile pigments. Bile salts emulsify fats in the small intestine.

bilirubin (*bil*-ee-**roo**-bin) A red bile pigment that gives the feces their characteristic brown color. Bilirubin is produced by the breakdown of hemoglobin in the liver.

blind spot The area of the retina in which the optic nerve ends and which lacks photoreceptors.

blood The fluid circulating within the heart and blood vessels and that provides the main transport of substances throughout the body.

blood-brain barrier The barrier separating the blood from the brain that prevents many substances from entering the cerebrospinal fluid from the blood.

blood pressure The force exerted upon the walls of the blood vessels by the blood. A blood pressure measurement is a measure of pressure during ventricular contraction and ventricular relaxation.

blood vessel A tube transporting blood in a circulatory system. The major blood vessels are the arteries, capillaries, and veins.

body cavity A space of the body containing organs.

bolus (**boe**-lus) A rounded mass of food that has been moistened for swallowing.

bone A hard type of connective tissue containing calcium salts that makes up most of the skeletal system.

bony labyrinth Cavities within the temporal bone forming the chambers of the inner ear.

Bowman's capsule The expanded cup-like end of proximal nephron surrounding the glomerulus.

bradycardia (*brad*-i-**kar**-dee-ah) A slow heart rate of less than 60 beats per minute.

brain Nervous tissue in the cranial cavity that with the spinal cord makes up the central nervous system.

brain stem The elongated part of the brain located superior to the spinal cord that contains the medulla, pons, and midbrain.

Broca's area (**broe**-kaz) A part of the premotor area of the cerebrum involved with directing the formation of words.

bronchiole (**brong**-kee-ol) A small branch of a tertiary bronchus whose terminal branches (respiratory bronchioles) divide into alveolar ducts.

bronchitis (brong-**kye**-tis) An inflammation of the bronchi.

buccal (**buk**-al) Pertaining to the mouth or the cheek area.

buffer (**buf**-er) A substance that minimizes changes in pH.

bulbourethral gland (*bul*-boe-you-**ree**-thral) One of two glands located inferior to the prostate gland of the male, secreting an alkaline solution into the urethra during sexual excitation. It is also called Cowper's gland.

bursa (**bur**-sah) A small sac lined with synovial membrane and filled with fluid interposed between nearby body parts that move in relation to each other.

bursitis (bur-**sye**-tis) An inflammation of the bursa.

buttocks (**but**-okz) A pair of prominences of the lower back formed by the gluteal muscles.

calcaneus (kal-**kay**-nee-us) The heel bone.

calcitonin (*kal*-sih-**toe**-nin) A thyroid hormone that lowers calcium and phosphate levels in the blood by stimulating calcium absorption by bone and inhibiting the breakdown of bone.

calorie (**kal**-o-ree) A unit of heat that is used in the study of metabolism and is defined as the amount of heat required to raise the temperature of 1 kilogram of water 1 degree Celsius.

calyx (**kayl**-ikz) A process of the renal pelvis of the kidney. *Plural,* calyces.

cancer (**kan**-ser) A malignant tumor in which cells multiply uncontrollably and invasively, infiltrating adjacent tissues and often spreading to other parts of the body. Also called carcinoma.

canine (**kay**-nine) The tooth between the incisors and the premolars in each quadrant of teeth.

capillary (**kap**-ih-lar-ee) The smallest blood vessel that permits exchanges to take place between the blood and body tissues.

carbohydrate (*kar*-boe-**hye**-drayt) An organic compound (e.g., sugar or starch) composed of carbon, hydrogen, and oxygen in which the numbers of hydrogen and oxygen atoms are in approximately 2:1 proportion.

cardiac (**kar**-dee-ak) Pertaining to the heart.

cardiac cycle The sequence of events occurring during one complete heartbeat.

cardiac muscle One of three types of muscle. Cardiac muscle is located within the heart.

cardiac output The volume of blood pumped by one ventricle in one minute. Cardiac output averages about 5.2 l/min at rest.

cartilage (**kar**-tih-lij) A specialized fibrous connective tissue that forms most of the temporary skeleton of the embryo. It also serves as the skeletal tissue for certain regions of the body such as the external ear and the tip of the nose.

castration (kas-**tray**-shun) Surgical removal of the gonads, especially the testes.

catabolism (kah-**tab**-o-lizm) The breaking-down phase of metabolism in which complex substances are broken down into simpler compounds with the release of energy.

catecholamine (*kat*-e-**kole**-ah-*mean*) A class of chemical compounds that includes the transmitter substances epinephrine, norepinephrine, and dopamine.

cation A positively charged ion.

cecum The blind sac that marks the first part of the large intestine.

cell The basic structural and functional unit of the body, consisting of organelles bounded by a cellular membrane, and usually microscopic in size.

cell body The part of a neuron, containing the nucleus, where most of the materials needed by the neuron are produced.

cell-mediated immunity The immunologic process whereby specially sensitized lymphocytes or T cells combine with antigens and destroy them. Also called cellular immunity.

cementum (se-**men**-tum) A bonelike substance forming the outer layer of the root of a tooth that attaches the root to the jaw bones.

central canal The circular canal running the length of the spinal cord.

central nervous system (CNS) The subdivision of the nervous system containing the brain and the spinal cord.

cephalic (se-**fal**-ik) Pertaining to, or directionally close to, the head.

cerebellum (*ser*-eh-**bel**-um) The deeply convoluted subdivision of the brain lying beneath the cerebrum that is concerned with the coordination of muscular movements. It is part of the metencephalon.

cerebral aqueduct (**ser**-eh-bral **ak**-we-dukt) The channel running through the midbrain that connects the third and fourth ventricles. It is also called the aqueduct of Sylvius.

cerebral cortex The outer part of the cerebrum, composed of gray matter and consisting mainly of nerve cell bodies.

cerebral palsy (**pal**-zee) Nonprogressive motor disorders caused by perinatal damage to the motor areas of the brain.

cerebrospinal fluid (CSF) (se-*ree*-broe-**spy**-nal) A clear fluid that circulates within the cavities of the central nervous system and within the subarachnoid space.

cerebrovascular accident (CVA) (se-*ree*-broe-**vas**-kyou-lar) Disorders of the blood vessels supplying the brain that result in damage to neural tissues of the brain. Also called a stroke.

cerebrum (se-**ree**-brum) The largest subdivision of the brain containing centers for learning, voluntary movement, and the interpretation of sensation.

cervical (**ser**-vih-kul) Pertaining to the neck or cervix.

cervical plexus (**plek**-sus) A network of the branches of anterior rami of cervical nerves C1–C4 that mainly supplies neck structures.

cervix (**ser**-viks) Neck or a constricted area of an organ, as in the cervix of the uterus.

chiasma (kye-**az**-mah) An X-shaped crossing, as in the optic chiasma formed by the crossing of the optic nerves.

cholesterol (koe-**les**-te-rol) The steroid that is a component of cell membranes and is used in the production of steroid hormones and bile salts.

cholinergic fiber (*koe*-lin-**er**-jik) A neuron releasing acetylcholine as its neurotransmitter.

cholinesterase (*koe*-lin-**es**-ter-ayz) An enzyme breaking down acetylcholine.

chondrocyte (**kon**-droe-site) A mature cartilage cell.

chordae tendineae (**kor**-dee **ten**-di-nee) Cords connecting the cardiac papillary muscles with the atrioventricular valves.

choroid (**koe**-royd) The black vascular coat of the eye between the sclera and the retina.

choroid plexus Specialized capillary network projecting from the pia mater into the ventricles of the brain, forming cerebrospinal fluid.

chromosome (**kroe**-mo-sowm) One of 46 discrete

rod-shaped bodies in the nucleus of a cell undergoing mitosis that contains genes composed of DNA.

chronic (**kron**-ik) Of a long duration or recurring frequently, as in a chronic disease.

chyme (kime) The semifluid mixture of partially digested food and gastric juices.

cilia (**sil**-ee-uh) Threadlike cellular organelles that project from the surface of some cells and by their movement can propel a stream of fluid.

ciliary muscle Smooth muscle of the ciliary body of the eye that functions in visual accommodation.

circle of Willis A circular anastomosis at the base of the brain.

circumcision (*ser*-kum-**sizh**-un) Removal of the prepuce (foreskin) of the penis.

circumduction (*ser*-kum-**duk**-shun) The movement of a limb in such a manner that its distal part describes a circle.

climax The time of greatest intensity, as in sexual response or the course of a disease.

clitoris (**kli**-to-ris) A small erectile organ located at the top of the vulva which serves as the center of sexual sensation in the female.

clot A semisolid mass. A blood clot results from a cascade of biochemical reactions ending in the conversion of fibrinogen into fibrin.

coccyx (**kok**-six) The bone formed by the fusion of the four coccygeal vertebrae at the inferior end of the vertebral column.

cochlea (**koke**-lee-ah) The spirally shaped portion of the temporal bone that houses the membranous labyrinth used in the sense of hearing.

coenzyme A small, nonprotein molecule essential for an enzyme to operate.

coitus (**koe**-i-tus) The act of copulation or sexual intercourse in which the penis is inserted into the vagina.

collagen (**kol**-a-jen) A fibrous protein found in collagen fibers that is the principal support of many connective tissues.

colon The part of the large intestine consisting of the ascending, transverse, descending, and sigmoid sections.

color blindness An abnormal perception of one or more colors caused by the absence of one or more of the photopigments in the cones.

commissure (**kom**-i-shyour) A joining site between corresponding parts as in the eyelids or lips.

common bile duct The duct formed by the union of the common hepatic duct with the cystic duct which takes bile to the duodenum.

compact bone Dense skeletal tissue that has tightly joined layers.

complement A sequence of proteins in plasma and other body fluids activated by an antigen-antibody complex, functioning in destroying invading pathogens.

compound In chemistry, a substance composed of two or more chemically united elements in definite proportion.

conception The process of fertilization and the subsequent establishment of pregnancy.

concha (**kong**-kah) Skull bones with a shell-like shape.

condyle (**kon**-dial) A rounded projection on a bone.

cone The photoreceptors of the retina of the eye involved in color vision.

congenital (kon-**jen**-i-tal) Refers to a condition existing before or at birth.

conjunctiva (*kon*-junk-**tye**-vah) The membrane covering the eyeball and eyelids.

connective tissue A diverse group of tissues that support and protect the organs of the body and hold body parts together; characterized by a large proportion of intercellular substance through which its cells are scattered.

contralateral (*kon*-trah-**lat**-er-al) Referring to the opposite side of the body or a body part.

cornea (**kor**-nee-ah) The transparent anterior portion of the outer covering of the eyeball.

coronal plane (koe-**roe**-nal) A plane running vertical to the ground and dividing the body into anterior and posterior parts. Also called a frontal plane.

coronary (**kor**-o-na-ree) Pertaining to the heart.

coronary artery disease A disorder in which the cardiac muscle receives an inadequate amount of blood because of a disruption of its blood supply.

coronary sinus A large vein on the posterior side of the heart that drains smaller coronary veins and empties into the right atrium.

corpus callosum (kal-**loe**-sum) The largest cerebral commissure that connects the cerebral hemispheres.

corpus luteum (**loo**-tee-um) The yellow endocrine body that develops from the ruptured follicle after ovulation and secretes progesterone and estrogens.

cortex (**kor**-teks) The outer portion of an organ, as in the adrenal cortex or outer part of the cerebrum.

cortisol (**kor**-ti-sol) Principal glucocorticoid secreted by the adrenal cortex.

costal cartilage (**kos**-tal **kar**-ti-lij) The hyaline cartilage forming the articulation of the first 10 ribs to the sternum or each other.

cranial nerves The 12 pairs of nerves emerging from the brain that transmit information directly between certain sensory receptors and the brain and between the brain and certain effectors.

cranium (**kray**-nee-um) The bones of the skull case, including the frontal, parietal, temporal, occipital, ethmoid, and sphenoid bones.

creatine phosphate An intermediate energy-transfer compound occurring mainly in muscles.

cretinism (**kree**-tin-izm) A condition in which a person is dwarfed and mentally retarded by severe deficiency of thyroid hormones during childhood.

Cushing's syndrome A condition caused by abnormally large amounts of glucocorticoids; characterized by edema, an abnormal deposition of fat to the face and trunk, and an increased susceptibility to infection.

cutaneous (kyou-**tay**-nee-us) Referring to the skin.

deamination The removal of an amino group from an amino acid.

decibel (**des**-i-bel) A unit of measurement of sound intensity.

deciduous teeth (dee-**sid**-you-us) The primary teeth or the first set of human dentition. Also called the milk or baby teeth.

dehydration (*dee*-hi-**dray**-shun) The condition due to excessive water loss from the body or its parts.

dendrite (**den**-dryt) A short branch of a neuron that receives nerve impulses and conducts them to the cell body.

dentin (**den**-tin) The layer forming the body of the tooth; lies under the enamel and cementum and encloses the pulp.

depolarization (dee-*poe*-lar-i-**zay**-shun) Decreasing the electrical voltage across a plasma membrane or neutralizing its polarity.

dermis (**der**-mis) The thick layer of skin composed of irregular dense connective tissue that is located beneath the epidermis.

descending colon The section of the large intestine located between the transverse colon and sigmoid colon.

dextrin (**dek**-strin) A small polysaccharide containing several glucose molecules.

diabetes insipidus (*dye*-ah-**bee**-teez in-**sip**-i-dus) A disease resulting from insufficiency of antidiuretic hormone (ADH) and characterized by the production of large volumes of urine.

diabetes mellitus (**mel**-ih-tus) A disease resulting from insulin deficiency in which there is an excessive amount of glucose in the blood and an excessive volume of urine is produced.

dialysis (dye-**al**-ih-sis) The diffusion of solutes through a selectively permeable membrane, resulting in separation of solutes.

diaphragm (**dye**-ah-fram) The muscle separating the thoracic cavity from the abdominal cavity. It functions in breathing.

diaphysis (dye-**af**-ih-sis) The shaft of a long bone.

diarthroses (*dye*-ar-**throe**-seez) Joint articulations in which the bones are freely movable. Also called synovial joints.

diastole (dye-**as**-toe-lee) The time during the cardiac cycle in which the ventricles are relaxing.

diencephalon (*dye*-en-**sef**-a-lon) The part of the prosencephalon (forebrain) of the brain that primarily consists of the thalamus and the hypothalamus.

diffusion (dif-**you**-zhun) The net movement of solvent or solute molecules from a higher concentration to a lower concentration, resulting in the tendency of a molecular mixture to attain a uniform composition throughout.

digestion (di-**jes**-chun) The process of mechanical or chemical breaking-down of food into molecules small enough to be absorbed.

digestive system The digestive tract and the accessory digestive structures.

distal (**dis**-tal) Farther from the midline or point of attachment to the trunk.

diuretic (dye-you-**ret**-ik) A substance that inhibits the reabsorption of water and thus increases urine output.

DNA Abbreviation for deoxyribonucleic acid. The basic storage molecule for genetic information. DNA is a nucleic acid whose pentose sugar is deoxyribose and whose bases are adenine, thymine, guanine, and cytosine.

duodenum (*doo*-o-**dee**-num) The first portion of the small intestine.

dura mater (**dyoo**-ra **may**-ter) The outer meninx of the central nervous system.

edema (e-**dee**-mah) An abnormal accumulation of fluid in the tissues.

efferent (**ef**-er-ent) Indicates movement *away* from a structure.

efferent arteriole The blood vessel taking blood away from the glomerulus.

ejaculation (e-*jak*-yoo-**lay**-shun) The reflex expulsion of semen from the penis.

ejaculatory duct (e-**jak**-yoo-lah-*toe*-ree) The tube transporting sperm from the vas deferens to the urethra.

electrocardiogram (ECG or EKG) (e-*lek*-troe-**kar**-

dee-o-gram) A graphic recording of the electrical changes occurring during the cardiac cycle.

electroencephalogram (EEG) (e-*lek*-troe-en-**sef**-ah-loe-gram) A graphic recording of the electrical changes associated with the activity of the cerebral cortex.

electrolyte (ee-**lek**-troe-lite) A compound that dissociates into ions when dissolved in water.

element Any one of the more than 100 pure chemical substances that in combination make up chemical compounds.

elimination The ejection of waste products, especially undigested food remnants from the digestive tract.

emphysema (*em*-fih-**see**-mah) A disease in which air accumulates in the respiratory passageways because of decreased alveolar elasticity.

emulsification (ee-*mul*-si-fi-**kay**-shun) The breaking down of large fat droplets into smaller ones.

enamel (e-**nam**-el) The bony outer covering of the crown of the tooth.

endocardium (en-doe-**kar**-dee-um) The inner layer of the heart wall, consisting of an endothelial lining resting upon connective tissue.

endocrine gland (**en**-doe-krin) A ductless gland that secretes hormones.

endocrinology (*en*-doe-kri-**nol**-o-jee) The study of the endocrine glands and their hormones.

endogenous (en-**doj**-e-nus) Produced within the body or due to internal causes.

endolymph (**en**-doe-*lymf*) The fluid of the membranous labyrinth of the ear.

endometrium (*en*-doe-**mee**-tree-um) The inner mucous membrane lining the uterus.

endomysium (*en*-doe-**meez**-ee-um) The connective tissue covering each muscle cell.

endoneurium (*en*-doe-**nyoo**-ree-um) The connective tissue covering a neuron.

endoplasmic reticulum (*en*-doe-**plaz**-mik re-**tik**-yoo-lum) An intracellular system of membranes continuous with the plasma membrane and functioning in transporting material through the cell, storage, synthesis, and packaging.

endorphin (en-**dor**-fin) A peptide in the central nervous system that affects pain perception and other aspects of behavior.

endosteum (en-**dos**-tee-um) The thin layer of connective tissue lining the marrow cavity of a bone.

endothelium (*en*-doe-**thee**-lee-um) The simple epithelial tissue that lines the cavities of the heart and of the blood and lymphatic vessels.

enkephalin (en-**kef**-ah-lin) A peptide of the nervous system that affects pain perception.

enzyme (**en**-zime) An organic catalyst, usually a protein, that promotes or regulates a biochemical reaction.

eosinophil (*ee*-o-**sin**-o-fil) A type of white blood cell with a granular cytoplasm.

epididymis (*ep*-i-**did**-i-mis) A coiled tube that receives sperm from the testes and conveys it to the vas deferens.

epidural space (*ep*-ih-**doo**-ral) Space between the wall of the vertebral canal and the dura mater surrounding the spinal cord.

epiglottis (*ep*-ih-**glot**-is) Cartilage guarding the superior opening into the larynx.

epimysium (*ep*-ih-**miz**-ee-um) The fibrous connective tissue that envelops muscles.

epinephrine (*ep*-ih-**nef**-rin) Hormone secreted by the adrenal medulla. Its actions are similar to those produced by stimulation of the sympathetic nervous system. Also known as adrenaline.

epineurium (*ep*-ih-**nyoo**-ree-um) Outermost connective tissue covering that surrounds a peripheral nerve.

epiphyseal plate (*ep*-ih-**feez**-eal) Cartilage plate separating the epiphysis from the diaphysis in growing long bones.

epiphysis (eh-**pif**-ih-sis) One end of a long bone. The two epiphyses are connected by the shaft or diaphysis.

epithelial tissue (*ep*-ih-**thee**-lee-uhl) Tissue of which glands and the external layer of the skin are formed. This tissue also lines the hollow organs, blood vessels, and the orifices leading to the surface of the body. Epithelial tissue is classified according to the number of cell layers present and the shape of the superficial cells.

erection (ee-**rek**-shun) Engorgement of the spongy erectile tissue of the penis or clitoris, resulting in enlargement and stiffening of the organ.

erythrocyte (eh-**rith**-roe-site) A red blood cell.

erythropoiesis (eh-*rith*-roe-poy-**ee**-sis) The formation of red blood cells or erythrocytes.

erythropoietin (eh-*rith*-roe-**poy**-ih-tin) Hormone that stimulates erythropoiesis or red blood cell formation. Formed from a protein in the blood plasma.

esophagus (eh-**sof**-ah-gus) A portion of the digestive tract, consisting of a hollow muscular tube that interconnects the pharynx and the stomach.

essential amino acids Amino acids that cannot be synthesized by the body in appropriate amounts and therefore need to be acquired through one's diet. There are 10 essential amino acids.

estradiol (*es*-trah-**die**-ol) Most potent of the naturally occurring estrogens in humans.

estrogens (**es**-trow-jens) Female sex hormones produced by the ovaries. Function in the development and maintenance of the female reproductive organs as well as secondary sex characteristics. Estrogens also play roles in protein anabolism and in fluid and electrolyte balance. Also produced by the testes in the male.

eustachian tube (yoo-**stay**-key-an) Tube connecting the middle ear with the pharynx. Also called the auditory tube.

eversion (eh-**ver**-zhun) Elevation of the lateral border of the foot such that the sole of the foot is directed laterally.

excretion (eks-**kree**-shun) Ejection of metabolic waste products from individual cells, tissues, or the body as a whole.

exocrine gland (**ek**-so-krin) A type of gland that secretes its products into ducts that open onto a free surface. Opposite of endocrine.

expiration (*eks*-pih-**ray**-shun) The process of moving air from the lungs into the atmosphere. Also called exhalation.

extension An angular form of movement resulting in an increase in the angle between adjoining bones; the opposite of flexion.

exteroceptor (*eks*-ter-oh-**sep**-tor) Receptor specialized for receiving stimuli from the external environment.

extracellular (*eks*-trah-**sell**-you-lar) Outside a cell.

extracellular fluid (ECF) Fluid, such as plasma and interstitial fluid, that is located outside the body's cells.

eyeball The ball-shaped part or globe of the eye.

face Anterior region of the head.

facet (**fas**-et) Small planar surface on a bone serving as an articular surface for another bone.

fallopian tube (fal-**low**-pee-an) Also called uterine tube. Passageway through which either the zygote or secondary oocyte reaches the uterine cavity.

fascia (**fash**-ee-ah) Fibrous tissue forming the investing layer for muscles and various organs of the body.

fascicle (**fas**-ih-kul) A small grouping of nerve or muscle fibers surrounded by a connective tissue envelope.

fat Adipose tissue. Normally existing as a liquid at body temperature. Composed of fatty acids combined with glycerol.

feces (**fee**-seez) Bodily waste excreted from the anus.

feedback Mechanism by which a form of output is utilized as input in order to exert some degree of control over a specific process. Classified as positive and negative feedback. Such mechanisms are used by most of the body's systems in an attempt to maintain homeostasis.

fertilization Union of an ovum and sperm to form a single-cell zygote.

fetus (**fee**-tus) During intrauterine life, the term applied to the new individual starting at the end of the embryonic period; that is, at the end of the eighth week of gestation.

fever (**fee**-vur) Condition in which the body temperature is elevated above normal. Normal body temperature is 37°C or 98.6°F.

fibrillation (fih-brih-**lay**-shun) Contraction of cardiac muscle at an extremely high rate and in an uncoordinated fashion. Little or no blood is actually pumped by the heart.

fibrin (**fye**-brin) The protein formed by the action of thrombin on fibrinogen during normal clotting of blood.

fibrinogen (fye-**brin**-oh-jin) Plasma protein converted to fibrin when acted upon by thrombin. Also called factor I.

fibroblast (**fye**-bro-blast) A large cell common to connective tissue that produces the fibers of the connective tissue.

fibrocartilage A specific type of cartilage containing numerous collagen fibers in its amorphous matrix. Its characteristics are intermediate between those of hyaline cartilage and dense ordinary connective tissue.

fissure (**fish**-yoor) Structure characterized as a groove or slit between two adjacent structures. Fissures may be either normal or abnormal in their occurrence. For example, the longitudinal fissure partially separates the two cerebral hemispheres.

fixator (**fick**-say-tor) A muscle that by its action tends to fix a body part in position or to limit its range of motion.

flagellum (fla-**jel**-um) A whiplike cellular organelle utilized in movement, e.g., by sperm cells.

flexion An angular form of movement that reduces the angle between the adjoining bones.

follicle-stimulating hormone (FSH) Hormone that is secreted by the anterior lobe of the pituitary gland. Its action stimulates development of the ovarian follicles in the female and spermatogenesis in the male. It also stimulates the ovarian follicles to produce and secrete estrogens.

fontanelle (fon-tah-**nell**) A gap or interval between adjacent bones that is typically covered by membranous tissue until the bones have completed their growth. Examples include the anterior and posterior fontanelles of the fetal skull.

foramen (foe-**ray**-men) A perforation or opening, especially within a bone.

forearm (**four**-arm) The region of the upper limb located between the elbow proximally and the wrist distally.

foreskin The prepuce of the penis, which is removed during the process of circumcision.

fossa (**foes**-ah) A depression or hollow located below the surface level of a structure or part of structure. For example, the fossa ovalis of the heart and the subscapular fossa. *Plural,* fossae.

fovea (**foe**-vee-ah) The location of the sharpest vision within the retina.

frontal plane Plane or section directed perpendicular to the midsagittal plane of the body and dividing the body into anterior and posterior parts. Also called a coronal plane or section.

fundus (**fun**-dus) In a hollow organ, that part located farthest from its opening or exit. Examples include the fundus of the stomach and the fundus of the uterus.

gallbladder Small, pouchlike organ located on the visceral aspect of the liver. It serves to store bile. The cystic duct conveys bile to and from this organ.

gamete (**gam**-eet) A sperm or ovum.

gamma globulins A group of plasma proteins that serve as antibodies or substances providing immunity against disease.

ganglion (**gang**-lee-on) A group of nerve-cell bodies usually located outside of the central nervous system.

gastric glands (**gas**-trik) Tiny glands located within the wall of the stomach that secrete gastric juice.

gastrin Hormone released by the stomach mucosa in response to stretching or the presence of substances such as caffeine and partially digested proteins. Its action stimulates the release of gastric juice from the gastric glands.

gastrointestinal tract That portion of the digestive tract located inferior to the diaphragm. Also called the GI tract.

gene That portion of a chromosome that contains the biological information for a specific trait. The gene represents the biological unit of heredity.

genetics (jeh-**net**-iks) The branch of biology that is concerned with the study of heredity.

genitalia (*jen*-ih-**tal**-ee-ah) The reproductive organs of the male and female.

gigantism Clinical condition occurring when the anterior pituitary secretes excessive amounts of growth hormone during childhood.

gland A cell, tissue, or organ that discharges a substance used by or eliminated from the body.

glial cells Non-neuronal cellular elements of nervous tissue. They provide physical and functional support to adjacent neurons.

gliding joint Type of synovial joint in which the participating bones possess flat articulating surfaces, allowing only side-to-side and back-and-forth movement. Examples include joints between the carpal bones.

globulin A class of proteins; one of the plasma protein fractions.

glomerulus (glo-**mer**-yoo-lus) The tuft of capillaries located within Bowman's capsule of the kidney tubule. Also applies to any spherical mass of blood vessels or nerves.

glottis (**glot**-iss) The two vocal folds located immediately superior to the vocal cords.

glucagon (**gloo**-kuh-gon) Hormone released by the islets of Langerhans of the pancreas. Its action elevates the level of blood sugar.

glucocorticoid hormones (*gloo*-koe-**kor**-tih-koyd) Class of hormones secreted by the adrenal cortex that affects glucose metabolism; the principal glucocorticoid is called cortisol.

glucose (**gloo**-kose) Monosaccharide occurring in blood plasma; it serves as the principal cellular fuel of the body.

glucosuria (*gloo*-koe-**soo**-ree-uh) Condition characterized by the presence of glucose in the urine.

glycogen (**gly**-ko-jen) Polysaccharide carbohydrate resembling starch occurring in many tissues, particularly the liver and skeletal muscles.

goiter Any abnormal enlargement of the thyroid gland. Such a condition may be associated with either hyposecretion or hypersecretion of thyroid hormone. Endemic goiter is caused by dietary iodine deficiency.

Golgi complex (**goal**-jee) A specialized cellular organelle composed of a set of cytoplasmic membranes associated with cellular secretion and the production of lysosomes. Also called Golgi apparatus.

gonad (**go**-nad) Generalized term for ovary or testis; an organ that produces gametes.

gonadotropic hormone (*gon*-ad-oh-**trow**-pik) Hormone involved in the regulation of gonadal function.

graafian follicle A mature ovarian follicle. Normally only one follicle matures each month in the human female. Those in which the maturation process is terminated early deteriorate and are known as atretic follicles.

graft rejection An effective immune response launched against a graft when the host's immune system regards the graft as foreign.

gray matter Those portions of the central nervous system consisting of large masses of cell bodies, dendrites of association and efferent neurons, and unmyelinated axons.

greater omentum (oh-**men**-tum) Large double fold of peritoneum attached to the duodenum, the greater curvature of the stomach, and a portion of the large intestine. It contains large deposits of adipose and lymphatic tissue.

greater vestibular glands (ves-**tib**-yoo-lar) Mucus-secreting glands that open onto each side of the vaginal orifice. Their secretion helps provide lubrication during sexual intercourse. They are especially vulnerable to infections. Also called Bartholin's glands.

groin (groyn) Depression located at the junction of the anterior aspect of the thigh with the trunk.

growth hormone An anterior pituitary hormone that stimulates body growth. Also called somatotropin.

guanine One of the four nitrogen-containing bases of DNA.

gustatory (**gus**-tah-*toe*-ree) Of or pertaining to the sense of taste.

gyrus (**jye**-rus) A convolution of the cerebral cortex. *Plural,* gyri.

hair follicle (**fol**-ih-kul) An epithelial ingrowth of the epidermis that moves down into the dermis and surrounds the hair.

hamstrings Group of posterior thigh muscles consisting of the biceps femoris, semitendinosus, and semimembranosus.

hard palate (**pal**-at) The more anterior hard portion of the roof of the mouth, formed by the fusion of portions of the maxillae and palatine bones.

haversian system Lamellar bone deposited in concentric rings around a centrally located blood vessel. The system has a general spindle-shaped configuration and is also called an osteon.

heart murmur Abnormal heart sound resulting from turbulent blood flow of sufficient magnitude to make vibrations occur.

heart rate The number of times the heart beats in one minute; normally this is about 72 beats per minute in the adult.

heart sounds Characteristic sounds of the heartbeat typically heard with the assistance of a stethoscope. Specific sounds result from closure of specific valves.

helper T cells Differentiated T lymphocytes that play a role in the stimulation of B lymphocytes.

hematocrit (hee-**mat**-o-krit) Percentage of red blood cells present in the total blood volume. The determination of this value is a routine clinical blood test.

hemoglobin (*bee*-moh-**glo**-bin) The respiratory pigment of red blood cells that has the property of taking up oxygen or releasing it.

hemorrhage (**hem**-or-ij) Escape of blood from the blood vessels; typically referring to excessive bleeding.

hepatic (he-**pat**-ik) Of or pertaining to the liver.

hepatic portal system System of veins returning blood from the digestive tract to the liver where a second set of exchange vessels (capillaries or sinusoids) is present.

heredity (heh-**red**-ih-tee) The transfer of biological information from parent to offspring.

hilus of kidney (**high**-lus) Region on the concave border of the kidney where the ureter and blood vessels are attached.

histamine (**hiss**-tah-meen) A substance released from a variety of cells in response to injury. Histamine produces vasodilation, bronchiolar constriction, and increased permeability of the blood vessels.

histology (hiss-**tol**-oh-jee) The study of tissues.

holocrine gland (**hole**-oh-krin) Specific type of gland, such as a sebaceous gland, in which the secretory product consists not only of the excretory product, but of the cell itself.

homeostasis (*ho*-mee-oh-**stay**-sis) The automatic tendency to maintain a relatively constant internal environment within the body. Also called homeodynamics.

horizontal plane Anatomical plane that parallels the ground. It divides the body into inferior and superior portions. Also called a transverse plane.

hormone (**hoar**-moan) Chemical messenger that helps regulate the activity of other tissues and organs. Secreted by endocrine or ductless glands.

human chorionic gonadotropin (HCG) (*ko*-ree-on-ik *gon*-ah-do-**trow**-pin) Hormone secreted by cells of the trophoblast (a membrane surrounding the embryo) that signals the corpus luteum that pregnancy has begun.

human immunodeficiency virus (HIV) A retrovirus responsible for the deadly disease called acquired immune deficiency syndrome (AIDS). The virus rapidly infects helper T cells, resulting in irreversible defects in immunity.

hyaline (**high**-ah-line) Clear, glassy, apparently without structure. Hyaline cartilage is a clear cartilage, without large fibers, that occurs in synovial joints.

hydrogen bond (**high**-droe-jen) A very weak chemical bond formed between an already bonded hydrogen atom and a negatively charged atom such as oxygen or nitrogen.

hydrolysis (high-**drol**-ih-sis) A chemical reaction involving water in which a large molecule is usually broken down into smaller products with the addition of water.

hydrophilic (*high*-droe-**fil**-ik) Attracted to water.

hydrophobic (*high*-droe-**fo**-bik) Repelled by water.

hymen (**high**-men) A fold of membrane that partially covers the external opening of the vagina.

hypertension (*high*-pur-**ten**-shun) Elevated blood pressure.

hypertonic (*high*-pur-**ton**-ik) Having an osmotic pressure or solute concentration greater than that of some other solution that is taken as a standard.

hyperventilation (*high*-pur-*ven*-tih-**lay**-shun) Abnormally rapid, deep breathing.

hypoglycemia (*high*-poe-gly-**see**-mee-ah) Reduction in the blood-glucose level to below normal.

hypothalamus (*high*-poe-**thal**-ah-mus) A portion of the brain that functions in the regulation of the pituitary gland, the autonomic nervous system, emotional responses, body temperature, water balance, and appetite; located inferior to the thalamus.

hypothyroidism (*high*-poe-**thigh**-royd-izm) A condition of deficient thyroid gland activity. Characterized by a decreased thyroid gland activity, resulting in a decreased basal metabolic rate, lethargy, and increased sensitivity to cold temperatures.

hypotonic (high-poe-**ton**-ik) Referring to a solution whose osmotic pressure or solute content is less than that of some standard of comparison.

hypoxia (high-**pock**-see-ah) Oxygen deficiency.

ileum (**il**-ee-um) The terminal portion of the small intestine extending from the jejunum to the cecum.

immune (ih-**mewn**) **response** Any reaction designed to defend the body against pathogens or other foreign substances.

immunity (ih-**mew**-nih-tee) The ability to resist and overcome infection or disease; nonsusceptibility to the pathogenic effects of foreign microorganisms or to the toxic effect of antigenic substances.

immunization (*im*-yoo-nih-**zay**-shun) The process of inducing active immunity by the injection of a vaccine.

immunoglobulins (*im*-yoo-no-**glob**-yoo-lins) Antibodies produced by plasma cells in response to antigenic stimulation. The five classes of immunoglobulin include IgG, IgA, IgM, IgD, and IgE.

immunology (*im*-yoo-**nol**-oh-jee) The study of the body's specific defense mechanisms.

immunosuppression Inhibition of the body's ability to mount an effective immune response. Immunosuppression may be due to certain drugs or exposure to ionizing radiation.

implantation (*im*-plan-**tay**-shun) Attachment, penetration, and embedding of the blastocyst within the uterine wall, occurring 7 or 8 days following fertilization.

impotence (**im**-poe-tence) Chronic inability to sustain an erection; often caused by psychological factors. It may also be the result of motor nerve paralysis or spinal cord lesions.

infancy (**in**-fan-see) That period of postnatal development extending from the end of the neonatal period to the time when the individual is able to assume an erect posture. Some physicians consider the period of infancy to encompass the first 2 years of life.

infarct (**in**-farkt) A localized area of dead tissue caused by an inadequate blood supply and the resulting oxygen deprivation.

inferior (in-**fe**-ree-or) Anatomic directional term describing a structure located below, or directed downward, as compared to another structure or part.

inferior vena cava Large vein returning blood to the right atrium from the abdominopelvic structures and the lower limbs.

inflammation (*in*-flah-**may**-shun) The response of the body tissues to injury or infection, characterized clinically by heat, swelling, redness, and pain, and physiologically by increased vasodilation and capillary permeability.

ingestion (in-**jes**-chun) The process of eating; taking substances into the mouth and swallowing them.

inguinal canal (**ing**-gwih-nal) One of the two passageways that serve to connect the scrotal and abdominal cavities. The testes descend into the scrotum by way of the inguinal canals.

inhalation See **inspiration**.

inner ear Portion of the ear within the temporal bone consisting of the osseous labyrinth, the membranous labyrinth, and the cochlea.

insertion (in-**sir**-shun) The more movable point of attachment of muscle to bone; contrasts with the origin or less movable point of attachment of muscle to bone.

inspiration (*in*-spih-**ray**-shun) The drawing of air into the lungs.

insulin (**in**-suh-lin) A hormone released by the islets of Langerhans of the pancreas that facilitates diffusion of glucose into cells.

integration (*in*-teh-**gray**-shun) The process of sorting and interpreting neural impulses in order to determine an appropriate response.

integumentary system A body system consisting of the skin, its glands, nails, and hair.

interatrial septum (*in*-ter-**a**-tree-uhl) Wall located between the right and left atria of the heart.

intercellular Between the cells of a structure.

interferons (*in*-ter-**feer**-ons) Proteins secreted by certain cells when the body is invaded by viruses or other intracellular parasites. This group of proteins stimulates other cells to produce antiviral proteins.

interleukins (*in*-ter-**loo**-kins) Peptides produced by various cells of the body's immune system. These substances play important regulatory roles in the body's defense mechanisms.

interneuron An association neuron; one that links sensory and motor neurons within the central nervous system.

interoceptor (*in*-ter-o-**sep**-tor) A sensory receptor that transmits information from the viscera to the central nervous system.

interphase (**in**-ter-faze) The period in the life of a cell in which there is no mitotic division.

interstitial (*in*-ter-**stish**-al) Located between parts or cells.

interstitial cells Cells located in groups between the seminiferous tubules in the testes; produce the male hormone, testosterone. Also called the interstitial cells of Leydig.

interstitial fluid Fluid located between cells or body parts; tissue fluid.

interventricular septum (*in*-ter-ven-**trik**-yoo-lar) That portion of the heart wall located between the two ventricles.

intervertebral disc (*in*-ter-**ver**-teh-brahl) Fibrocartilaginous disc located between two adjacent vertebral bodies.

intracellular (*in*-trah-**sell**-yoo-lar) Located within the cell, as in the case of intracellular fluid.

intramembranous bone formation One type of bone formation in which a primitive connective tissue precedes bone development. As in endochondral bone formation, the connective tissue is replaced by bone itself.

inversion (in-**ver**-zhun) Elevation of the medial border of the foot such that the sole or plantar aspect is directed medially.

ion (**eye**-on) A charged atom or group of atoms.

(The electric charge results from gain or loss of electrons.)

ionic bond Type of bond formed when one atom donates an electron to another atom. Also called an electrovalent bond.

ionization (*eye*-on-eye-**zay**-shun) The dissociation of a substance (acid, base, salt) in solution into ions.

ipsilateral (*ip*-sih-**lat**-er-al) Pertaining to the same side of the body.

iris (**eye**-ris) The visible, colored, circular disc of the eye that functions to control the amount of light entering the eye.

ischemia (is-**kee**-me-ah) Deficiency of blood to a body part due to functional constriction or actual obstruction of a blood vessel.

ischemic heart disease Heart disease resulting from coronary artery narrowing.

ischium (**is**-kee-um) The dorsal and inferior portion of the hip bone.

islets of Langerhans (**eye**-lits of **Lahng**-er-hanz) The endocrine portion of the pancreas; alpha cells of the islets release glucagon while beta cells secrete insulin. These hormones regulate the blood-sugar level.

isometric (*eye*-so-**met**-rik) Maintaining the same measure or length. In muscle physiology, a contraction that produces no change in the length of the muscle.

isotonic (*eye*-so-**ton**-ik) 1. A solution having the same solute concentration or osmotic pressure as some other solution to which it is compared. Also a solution in which body cells can be immersed without a net flow of water across the semipermeable plasma membrane. 2. A form of muscle contraction in which the length but not the tension of the muscle changes.

jejunum (jeh-**joo**-num) The middle portion of the small intestine located between the duodenum and the ileum.

joint The site of junction or union between two or more bones of the skeleton. Also called an articulation.

juxtaglomerular cells (*juks*-tah-glo-**mer**-yoo-lar) A cuff of specialized cells located around the afferent arteriole of the glomerulus.

keratin (**ker**-ah-tin) An insoluble protein found in epidermis, hair, nails, and other horny tissues.

ketone bodies (**key**-tone) Compounds such as acetone, beta hydroxybutyric acid, and acetoacetic acid that are produced during fat metabolism.

ketosis (kee-**tow**-sis) Abnormal condition marked by an elevated concentration of ketone bodies in the body fluids and tissues; a complication of diabetes mellitus and of starvation.

kidney (**kid**-nee) One of two organs of the urinary system responsible for the production of urine. Function in the regulation of fluid volume and composition. Located in a retroperitoneal position on the posterior abdominal wall in the lumbar region.

kilocalorie (**kil**-oh-*kal*-oh-ree) Quantity of heat required to elevate the temperature of 1 kg of water 1°C; also the unit of measurement of the basal metabolic rate.

labia (**lay**-bee-ah) The liplike borders of the vulva.

labor Strong contractions of the uterus that occur with increasing frequency and intensity during the latter part of pregnancy. Labor is divided into three distinct stages.

labyrinth (**lab**-ih-rinth) The system of intercommunicating canals and cavities that make up the inner ear.

lacteal (**lak**-tee-al) One of the many lymphatic vessels in the intestinal villi that absorb fat; during absorption they appear white and milky from the absorbed fat.

lactic acid (**lak**-tik) Compound generated from glycogen during anaerobic energy metabolism. Its accumulation in muscle produces the sensation of fatigue, and oxygen is required for its elimination.

lactose (**lak**-tose) A disaccharide composed of one molecule of glucose and one molecule of galactose.

lacunae (la-**koo**-nee) Small, isolated spaces, each containing an osteoblast.

laryngopharynx (lah-*ring*-oh-**far**-inks) One of three divisions of the pharynx.

larynx (**lar**-inks) The organ at the superior end of the trachea that contains the vocal cords, located between the pharynx and trachea.

lateral (**lat**-er-al) Positional term designating a location away from the midline of the body or one of its organs or parts.

leg That portion of the lower limb located between the knee and the ankle.

lens Transparent structure responsible for focusing images upon the retina. Differential focusing of near and far objects is related to the lens's ability to alter its shape.

lesion (**lee**-zhun) Any local damage to tissue or loss of function of a part; may be the result of injury or disease.

lesser omentum (oh-**men**-tum) The peritoneal fold connecting the liver with the lesser curvature of the stomach and the duodenum.

lesser vestibular glands (ves-**tib**-yoo-lar) Mucus-producing glands whose ducts open into the female vestibule near the external urethral orifice.

leukemia (loo-**key**-mee-ah) A form of cancer in which any one of the kinds of white blood cells proliferates wildly in the bone marrow; may be either of an acute or chronic nature.

leukocyte (**loo**-ko-site) A white blood cell.

ligament (**lig**-ah-ment) Strong connective tissue cord, or band, that unites bones.

lipid Any of a group of organic compounds that are insoluble in water but soluble in fat solvents such as alcohol; they serve as a storage form of fuel and an important constituent of cellular membranes.

lobe A well-defined portion of any organ, especially of the brain, lungs, and glands.

lumen (**loo**-men) The space within a tubelike structure such as a blood or lymphatic vessel or intestine.

luteinizing hormone (LH) (**loo**-tee-in-*eye*-zing) Hormone secreted by the anterior lobe of the pituitary gland. Serves to stimulate ovulation and progesterone secretion by the corpus luteum. Helps prepare the mammary glands for milk secretion. In males, LH stimulates the testes to secrete testosterone.

lymph (limf) The fluid within the lymphatic vessels that is collected from the interstitial fluid and ultimately returned to the circulatory system.

lymphatic (lim-**fat**-ik) Of or pertaining to lymph. Also one of several large lymph vessels that unite to form the right and left lymphatic ducts.

lymph node A mass of lymphatic tissue surrounded by a connective tissue capsule; filters lymph and produces lymphocytes.

lymph nodules Small masses of lymphatic tissue without a connective tissue capsule. Found scattered throughout loose connective tissue, especially beneath moist epithelial membranes, and produce lymphocytes.

lymphocyte (**lim**-foe-site) A small mononuclear white blood cell. This class of cells includes the T and B lymphocytes, large agranular lymphocytes, and natural killer (NK) cells.

lysosome (**lye**-so-sowm) A cytoplasmic organelle containing lytic enzymes and surrounded by a membrane.

macrophage (**mak**-roe-faje) A large phagocytic cell capable of ingesting and digesting bacteria and cellular debris.

mammary gland (**mam**-er-ee) An organ of the female that produces and secretes milk, providing nutrition for the young; it develops as a modified sweat gland.

mammography (mam-**og**-rah-fee) A soft-tissue radiological study of the breast.

manubrium (mah-**noo**-bree-um) Superior portion of the sternum.

mast cell A specialized type of cell present in connective tissue; it contains histamine and is important in allergic reactions.

meatus (mee-**ay**-tus) A passageway or opening.

medial (**me**-dee-al) Directional term meaning nearer to the midline of the body or structure.

median plane A vertical plane situated at a right angle to a frontal or coronal plane and dividing the body into right and left halves.

mediastinum (*mee*-dee-as-**tie**-num) Region between the lungs that holds several organs.

medulla (meh-**dull**-ah) The inner portion of an organ such as the kidney.

medulla oblongata (*ob*-lon-**ga**-tah) The most inferior aspect of the brain stem; connects the brain with the spinal cord.

meiosis (mi-**oh**-sis) Reduction division; the special type of cell division by which gametes are produced.

melanin (**mel**-ah-nin) A group of dark pigments produced by certain cells (melanocytes) in the epidermis of the skin.

membrane bones Bones of the body that develop by intramembranous formation, for example, the parietal bones of the cranium.

memory B cells Activated B cells that do not differentiate into plasma cells. They continue to produce small quantities of antibody long after an infection has been overcome.

meninges (meh-**nin**-jeez) The three membranes that envelop the brain and spinal cord: the dura mater, arachnoid, and pia mater.

meniscus (meh-**nis**-kus) Articular disc found in certain types of synovial joints and consisting almost entirely of fibrocartilage.

menopause (**men**-oh-pawz) The period during which menstruation ceases in the human female, usually at about age 50.

menstrual cycle (**men**-stroo-al) Series of physiological changes resulting in preparation of the uterine lining for the reception of a fertilized ovum. Occurs on approximately a monthly basis in the nonpregnant female.

menstruation (*men*-stroo-**ay**-shun) The monthly discharge of blood and degenerated uterine lining in the human female; marks the initiation of each menstrual cycle.

mesentery (**mez**-en-terr-ee) A fold attaching various organs to the body wall, especially the peritoneum connecting the intestine to the posterior abdominal wall.

mesocolon (*mez*-oh-**ko**-lon) A fold of peritoneum connecting a portion of the colon to the posterior abdominal wall.

metabolism (meh-**tab**-oh-liz-um) All the chemical processes that take place within the body.

metaphase (**met**-ah-faze) Stage of mitosis characterized by pairs of chromatids lining up along the equator of the cell.

metaphysis (meh-**taf**-ih-sis) Region of growing long bone between the epiphyses and the diaphysis.

metastasis (meh-**tas**-tah-sis) The transfer of a disease such as cancer from one organ or part to another not directly connected to it.

microvilli (*my*-krow-**vill**-ee) Minute projections of the plasma membrane that increase the surface area of the cell; present mainly in cells concerned with absorption and secretion such as those lining the intestine.

micturition (*mik*-tu-**rish**-un) Urination; the passage of urine from the urinary bladder.

midbrain That portion of the brain that is situated between the pons and the diencephalon. Also referred to as the mesencephalon.

mineralocorticoids (*min*-er-al-oh-**kor**-tih-koyds) A class of hormones produced by the adrenal cortex that regulates mineral metabolism and, indirectly, fluid balance. The principal mineralocorticoid is called aldosterone.

mitochondria (*my*-tow-**kon**-dree-ah) Cellular organelles that are the site of most cellular respiration; sometimes they are referred to as the power plants of the cell.

mitosis (my-**tow**-sis) Division of the cell nucleus resulting in the distribution of a complete set of chromosomes to each end of the cell. Cytokinesis (actual division of the cell itself) usually occurs during the telophase stage of mitosis, giving rise to two daughter cells.

mitral valve Alternative term for the left atrioventricular or bicuspid valve.

molecule (**mol**-eh-kewl) A chemical combination of two or more atoms that form a specific chemical substance.

monocyte (**mon**-oh-site) A white blood cell; a large phagocytic nongranular leukocyte that enters the tissues and differentiates into a macrophage.

monoglyceride (*mon*-oh-**gliss**-er-ide) A fat that contains only one fatty acid per molecule.

mucosa (mew-**ko**-sah) A mucous membrane; for example, the lining of the gastrointestinal tract.

mucus (**mew**-kus) A sticky secretion produced by certain glandular cells (e.g., goblet cells), especially in the lining of the gastrointestinal and respiratory tracts. It serves to lubricate body parts and trap particles of dirt or additional contaminants. The adjectival form is spelled as mucous.

muscle (**mus**-ul) An organ that produces movement by contraction.

muscle tissue A tissue composed of cells specialized for contraction; three main types are skeletal, smooth, and cardiac.

muscle tone The incomplete but sustained contraction of a portion of a skeletal muscle.

mutation A change in one of the bases of a DNA strand, resulting in an alteration of the genetic information.

myelin (**my**-eh-lin) The white fatty substance forming a sheath around certain nerve fibers, which are then called myelinated fibers.

myocardium (*my*-oh-**kar**-dee-um) Cardiac muscle fibers forming the greatest mass of the heart wall. Fibers are intricately branched and interwoven and their rhythmical contraction is responsible for pumping of the blood.

myofibril (*my*-oh-**fye**-bril) Any threadlike organelle found in the cytoplasm of striated and cardiac muscle that is responsible for contraction.

myofilament (*my*-oh-**fil**-ah-ment) One of the filaments making up the myofibril; the structural unit of muscle proteins in a muscle cell.

myosin (**my**-oh-sin) A protein that, together with actin, is responsible for muscle contraction.

nail The hard cutaneous plate situated on the dorsal aspect of the distal region of each digit of the hand or foot.

nares (**nay**-reez) The external openings of the nose; also referred to as the nostrils.

nasopharynx (*nay*-zo-**far**-inks) One of three divisions of the pharynx.

natural killer (NK) cells Specific cells of the body's immune system that recognize and kill body cells altered by viruses.

neonate Term applied to the newborn infant.

neoplasm (**nee**-oh-plazm) A tumor; new and abnormal growth of cells or tissues.

nephron (**nef**-ron) The functional and microscopic anatomical unit of the kidney.

nerve (nerv) A large bundle of axons (or dendrites) wrapped in connective tissue, which conveys impulses between the central nervous system and some other part of the body.

neuron (**new**-ron) A nerve cell; an impulse-conducting cell of the nervous system that typically consists of a cell body, dendrites, and an axon.

neutrophil (**new**-tro-fil) A type of granular leukocyte.

norepinephrine (*nor*-ep-ih-**nef**-rin) 1. A neurotransmitter substance. 2. A hormone produced by the adrenal medulla.

nucleic acids (new-**klee**-ik) DNA or RNA; a very large compound composed of carbon, oxygen, hydrogen, nitrogen, and phosphorus arranged in molecular subunits called nucleotides. Nucleic acid codes information specifying the structure and function of the organism.

nucleolus (new-**klee**-oh-lus) Spherelike organelle located within the nucleus and containing DNA, RNA, and protein; is not surrounded by a membrane; plays role in the synthesis and storage of ribosomal RNA.

nucleotide (**new**-klee-oh-tide) A unit of the backbone of DNA consisting of the sugar deoxyribose, one phosphate group, and one nitrogen-containing base, either adenine, thymine, guanine, or cytosine.

nucleus (**new**-klee-us) 1. The core of an atom which contains the protons and neutrons. 2. A cellular organelle containing DNA and serving as the control center of the cell. 3. A mass of nerve cell bodies in the central nervous system concerned with a particular function.

nutrients (**new**-tree-ents) The chemical substances present in food that are utilized by the body as components for synthesizing needed materials and for fuel.

nutrition (new-**trish**-un) The utilization of food by an organism; nourishment.

obesity (oh-**bees**-ih-tee) The condition of being extremely overweight.

oocyte (**oh**-oh-site) A developing egg cell in either the primary or secondary stage.

opposition Type of movement unique to the thumb. This movement is a combination of rotation and adduction.

optic (**op**-tik) Of or pertaining to the eye or vision.

optimum (**op**-ti-mum) Most favorable; optimum conditions are the most favorable conditions under which a particular function can occur.

orbit (**or**-bit) The bony chamber that houses the eye and has a shape similar to a truncated pyramid.

organ (**or**-gan) A differentiated part of the body made up of tissues and adapted to perform a specific function or group of functions.

organelle One of many specialized parts of an individual cell. Examples include mitochondria, Golgi apparatus, nucleus, and the plasma membrane.

organ of Corti The cochlear organ that contains the special sensory receptors for hearing.

orgasm (**or**-gazm) The culmination of sexual excitement including ejaculation for the male and involuntary contraction of the perineal muscles in both sexes. Incorporates a host of sensory and cardiovascular responses as well.

orifice (**or**-ih-fis) The entrance or outlet of any body cavity.

origin (**or**-ih-jin) The more fixed end of attachment of a muscle to a bone; the end opposite the insertion.

oropharynx (*or*-oh-**far**-inks) The part of the pharynx between the soft palate and the upper edge of the epiglottis.

osmosis (oz-**mow**-sis) The passage of water molecules through a selectively permeable membrane in response to solute concentrations.

osmotic pressure The pressure necessary to stop the flow of water across a selectively permeable membrane; depends on the relative concentrations of the two solutions on either side of the membrane.

osseous (**os**-ee-us) Bony.

ossicle (**os**-ih-kul) A small bone, especially one of the three bones of the middle ear (malleus, incus, stapes).

ossification (*os*-ih-fih-**kay**-shun) Formation of bone; also called osteogenesis.

osteoblast (**os**-tee-oh-*blast*) A cell that produces bone.

osteoclast (**os**-tee-oh-*klast*) A large, multinuclear cell that resorbs, or breaks down, bone.

osteocyte (**os**-tee-oh-*site*) An osteoblast that has become embedded within the bone matrix and occupies a lacuna.

osteon (**os**-tee-on) The basic unit of structure of compact bone consisting of concentric rings of lamellae arranged around a central (haversian) canal. Also called a haversian system.

osteoporosis (*os*-tee-oh-poe-**row**-sis) A disease in which there is a severe reduction in bone mass; most common bone disease.

oval window of ear Opening between the middle and inner ear on which the stapes rests.

ovarian ligament The cord of connective tissue that attaches the ovary to the uterus.

ovary (**oh**-var-ee) The female gonad; produces ova and sex hormones, principally estrogens and progesterone.

ovulation (*oh*-vu-**lay**-shun) The discharge of the ovum (actually a secondary oocyte) from the mature (graafian) follicle into the pelvic cavity.

ovum (**oh**-vum) Egg cell; the female gamete.

oxidation (oks-ih-**day**-shun) The removal of electrons, or loss of hydrogen, from a compound. The oxidation of glucose is called cellular respiration.

oxygen debt The amount of oxygen needed to oxidize the lactic acid produced during exercise.

oxyhemoglobin (*ok*-see-**he**-mow-glow-bin) Hemoglobin combined with oxygen; the form in which oxygen is transported in the body.

oxytocin (*ok*-see-**toe**-sin) A hormone produced by the hypothalamus and released by the posterior lobe of the pituitary gland; stimulates contraction of uterus and release of milk from lactating breast.

pacinian corpuscle Encapsulated, onion-shaped tactile receptor that responds to heavy pressure and vibration.

palate (**pal**-at) The roof of the mouth; the horizontal partition separating the oral and nasal cavities.

pancreas (**pan**-kree-as) A large, elongated gland located behind the stomach, between the spleen and duodenum. Composed of both exocrine tissue (secretes pancreatic juice) and endocrine tissue (secretes insulin and glucagon).

pancreatic duct A single tube that joins the common bile duct, forming a single duct that passes into the wall of the duodenum.

papilla (pa-**pil**-ah) A small, nipple-like mound, for example, the papilla at the base of each hair follicle.

parasympathetic division (*par*-ah-*sim*-pah-**thet**-ik) One of the two subdivisions of the autonomic nervous system; the craniosacral portion of the autonomic nervous system. Its general effect is to conserve and restore energy in the body.

parathyroid glands (*par*-ah-**thy**-royd) Small endocrine glands located within the connective tissue surrounding the thyroid gland; they secrete parathyroid hormone.

parathyroid hormone (PTH) A hormone secreted by the parathyroid glands that regulates calcium and phosphate concentrations in the blood.

parietal (pa-**rye**-eh-tal) 1. Pertaining to the walls of an organ or cavity. 2. Pertaining to the parietal bone of the skull.

parotid glands (pah-**rot**-id) The largest of the three main pairs of salivary glands, located on either side of the face, just inferior and anterior to the ears.

parturition (*par*-too-**rish**-un) The process of giving birth to a child; delivery of a baby.

patellar reflex (pah-**tell**-ar) Involuntary contraction of the quadriceps muscle and jerky extension of the leg when the patellar ligament is sharply tapped.

pathogen (**path**-o-jen) Any disease-producing organism or agent.

pectoral (**pek**-to-ral) Pertaining to the chest or breast.

pelvic cavity (**pel**-vik) Inferior portion of the abdominopelvic cavity; contains the urinary bladder, sigmoid colon, rectum, and internal female and male reproductive structures.

pelvis (**pel**-vis) Any basinlike structure, for example, the basinlike structure formed by the hip bones, the sacrum, and the coccyx.

penis (**pee**-nis) The external male organ that functions in urination and in copulation.

pepsin (**pep**-sin) A protein-digesting enzyme that is the main digestive component of gastric juice.

peptide (**pep**-tide) A compound composed of two or more amino acids; peptides form the constituent parts of proteins.

pericardial cavity (*per*-ih-**kar**-dee-al) Potential space between the visceral and parietal layers of the serous pericardium.

pericardium (*per*-ih-**kar**-dee-um) The loose-fitting sac enclosing the heart, composed of an outer fibrous layer and an inner serous layer.

perilymph (**per**-ih-limf) The fluid contained between the bony and membranous labyrinths of the inner ear.

perimysium (*per*-ih-**mis**-ee-um) Connective tissue that surrounds the fascicles (bundles) of skeletal muscle fibers.

perineum (*per*-ih-**nee**-um) The diamond-shaped region bounded by the coccyx, symphysis pubis, and ischial tuberosities.

periosteum (*per*-ee-**os**-tee-um) The connective tissue membrane covering bones; possesses bone-forming potential.

peripheral nervous system (PNS) That portion of the nervous system consisting of the receptors, the nerves that link receptors with the central nervous system (CNS), and the nerves that link the CNS with the effectors.

peristalsis (*per*-ih-**stal**-sis) Waves of muscle contractions along the wall of a tube such as the digestive tract.

peritoneum (*per*-ih-tow-**nee**-um) The largest serous membrane of the body; lines the walls of the abdominal and pelvic cavities (parietal peritoneum) and covers the contained viscera (visceral peritoneum).

peritonitis (*per*-ih-tow-**nie**-tis) Inflammation of the peritoneum.

pH A symbol of the measure of the acidity or alkalinity of a solution. The pH scale extends from 0 to 14, with 7 being neutral; values lower than 7 indicate increasing acidity, and values higher than 7 indicate increasing alkalinity.

phagocytosis (*fag*-oh-sigh-**toe**-sis) Engulfing and ingestion of microorganisms, other cells, or foreign particles by cells.

phalanx (**fay**-lanks) The bone of a toe or finger. *Plural,* phalanges (fay-**lan**-jeez).

pharynx (**far**-inks) The throat; a tube that begins at the internal nares and extends part way down the neck, communicating with the mouth and opening into the esophagus posteriorly and into the larynx anteriorly.

photoreceptor (*fo*-tow-re-**sep**-tor) A neural receptor sensitive to light.

physiology (*fiz*-ee-**ol**-oh-jee) Science that deals with the functions of the living organism and its parts.

pia mater (**pee**-ah **may**-ter) The inner of the three meninges (membranes) covering the brain and spinal cord.

pineal gland (**pin**-ee-al) The cone-shaped gland attached by a stalk to the posterior wall of the third ventricle.

pinna (**pin**-ah) The projecting part of the external ear composed of elastic cartilage and covered with skin.

pituitary gland (pih-**too**-ih-*terr*-ee) An endocrine gland attached by a stalk to the hypothalamus of the brain; secretes a variety of hormones influencing a wide range of physiologic processes. Sometimes called the master gland. Also called the hypophysis.

placenta (plah-**sen**-tah) The organ of exchange between mother and developing fetus.

plasma (**plaz**-muh) The fluid portion of blood consisting of a pale yellowish fluid containing proteins, salts, and other substances.

plasma cell A differentiated, functioning B lymphocyte; produces antibodies.

plasma membrane Cell membrane; outer, limiting membrane of the cell that separates the cell from its external environment.

platelet (**plate**-let) A blood platelet or thrombocyte; a cell fragment suspended in the plasma that functions in blood clotting.

pleura (**ploor**-ah) The serous membrane that surrounds the lungs (visceral pleura) and lines the walls of the thoracic cavity (parietal pleura).

pleural cavity Potential space between the visceral and parietal pleura.

plexus (**plex**-us) A network of veins or nerves.

polysaccharides (*pol*-ee-**sak**-uh-rides) Carbohydrates consisting of three or more, usually many, sugar units chemically combined to form a large molecule.

polyunsaturated fat A fat that contains two or more double bonds between its carbon atoms. Most vegetable oils are polyunsaturated.

polyuria (*pol*-ee-**yoo**-ree-ah) Excessive excretion of urine.

pons (ponz) That part of the brain stem that forms a bridge between the medulla and the midbrain, anterior to the cerebellum; connects various other parts of the brain.

positron emission tomography (PET) A nuclear medicine imaging technique similar to computed tomography (CT) that produces a cross-sectional image of the distribution of radioactivity in a slice through the subject a few centimeters thick.

posterior (pos-**teer**-ee-or) Toward or at the back of the body; dorsal.

postganglionic neuron (*post*-gang-glee-**on**-ik) Neuron located distal to a ganglion. The second efferent neuron in an autonomic pathway.

postsynaptic neuron (*post*-sin-**ap**-tik) A neuron that transmits action potentials away from a synapse.

preganglionic neuron (*pre*-gang-glee-**on**-ik) Neuron located proximal to a ganglion. The first efferent neuron in an autonomic pathway; synapses with a postganglionic neuron.

pregnancy The condition of having a developing embryo or fetus in the body.

prepuce (**pre**-pyoos) The loose-fitting skin covering the glans of the penis or clitoris. Also referred to as the foreskin.

presynaptic neuron (*pre*-sin-**ap**-tik) A neuron that transmits action potentials toward a synapse.

prevertebral ganglion (pre-**vert**-eh-bral) A mass of cell bodies of postganglionic sympathetic neurons located close to blood vessels. Also called collateral ganglion.

primary motor area A region within the precentral gyrus of the frontal lobe of the cerebrum that controls skeletal muscles. Also called the motor cortex.

progesterone (pro-**jes**-ter-own) A steroid sex hormone secreted by the corpus luteum (in the ovary) and by the placenta; stimulates thickening of the endometrium of the uterus and helps prepare the mammary glands for milk secretion.

prolactin (pro-**lak**-tin) A hormone secreted by the anterior lobe of the pituitary gland that stimulates lactation (milk production). Also called lactogenic hormone.

prolapse (**pro**-laps) The downward displacement, or falling down, of a part or organ.

proliferation (pro-*lif*-er-**a**-shun) Multiplication of new parts, especially cells.

pronation (pro-**nay**-shun) The act of assuming the prone (lying face-downward) position. Applied to the hand, the turning of the palm of the hand downward (posteriorly).

prophase (**pro**-faze) The first stage of cell replication in either mitosis or meiosis.

proprioceptors (*pro*-pre-oh-**sep**-tors) Mechanoreceptors located within the skeletal muscles, tendons, joints, and inner ear that send sensory information to the brain allowing us to know the location of one body part in relation to another, the degree of joint flexibility, the degree of muscle contraction and tendon stress, and head and body position during movement.

prostaglandins (PG) (*pros*-tah-**glan**-dins) A group of fatty acids released by many different tissues that affect the action of certain hormones and have a wide range of physiological effects.

prostate gland (**pros**-tate) A gland in the male that surrounds the neck of the bladder and the urethra and secretes an alkaline fluid that is a component of semen.

protein (**pro**-teen) A complex organic compound composed of chemically linked amino acid subunits; contains carbon, hydrogen, oxygen, nitrogen, and sulfur.

prothrombin (pro-**throm**-bin) An inactive protein synthesized by the liver, present in the plasma, and converted to thrombin during blood clotting.

proximal (**prok**-sih-mal) Nearer to the center of the body or to the point of attachment or origin.

pseudostratified epithelium (*soo*-dow-**strat**-ih-fide) Refers to an epithelial tissue that appears to be stratified (layered) but is not.

puberty (**pyoo**-ber-tee) The period during which the secondary sex characteristics begin to develop and the individual becomes capable of sexual reproduction. Girls usually reach puberty between ages 11 and 13, and boys between 13 and 15.

pudendum (poo-**den**-dum) The female external reproductive structures. Also called vulva.

pulmonary (**pul**-mow-*ner*-ee) Pertaining to the lungs.

pulmonary circulation The circuit of blood flow

between the heart and lungs. The flow of oxygen-poor blood from the right ventricle to the lungs where it is oxygenated and the return of the oxygen-rich blood from the lungs to the left atrium.

pulp cavity A cavity within the tooth filled with pulp, a connective tissue containing blood vessels, nerves, and lymphatics.

pulse The rhythmic expansion and recoil of the elastic arteries each time the left ventricle pumps blood into the aorta. The pulse rate corresponds to the heart rate.

pupil The opening in the center of the iris through which light enters the eye.

Purkinje fibers (per-**kin**-jee) Modified cardiac muscle fibers concerned with conducting impulses through the heart.

pus The liquid product of inflammation that contains white blood cells and debris of dead cells.

pyloric sphincter (pie-**lor**-ik) A thick ring of muscle that serves as a gate, closing the opening of the stomach into the duodenum.

pyramid (**pir**-a-mid) A pointed or cone-shaped structure. 1. Pyramids of the medulla oblongata are two prominent bulges of white matter on the ventral side of the medulla containing descending fibers of the pyramidal tracts that pass from the cerebrum to the spinal cord. 2. Renal pyramids are conical masses that make up the medulla of the kidney.

pyramidal tracts (pih-**ram**-i-dal) Groups of descending tracts arising in the cerebral cortex, crossing in the pyramids of the medulla, and extending into the spinal cord; provide for control of skilled voluntary movement.

ramus (**ray**-mus) A general term for a branch of a nerve, artery, or vein.

rapid eye movement (REM) sleep A stage of sleep characterized by rapid movement of the eyes and a brain wave pattern similar to that of an awake individual.

receptor (re-**sep**-tor) 1. A sensory structure that responds to specific stimuli such as light, sound, touch, pressure, or change in position. 2. A specific chemical grouping (usually a protein) on a cell surface that may combine with a specific chemical such as a neurotransmitter or hormone.

rectum (**rek**-tum) The distal portion of the large intestine, extending from the sigmoid colon to the anus.

reflex (**re**-flex) A predictable, automatic sequence of stimulus-response usually involving a reflex arc (pathway) consisting of at least three neurons: a sensory neuron, an association neuron, and a motor neuron.

refractory period (re-**frak**-to-ree) The time period during which a neuron cannot respond to a stimulus that is usually sufficient to result in an action potential.

renal (**ree**-nul) Pertaining to the kidney.

renal pelvis The funnel-shaped expansion of the upper end of the ureter into which the renal calices open.

renin (**reh**-nin) A proteolytic enzyme synthesized by the juxtaglomerular cells of the kidney; it plays a role in the regulation of blood pressure.

respiration (*res*-pih-**ray**-shun) The exchange of oxygen and carbon dioxide between the atmosphere and the body cells, including inspiration and expiration, diffusion of gases between the alveoli and blood, transport of oxygen and carbon dioxide, and cellular respiration.

resting potential The membrane potential of an inactive neuron; the inside of the cell is negative relative to the outside.

reticular activating system (RAS) (reh-**tik**-yoo-lur) An action system of the brain responsible for the overall extent of CNS activity including wakefulness, attentiveness, and sleep; the system of neurons of the reticular formation that project to higher centers.

retina (**ret**-ih-na) The inner coat of the eyeball; composed of light-sensitive neurons including the rods and cones.

retroperitoneal (*reh*-trow-*per*-ih-tow-**nee**-al) External to the peritoneal lining of the abdominal cavity; behind the peritoneum.

Rh system A system of blood types with at least eight different kinds of Rh antigens, each referred to as an Rh factor.

rhodopsin (row-**dop**-sin) A photosensitive pigment in the retinal rods.

ribonucleic acid (RNA) Functions mainly in the expression of the cell's genetic information. It is a single-stranded nucleic acid whose pentose sugar is ribose and whose bases are adenine, uracil, guanine, and cytosine. (Varieties are messenger RNA, transfer RNA, ribosomal RNA.)

ribosome (**rye**-bo-sowm) Organelle containing RNA that may be attached to the ER and that functions in protein synthesis.

rickets (**rik**-ets) A condition affecting children in which vitamin D deficiency leads to altered calcium metabolism and disturbance of ossification of bone; bones become soft and deformed.

right lymphatic duct A lymphatic vessel that drains lymph from the upper right side of the body and empties it into the right subclavian vein.

rods Photoreceptors in the retina that are stimulated by low light intensities. There are more than 100 million rods in each eye.

roentgenogram (**rent**-gen-oh-*gram*) An x-ray; a film produced by taking pictures of internal structures by passage of x-rays through the body.

root canal The narrow extension of the pulp cavity that lies within the root of a tooth.

rotation The process of turning around an axis. Moving a bone around its own axis.

saccule (**sak**-yool) One of two sacs in the membranous labyrinth within the vestibule of the inner ear; the saccule is connected to the other sac, the utricle, by the endolymphatic duct.

sacral plexus (**say**-kral) The network formed by the anterior branches of spinal nerves L4 through S3.

saddle joint A synovial joint in which the articular surfaces of both bones are saddle shaped.

sagittal plane (**sadj**-ih-tul) A section or plane through the body that divides the body into right and left parts. The term may also be applied to an organ or other body part.

saliva The enzyme-containing secretion of the salivary glands.

salivary amylase (**sal**-ih-ver-ee **am**-ih-lase) An enzyme in saliva that initiates the digestion of starch, mainly in the mouth.

salivary glands Glands that secrete saliva into the mouth. The major ones are the paired parotid, submaxillary, and sublingual glands.

sarcolemma (*sar*-koe-**lem**-ma) The plasma membrane of a muscle cell, especially of a skeletal muscle.

sarcomere (**sar**-koe-mere) The contractile unit of a muscle cell extending from one Z band to the next along the length of the myofibril.

sarcoplasm (**sar**-koe-plazm) The cytoplasm of a muscle cell.

saturated fat A fat that contains no double bonds between any of its carbon atoms; each carbon is bonded to the maximum number of hydrogen atoms. Saturated fat is found in animal foods such as meat, milk, dairy products, and eggs.

Schwann cell (shvon) A type of glial cell found in the peripheral nervous system that forms the myelin sheath and cellular sheath of a nerve fiber by wrapping itself around the fiber.

sclera (**skleh**-rah) The tough, white outer coat of the eyeball; continuous anteriorly with the cornea and posteriorly with the covering of the optic nerve.

scrotum (**skrow**-tum) A skin-covered pouch that contains the testes and their accessory structures.

sebaceous gland (see-**bay**-shus) An exocrine gland in the dermis of the skin that secretes sebum, an oily material that lubricates the skin surface; its duct opens into a hair follicle. Also called oil gland.

sebum (**see**-bum) The oil secretion of the sebaceous glands.

secondary sex characteristics Characteristic male or female features (not directly involved in sexual reproduction) that develop at puberty in response to sex hormones such as shape of body, muscle development, pubic hair, and pitch of voice.

secretion (se-**kree**-shun) 1. The process by which a cell releases a specific product. 2. Any substance produced by secretion, for example, saliva produced by the cells of the salivary glands.

sella turcica (**sel**-ah **tur**-sih-kah) The depression on the upper surface of the sphenoid bone that houses the pituitary gland.

semen (**see**-men) Fluid discharged at ejaculation in the male, consisting of sperm and the secretions of the seminal vesicles, prostate gland, and bulbourethral glands. Also called seminal fluid.

semicircular canals The three channels located in the bony labyrinth of the inner ear that contain receptors for dynamic equilibrium.

semicircular ducts The three extensions of the membranous labyrinth of the inner ear that are located within the bony semicircular canals. Contain the cristae that function in dynamic equilibrium.

semilunar valve (*sem*-ee-**loo**-nar) A valve between each ventricle and the great artery into which it pumps blood; consists of flaps shaped like half-moons.

seminal vesicles (**sem**-ih-nul **ves**-ih-kuls) Glands that secrete a major portion of the semen into the ejaculatory ducts.

seminiferous tubules (*sem*-ih-**nif**-ur-us) The tubules within the testes where sperm cells are produced.

sensation A feeling; awareness of sensory input.

sensory areas of cerebrum Areas in the cerebrum that receive and interpret information from the sense receptors.

septum (**sep**-tum) A wall dividing a body cavity.

serosa (ser-**oh**-sah) Any serous membrane. Serous membranes line the pleural, pericardial, and peritoneal cavities.

serum (**see**-rum) The clear portion of blood that

remains after the solid components (cells and platelets) have been separated out.

sesamoid bone (**ses**-ah-moyd) A small bone that typically occurs in a tendon subject to stress or pressure; it does not form a joint directly.

sex chromosomes The X and Y chromosomes. Females have two X chromosomes, whereas males have one X and one Y chromosome.

sigmoid colon (**sig**-moyd **koe**-lon) The distal S-shaped part of the colon from the level of the iliac crest to the rectum.

sinoatrial (SA) node (*sigh*-no-**ay**-tree-al) Pacemaker of the heart; a mass of cardiac muscle specialized for conduction, located in the posterior wall of the right atrium near the opening of the superior vena cava.

sinus (**sigh**-nus) A cavity or channel such as the air cavities in the cranial bones (paranasal sinuses) or dilated channels for venous blood.

sinusoids (**sigh**-nuh-soyds) Tiny blood vessels (slightly larger than capillaries) found in certain organs such as the liver and spleen.

skeletal muscle An organ specialized for contraction, composed of striated (striped) muscle fibers (cells), surrounded and supported by connective tissue; stimulated by somatic efferent (motor) neurons.

skin The outer covering of the body; consists of two main layers, epidermis and dermis; the largest organ of the body. The skin and its associated structures, such as hair and sweat glands, make up the integumentary system.

skull The bony framework of the head consisting of the cranium and facial skeleton.

small intestine The region of the digestive tract that extends from the stomach to the large intestine; it is a long, coiled tube consisting of the duodenum, jejunum, and ileum.

smooth muscle A tissue specialized for contraction, composed of smooth (non-striated) muscle fibers (cells) located in the walls of hollow organs such as the intestine or uterus; innervated by a visceral efferent neuron.

sodium-potassium pump An active transport system located in the plasma membrane that uses the energy from ATP to transport sodium out of the cell and potassium into the cell; functions to maintain the concentrations of these ions at homeostatic levels.

soft palate (**pal**-at) The posterior portion of the roof of the mouth; a muscular partition lined with mucous membrane that extends from the palatine bones to the uvula.

solute (**sol**-yoot) The substance that is dissolved in a liquid (solvent) to form a solution.

solution A liquid (solvent) in which is dissolved one or more substances (solutes).

solvent (**sol**-vent) A liquid that dissolves another substance (solute) to form a solution without chemical change in either.

somatic nervous system (so-**mat**-ik) The part of the peripheral nervous system that keeps the body in adjustment with the external environment; includes the sensory receptors on the body surface and within the muscles, the nerves that link them with the central nervous system (CNS), and the efferent nerves that link the CNS with the skeletal muscles.

somesthetic (*sow*-mes-**thet**-ik) Pertaining to sensations and sensory structures of the body.

sperm cell Male gamete (sex cell) that combines with an ovum in sexual reproduction to produce a new individual. Also called spermatozoon.

spermatic cord (sper-**mat**-ik) The male reproductive structure extending from the abdominal inguinal ring to the testis; includes the vas deferens, testicular artery, veins, nerves, cremaster muscle, and connective tissue.

sphincter (**sfink**-ter) A circular muscle that constricts a passageway or orifice.

sphygmomanometer (*sfig*-mow-mah-**nom**-eh-ter) An instrument for measuring arterial blood pressure.

spinal cord (**spy**-nal) The part of the central nervous system located in the vertebral canal and extending from the foramen magnum to the upper part of the lumbar region.

spinal ganglion Dorsal root ganglion; consists of the cell bodies of sensory neurons and is located along the dorsal root just before it joins the spinal cord.

spinal nerve Any of the 31 pairs of nerves that arise from the spinal cord and pass out between the vertebrae.

spleen The largest organ of the lymphatic system, located in the upper part of the abdominal cavity on the left side; filters blood and provides the opportunity for lymphocyte activation.

sprain Wrenching or twisting of a joint with partial rupture of its ligaments.

squamous epithelium (**skway**-mus) Epithelium consisting of flat, scalelike cells.

stenosis (steh-**no**-sis) Narrowing or contraction of a body passage or opening.

sterile (**ster**-il) 1. Not fertile; not producing young. 2. Aseptic; free from living microorganisms.

sterilization (**ster**-il-ih-**zay**-shun) The process of rendering an individual incapable of producing offspring; for example, vasectomy.

stimulus Any change in the environment that produces a response in a receptor or irritable tissue.

stomach (**stum**-ak) The curved, muscular, saclike part of the digestive tract between the esophagus and the small intestine; occupies the abdominal cavity just below the diaphragm.

stratum (**stray**-tum) *Plural,* strata. A sheetlike mass of tissue of fairly uniform thickness; used to designate distinct sublayers making up various tissues or organs; for example, the strata of the skin.

stressor Any factor that disturbs homeostasis, producing stress.

stroke volume The volume of blood pumped by one ventricle during one contraction.

subarachnoid space (*sub*-ah-**rak**-noyd) The space between the arachnoid and pia mater through which cerebrospinal fluid circulates.

subcutaneous (*sub*-kyoo-**tay**-nee-us) Beneath the skin.

subcutaneous layer The layer of loose connective tissue and adipose tissue beneath the skin.

subdural space (sub-**doo**-ral) The space between the dura mater and arachnoid.

sublingual glands (sub-**ling**-gwal) The paired salivary glands located in the floor of the mouth under the tongue.

submandibular glands (*sub*-man-**dib**-yoo-lar) The paired salivary glands located in the posterior region of the floor of the mouth posterior to the sublingual glands.

submucosa (*sub*-myoo-**koe**-sah) A layer of connective tissue located beneath a mucous membrane, as in the digestive tract.

substrate (**sub**-strate) Any substance upon which an enzyme acts.

sulcus (**sul**-kus) A groove or furrow; a linear depression as is found between the gyri of the brain.

superficial (*soo*-per-**fish**-al) Located on or near the body surface.

superior (sue-**peer**-ee-ur) Higher; refers to structures nearer the head than the feet.

superior vena cava (**vee**-nah **kay**-vah) Large vein that receives blood from parts of the body superior to the heart and returns it to the right atrium.

supination (*soo*-pih-**nay**-shun) The act of assuming the supine position, that is, lying on the back. Applied to the hand, the act of turning the palm upward.

suture (**soo**-cher) The fibrous joint between adjoining bones in the skull.

sweat (swet) Perspiration; the salty fluid, consisting mainly of water, excreted by the sweat glands in the skin.

sympathetic division (*sim*-pah-**thet**-ik) The thoracolumbar portion of the autonomic nervous system; its general effect is to mobilize energy, especially during stress situations; prepares body for fight-or-flight response.

symphysis (**sim**-fih-sis) A relatively immovable type of joint in which the two joining bones are firmly united by a plate of fibrocartilage.

symphysis pubis (**pyoo**-bis) A slightly movable cartilaginous joint between the pubic bones.

symptom (**simp**-tum) Any indication of disease perceived by the patient.

synapse (**sin**-aps) Junction between two neurons or between a neuron and an effector.

synaptic cleft (sin-**ap**-tik) The narrow gap that separates the axon terminal of one neuron from another neuron or from a muscle fiber. Neurotransmitter diffuses across the cleft to affect the postsynaptic cell.

synaptic knobs Tiny enlargements in the axon terminal that synthesize neurotransmitter and store it in synaptic vesicles.

synaptic vesicle Membrane-enclosed sac containing neurotransmitter; found in the synaptic knobs of axons.

synarthrosis (*sin*-are-**throw**-sis) An immovable joint; a joint in which the bones are tightly united by fibrous tissue.

syndrome (**sin**-drome) A combination of symptoms that occur together forming a pattern characteristic of a particular disorder.

synovial fluid (sih-**no**-vee-al) The transparent, viscous fluid secreted by the synovial membrane and found in joint cavities, bursae, and tendon sheaths.

synovial joint A fully movable or diarthrotic joint in which a synovial cavity is present between the two articulating bones.

systemic (sis-**tem**-ik) Affecting the body as a whole.

systemic circulation The circuit of blood vessels through which oxygen-rich blood flows from the left ventricle through the aorta to all of the organs of the body and oxygen-poor blood returns to the right atrium.

systole (**sis**-toe-lee) The phase of contraction of the heart during which blood is forced into the aorta and pulmonary artery.

systolic blood pressure (sis-**tol**-ik) The force exerted by the blood on arterial walls during ventricular contraction; about 120 mm Hg under normal conditions for a young adult.

T cell A T lymphocyte; a lymphocyte responsible for cell-mediated immunity. Subtypes include cytotoxic, memory, helper, and suppressor T cells.

tachycardia (*tak*-ih-**kar**-dee-ah) An abnormally

rapid heart rate, usually defined as more than 100 beats per minute.

tactile (**tak**-tile) Pertaining to the sense of touch.

target cell A cell whose activity is affected by a particular hormone.

tarsus (**tar**-sus) The seven bones that make up the ankle.

telophase (**tel**-oh-faze) The last of the four stages of mitosis and of the two divisions of meiosis; the cytoplasm usually divides during telophase, giving rise to two daughter cells.

tendinitis (*ten*-din-**i**-tis) Inflammation of tendons and tendon-muscle attachments; frequently associated with calcium deposits and may also involve the bursa around the tendon, causing bursitis.

tendon (**ten**-don) A cord of strong white fibrous tissue that connects a muscle to a bone.

testis (**tes**-tis) The male gonad; either of the paired glands located in the scrotum which produce sperm and the male sex hormone testosterone. Also called testicle. *Plural,* testes.

testosterone (tes-**tos**-teh-rone) The principal male sex hormone (androgen); produced by the interstitial cells in the testes; stimulates development of the male reproductive organs and secondary sex characteristics.

tetanus (**tet**-ah-nus) A fatal disease caused by the tetanus bacillus (*Clostridium tetani*) and characterized by muscle spasms and convulsions.

tetany (**tet**-ah-nee) 1. Steady contraction of a muscle without distinct twitching; continuous topic spasm of a muscle. 2. A syndrome characterized by muscle twitchings, cramps, and convulsions, caused by abnormal calcium metabolism.

thalamus (**thal**-uh-mus) A large oval structure composed of gray matter covered by a thin layer of white matter and located at the base of the cerebrum. The thalamus serves as a main relay center transmitting information between the spinal cord and the cerebrum.

thermoreceptor (*ther*-mow-ree-**sep**-tor) A receptor that detects changes in temperature.

thigh The part of the lower limb between the hip and the knee.

thoracic cavity (thow-**ras**-ik) The superior part of the ventral body cavity; contains the two pleural cavities, pericardial cavity, and mediastinum.

thoracic duct A lymphatic vessel that receives lymph and empties it into the left subclavian vein.

thorax (**thow**-rax) The chest.

thrombin (**throm**-bin) An enzyme formed by the activation of prothrombin that catalyzes the conversion of fibrinogen to fibrin.

thromboplastin (*throm*-bow-**plas**-tin) A complex of several phospholipids and a proteolytic enzyme released from damaged tissue; important in the clotting process.

thrombus (**throm**-bus) A blood clot formed within a blood vessel or within the heart.

thymus gland (**thy**-mus) A gland located in the upper mediastinum beneath the sternum that reaches its maximum development during puberty and plays a role in immunologic function throughout life.

thyroid gland An endocrine gland located in the front and sides of the neck just below the thyroid cartilage; its hormones are essential for normal growth and metabolism.

thyroid-stimulating-hormone (TSH) A tropic hormone secreted by the anterior lobe of the pituitary gland that stimulates the synthesis and secretion of hormones produced by the thyroid gland.

thyroxine (T$_4$) (thy-**rok**-sin) One of the hormones secreted by the thyroid gland; essential for normal growth and metabolism.

tissue (**tiss**-you) A group of closely associated similar cells that work together to carry out specific functions.

tongue A large muscular organ on the floor of the mouth that functions in chewing, swallowing, and speech.

tonsil (**ton**-sil) Aggregate of lymph nodules embedded in the mucous membrane in the throat region. The tonsils are located strategically to deal with pathogens that enter through the mouth or nose.

toxic (**tok**-sik) Poisonous; pertaining to poison.

trachea (**tray**-kee-ah) The air passageway extending from the larynx to the main bronchi. Also called windpipe.

tract A bundle of nerve fibers in the central nervous system.

transmission (trans-**mish**-un) Conduction of an action potential (neural impulse) along a neuron or from one neuron to another.

transverse colon (trans-**verse koe**-lon) The portion of the large intestine extending across the abdomen from the ascending to the descending colon.

trauma (**traw**-mah) A wound or injury, especially damage caused by external force.

tricuspid valve (try-**kus**-pid) The valve consisting of three flaps that guards the opening between the right atrium and right ventricle.

triiodothyronine (T$_3$) (*try*-i-o-dow-**thy**-row-nene) One of the thyroid hormones; essential for normal growth and metabolism.

tropic hormone (**trow**-pik) A hormone that helps to regulate another endocrine gland; for example, thyroid-stimulating hormone released by the pituitary regulates the thyroid gland.

trunk 1. The main part of the body to which the head and limbs are attached. 2. A large structure, such as a nerve or blood vessel, from which smaller branches arise, or which is formed by small branches.

tubular reabsorption The movement of a substance out of the renal tubule and into the peritubular capillaries.

tubular secretion The movement of a substance out of the peritubular capillaries and into the renal tubule.

tumor (**too**-mor) Neoplasm; a new growth of tissue in which cell multiplication is uncontrolled and progressive.

twitch Rapid, brief, jerky contraction of a muscle in response to a single stimulus.

tympanic membrane (tim-**pan**-ik) Thin, semitransparent membrane that stretches across the ear canal, separating the outer ear from the middle ear.

ulcer (**ul**-ser) An open lesion, or excavation, of a tissue produced by the sloughing of inflamed, dying tissue.

umbilical cord (um-**bil**-ih-kal) The long, ropelike structure that connects the fetus and placenta; contains the umbilical arteries and vein.

uremia (yoo-**ree**-me-ah) An excess in the blood of urea and other nitrogenous wastes, generally resulting from kidney malfunction. A sign of renal failure.

ureter (**you**-ree-ter) One of the paired tubes that conduct urine from the kidneys to the bladder.

urethra (you-**ree**-thruh) A muscular tube that conducts urine from the bladder to the exterior surface of the body.

urinalysis (*u*-rih-**nal**-ih-sis) Examination of the physical, chemical, and microscopic characteristics of urine used as an aid in the diagnosis of disease.

urinary bladder A muscular sac in the anterior floor of the pelvic cavity that serves as a storage sac for urine.

urine (**u**-rin) The fluid containing water, waste products, salts, and traces of other substances that is produced by the kidneys.

uterine tube (**you**-tur-in) One of the paired tubes attached to each end of the uterus; site of fertilization. Also called fallopian tube or oviduct.

uterus (**you**-tur-us) The womb; the organ that houses the embryo and fetus during development.

utricle (**u**-trih-kul) The larger of the two divisions of the membranous labyrinth of the inner ear.

uvula (**u**-vue-lah) A fleshy mass of tissue, especially the structure extending from the soft palate.

vacuole (**vac**-you-ole) A cavity enclosed by membrane and located in the cytoplasm.

vagina (vah-**jye**-nuh) The elastic, muscular tube extending from the cervix to the vestibule; receives the penis during sexual intercourse and serves as the birth canal.

vagus nerve (**vay**-gus) The tenth cranial nerve; each vagus nerve emerges from the medulla and innervates thoracic and abdominal organs; the main nerve of the parasympathetic system.

varicose veins (**var**-ih-kose) Swollen, distended veins usually located in the subcutaneous tissues of the leg.

vascular (**vas**-kyoo-lar) Pertaining to or containing many blood vessels.

vas deferens (**def**-ur-enz) One of the paired ducts that conveys semen from the epididymis to the ejaculatory duct.

vasectomy (vah-**sek**-tow-me) A sterilization procedure in which a portion of each vas deferens is removed.

vasoconstriction (*vas*-o-kon-**strik**-shun) The narrowing of blood vessels; refers especially to the narrowing of the arterioles.

vasodilation (*vas*-o-die-**lay**-shun) The widening of blood vessels; refers especially to the widening of arterioles.

vein (vane) A vessel that conducts blood from tissues back to the heart.

vena cava (**vee**-nah **kay**-vah) The superior or inferior vein that opens into the right atrium returning oxygen-poor blood to the heart.

ventral (**ven**-tral) Pertaining to the abdomen or anterior (front side) of the body; opposite of dorsal.

ventricle (**ven**-tri-kul) A small cavity or chamber, such as one of the cavities of the brain or heart.

venule (**ven**-yule) A small vein that collects blood from capillaries and delivers it to a larger vein.

vermiform appendix (**ver**-mih-form) A small appendage attached to the cecum.

vertebral canal (**ver**-teh-bral) The canal formed by the series of vertebral foramina together, containing the spinal cord.

vertebral column The spine; the rigid structure in the midline of the back, composed of the vertebrae.

vesicle (**ves**-ih-kul) A small sac containing fluid.

vestibule (**ves**-tih-byool) A small space or region at the beginning of a canal, for example, the vagina opens into a vestibule.

villus (**vil**-us) A small vascular projection from the free surface of a membrane, for example, intestinal villi project from the surface of the small intestine.

viscera (**vis**-ur-uh) The organs located within the body cavities.

visceral (**vis**-er-al) Pertaining to the organs or to the covering of an organ.

visceral peritoneum The inner layer of the serous membrane that covers the abdominal viscera.

vitamin (**vie**-tah-min) An organic compound essential in the diet in small amounts; acts as a coenzyme in metabolic reactions and is essential for normal growth and health.

vitreous humor (**vit**-ree-us **hyoo**-mor) A clear, jelly-like fluid that fills the posterior cavity of the eye lying between the lens and retina.

vocal cords The folds of mucous membranes in the larynx that vibrate to make vocal sounds during speaking. The inferior folds are called true vocal cords or vocal folds.

vulva (**vul**-vah) The external genital organs in the female. Also called pudendum.

white blood cells (WBC) Leukocytes.

white matter Nervous tissue composed mainly of myelinated nerve fibers; makes up the conducting portion of the brain and spinal cord.

wound A bodily injury caused by physical means, with disruption of the normal continuity of structures.

zygote (**zye**-goat) Fertilized ovum; the cell resulting from the fusion of male and female gametes.

INDEX

Note: Page numbers in *italics* refer to illustrations; page numbers followed by (t) refer to tables; **boldface** page numbers indicate definitions.

Abdomen, *13*, **271**
  external oblique muscle of, *19, 83, 84, 85,* 86(t)
    aponeurosis of, *85*
  internal oblique muscle of, *85*
    aponeurosis of, *85*
Abdominal aorta, 172, *173, 174,* 175(t), *231*
Abdominal cavity, *14,* 16, **271**
Abdominal region, 13
Abdominopelvic cavity, *14, 15,* 16, **271**
  quadrants of, *15,* 16–17
  regions of, *15,* 17
Abducens nerve, *110,* 111(t)
Abduction, 68(t), **271**
ABO blood types, 152, 154, *154,* 154(t), **271**
Abortion, **271**
Absorption, 211, 220–221, **271**
Accessory digestive glands, 211
Accommodation, **121**
Acetabulum, 56(t), *65*
Acetylcholine, 78, **271**
Achilles tendon, *84,* **271**
Acid(s), **271**
  amino, 4, **272**
    essential, **278**
    release of, in protein digestion, 220
  ascorbic, 224(t)
  deoxyribonucleic, 4, **277**
  folic, 224(t)
  lactic, 79, **284**
  nicotinic, 224(t)
  nucleic, 4, **286**
  pantothenic, 224(t)
  ribonucleic, 4, **290**
Acne, 43
Acquired immune deficiency syndrome (AIDS), **271**
Acromegaly, **271**
Acromion process, *53,* 56(t)
ACTH (adrenocorticotropic hormone), 133(t), 137, 141, *142,* **271**
Actin, **271**
Actin filaments, **78**
Action(s), muscular, 86(t)–88(t)
  parasympathetic, 116(t)
  reflex, **104,** *114*
    withdrawal as, 104, *104*
  sympathetic, 116(t)
Action potential, 78, **271**
Activating system, reticular, **290**
Active immunity, 196, **271**
Active transport, **29, 271**
Actual response, 93
Acupuncture, 126
Acute, **271**

Adam's apple, 201, **271**
Adduction, 69(t), **271**
Adductor longus muscle, *83,* 87(t)
Adductor magnus muscle, *19, 83, 84,* 87(t)
Adenoids, 183
Adenosine monophosphate (AMP), cyclic, 132
Adenosine triphosphate (ATP), 5, **271**
  and muscle contraction, 78–79
ADH (antidiuretic hormone), 98, 133(t), 136, 235–236, 242–243, **272**
Adipose (fat) tissue, *34,* 35, 43, **271**
  mammary, 253, *253*
  sympathetic actions on, 116(t)
Adolescence, 258
Adrenal cortex, 134(t), *140,* 140–141, *142,* **271**
Adrenal gland(s), 7, *18, 132,* 133(t)–134(t), 139–141, *140, 142,* **271**
Adrenal medulla, 133(t), 140, *140, 142,* **271**
  sympathetic actions on, 116(t)
Adrenocorticotropic hormone (ACTH), 133(t), 137, 141, *142,* **271**
Adulthood, 258
Adventitia, **271**
Aerobic, **272**
Afferent, **272**
Afferent arterioles, 232, *232,* 233, *233, 234,* **272**
Afferent nerves (sensory nerves), 92
Afferent neurons (sensory neurons), 109, 111, 113, **272**
  in reflexes, 104, *104, 114*
Afterbirth, **272**
Agglutination, 152, 154, **272**
Aging, 257–258
Agonist muscle (prime mover), 81, *81*
Agranular leukocytes, 150, *150*
AIDS (acquired immune deficiency syndrome), **271**
Air, dirty, 205–206
  exhaled, carbon dioxide in, 204, 205(t)
    nitrogen in, 205(t)
    oxygen in, 205(t)
  inhaled, 205–206
    carbon dioxide in, 205(t)
    nitrogen in, 205(t)
    oxygen in, 205(t)
Air-filled sinuses, 51, 51(t), 61, *200,* 201
Air movement, into and out of lungs, 202–204
Air sacs, pulmonary, 199, 201, *202*
  in gas exchange, 204, *204*
Air spaces, in middle ear, 122
Alarm reaction, 141

Albino, 44–45
Albumin, **272**
Aldosterone, 134(t), 141, 236, 244, **272**
Alimentary canal, **211, 272**
  wall of, 211, *212*
Alkaline, **272**
Allergen, **272**
Allergic reaction, to transfusion, 152
Allergy, **272**
All-or-none law, **272**
Alpha cells, 138, *139,* **272**
Alveolar gland, **272**
Alveolar process, 54(t), *214*
Alveolus (alveoli), **272**
  dental, *61,* 213
  pulmonary, 199, 201, *202*
    in gas exchange, 204, *204*
Amino acid(s), 4, **272**
  essential, **278**
  release of, in protein digestion, 220
Amnion, 255, *256,* **272**
AMP (adenosine monophosphate), cyclic, 132
Amphiarthrosis, 66, *67,* **272**
Amylase, pancreatic, 218, 219(t)
  salivary, 215, 218, 219(t), **291**
Anabolism, 5, *9,* **272**
Anaerobic, **272**
Anaerobic metabolism, 79
Anal canal, 222, **272**
Anal sphincters, 222
Anaphase, 31, *31,* **272**
Anaphylaxis, **272**
Anastomosis, **272**
  arterial, 177
Anatomical position, **11,** *11,* **272**
Anatomy, **1, 272**
Androgen, 141, **272**
Anemia, 150, **272**
  vitamin deficiency and, 224(t), 225(t)
Anesthetic injection, into subarachnoid space, 104
Angina, 126
Angiotensins, 181, **272**
Anion(s), 244, **272**
Ankle, *13*
  muscles of, 88(t)
Antagonist muscle, 81, *81,* **272**
Anterior, 11, **272**
Anterior cavity of eye, *120,* 121
Anterior cerebral artery (arteries), right, *176*
Anterior column of spinal cord, *101,* 102
Anterior communicating artery of cerebrum, *176*
Anterior lobe of pituitary gland, 133(t), *136,* 136–137

Anterior median fissure of spinal cord, *101*, 102
Anterior root (ventral root) of spinal nerve, 113, *113*, **272**
Anterior spinal artery, *176*
Anterior superior iliac spine, 57(t)
Anterior tubercle of atlas, *63*
Antibiotic, 151, **272**
Antibody (antibodies), 149, 152, 154, 154(t), 194, **272**
  antigen combinations with, 194, 196
  circulating, 194
  classes of, 194
  in breast milk, 196
  to Rh blood, 155
Antibody-mediated immunity, 194, *195*
Antidiuretic, **272**
Antidiuretic hormone (ADH), 98, 133(t), 136, 235–236, 242–243, **272**
Antigen(s), 152, 154, 154(t), **190**, **272**
  immunity following exposure to, 196
  T cell reaction to, 193, 194
Antigen-antibody complex, 194, 196
Antigen D, 154
Antihistamine, **273**
Anus, *8*, *210*, 222, *248*, *250*, *252*, **273**
Aorta, *17*, *161*, *165*, 172, *172*, **273**
  abdominal, 172, *173*, *174*, 175(t), *231*
  arch of, *17*, *18*, *160*, 172, *173*, *174*, 175(t)
  ascending, *160*, 172, *174*, 175(t)
  branches of, *174*, 175(t)
  CT appearance of, *20*
  descending, *17*, *160*, *174*
  parietal branches of, 175(t)
  thoracic, 172, *174*, 175(t)
  visceral branches of, 175(t)
Aortic arch, *17*, *18*, *160*, 172, *173*, *174*, 175(t)
Aortic valve, *161*, 162
Apatite, *49*
Apex of heart, *160*
Aponeurosis, of external oblique muscle of abdomen, *85*
  of internal oblique muscle of abdomen, *85*
Apparatus, juxtaglomerular, 233, *233*
Appendicitis, 222
Appendicular portion of body, 13, *13*
Appendicular skeleton, *50*
Appendix, *17*, *210*, 222, **295**
Aqueduct, cerebral, *97*, *103*, **275**
Aqueous humor, *121*, **273**
Arachnoid granulations, *102*, 103, *103*
Arachnoid membrane, *102*, **102**, *103*, 104, **273**
Arch, aortic, *17*, *18*, *160*, 172, *173*, *174*, 175(t)
  longitudinal, of foot, *66*
  posterior, of atlas, *63*
  pubic, *65*
  superciliary, *58*
  transverse, of foot, *66*
  zygomatic, *53*
Areola, 253, *253*, **273**
Arm, 13, *13*, **273**
  muscles of, 87(t)
Armpit, *13*
Arrector pili muscles, *42*, 44, **273**
Arterioles, 170, *170*, *171*, **273**
  afferent, 232, *232*, 233, *233*, *234*, **272**

Arterioles (*Continued*)
  efferent, 232, *232*, 233, *233*, *234*, **277**
  resistance of, to blood flow, 180
Artery (arteries), 7, 170, *170*, **273**. See also specific arteries, e.g., *Carotid artery.*
  expansion and recoil of, 179
  joining of, 177
  resistance of, to blood flow, 180
  walls of, 170, *171*
Arthritis, **273**
Articular cartilage, *48*, *49*, *70*
Articular processes of vertebrae, *62*, *63*, 64(t)
Articulation(s), 66, *67*, 68(t), 70–71, **283**. See also specific joints.
  movement at, 68(t)–70(t)
Ascending aorta, *160*, 172, *174*, 175(t)
Ascending colon, *16*, *17*, *210*, 222, **273**
Ascending tracts, in central nervous system, 102
Ascorbic acid (vitamin C), 224(t)
Association area, 96(t), 100, *101*, **273**
Association neurons, **273**
  in reflexes, 104, *104*, *114*
Asthma, **273**
Astigmatism, **273**
Atherosclerosis, **273**
Atlas (C1 vertebra), *19*, 55(t), *63*
  anterior tubercle of, *63*
  posterior arch of, *63*
  posterior tubercle of, *63*
Atom, 4, **273**
  nucleus of, **286**
ATP (adenosine triphosphate), 5, **271**
  and muscle contraction, 78–79
Atrial natriuretic factor, 143
Atrioventricular bundle, 163, *163*
Atrioventricular node, 163, *163*, **273**
Atrioventricular valve, *161*, 162, **273**
  opening and closing of, 164, *165*
Atrium (atria) of heart, *160*, **273**
  auricle of, *160*, *162*, **273**
  contraction and relaxation of, 164, *165*
  left, *161*, *163*, *173*
  right, *160*, *161*, *163*, *173*
Auditory association area, *101*
Auditory meatus, external, *59*, 121, *122*
  internal, *60*
Auditory ossicles, 55(t), 122, *122*, **273**
Auditory reflexes, 98
Auditory tube (eustachian tube), 122, *122*, **273**
Auricle, of atrium, *160*, *162*, **273**
  of ear, **273**
Autoimmune disease, **273**
Autonomic ganglion, **273**
Autonomic nervous system, 92, 98, 113–116, **273**
  parasympathetic division of, *114*, 115, **287**
    actions of, 116(t)
  sympathetic division of, *114*, 115, **293**
    actions of, 116(t)
Autonomic reflex, *114*
Axial portion of body, 13, *13*
Axial skeleton, *50*
Axilla, **273**
Axillary artery, *173*
Axillary lymph nodes, *182*
Axillary region, 13, *13*

Axis (body axis), 11
Axis (C2 vertebra), 55(t), *63*
  odontoid process of (dens axis), 55(t), *63*
Axon, 35, *36*, 92, 93, *93*, **273**
Azygos vein, 176(t)

Baby teeth, 214, *215*
Bacteria, in large intestine, 221, 222
Bacterial infection, 194
  defenses against, 190
    macrophages in, *191*, 192
  vs. viral infection, 150, 151
Ball-and-socket joint, *67*, 68(t), **273**
Baroreceptors, 180, 181, **273**
Barrier, blood-brain, **274**
Bartholin's glands (greater vestibular glands), 253, **281**
Basal ganglia, 99, **273**
Basal metabolic rate (BMR), **273**
Base, **273**
Basilar artery, *174*, *176*, 177
Basophil, 150, *150*, **274**
B cells (B lymphocytes), 192(t), 193, 194, *195*, **274**
  memory, 192(t), 194, **285**
B complex vitamins, 224(t)–225(t)
Belly, **274**
Benign, **274**
Beriberi, 224(t)
Beta cells, 138, 139, *139*, **274**
Beta receptor, **274**
Bicarbonate, 205
Biceps brachii muscle, 81, *81*, *83*, *84*, 87(t)
Biceps femoris muscle, *19*, *84*, 88(t)
Bicuspid (mitral) valve, *161*, 162, *162*, **274**
  stenosis of, 162
Bilateral, **274**
Bilateral symmetry, 10
Bile, 218, **274**
Bile duct, common, *217*, 218, **276**
  CT appearance of, *20*
Bile pigments, 230
Bilirubin, 218, **274**
Biotin, 225(t)
Birth, 257
Bitter taste, *124*, 125
Blackhead, 44
Bladder, *9*, *16*, *17*, *18*, 230, *231*, 236, *248*, *250*, **295**
  emptying of, 104, 236
Bleeding. See *Hemorrhage.*
Blind spot, **274**
Blood, 147–157, *148*, 170–181, **274**
  circulation of, 171–172, *172*, *173*
    pulmonary, 171–172, *172*, **289–290**
    systemic, 171, 172, *172*, **293**
      resistance in, 180
  loss of, 180
  oxygen-poor, *160*, 171, 172, *172*, *173*
  oxygen-rich, *160*, 171, 172, *172*, *173*
  regulation of calcium levels in, 134–135, *135*, 138
  regulation of glucose levels in, 138–139, *139*
Blood-brain barrier, **274**
Blood cell(s), *150*
  counting of, 152(t), 153(t)

Blood cell(s) (*Continued*)
  red, *148*, 149–150, *150*
  white, *26*, *27*, *148*, *150*, 150–151
    agranular, 150, *150*
    granular, 150, *150*
Blood clotting, *151*, 151–152
Blood clotting factors, 151
Blood count, complete, 152(t)
Blood flow, 179–181
  resistance to, *180*, 180–181
Blood pressure, **179**, **274**
  diastolic, 181
  factors affecting, 179–181, *180*
  measurement of, 181
  systolic, 181, **293**
Blood tests, 152(t)–153(t)
Blood transfusion, 152
Blood typing, 152, *154*, 154(t), 154–155
Blood vessels, 170, *170*, **274**. See also
    specific types.
  in inflammation, 190, *191*
  resistance to flow in, 180
  sympathetic actions on, 116(t)
  walls of, 170–171, *171*
Blood volume, 180
  and blood pressure, 180, *180*
  and urine volume, 235, *235*
BMR (basal metabolic rate), **273**
Body, 1–22
  cavities of, *14*, *15*, 15–17, **274**
  compounds in, 4
  defense mechanisms of, 189–198. See
    also *Defense mechanisms.*
  directions in, 10–12, *11*
  elements in, 2(t), 4
  levels of organization in, 2, *3*, 4
  organ systems of, *3*, 4–5, 5(t), *6–9*
  planes of, 12, *12*
  regions of, *13*, 13–15
Body axis, 11
Body cavities, *14*, *15*, 15–17, **274**
Body fluid, 241
Body movement, 68(t)–70(t)
Body systems (organ systems), *3*, 4–5,
    5(t), *6–9*
Body temperature regulation, 104
Bolus, **274**
  conversion of food to, 215
Bone(s), *48*, 49. See also specific bones,
    e.g., *Temporal bone.*
  development of, 49–50
  joints between, 66, *67*, 68(t), 70–71
    movement at, 68(t)–70(t)
  microscopic structure of, *50*
  skeletal, *52–53*, 54(t)–58(t)
Bone markings, 51(t)
Bone marrow, *48*, 49
  red, *48*, 49, 149
  yellow, *48*, 49
Bone marrow cavity, 49
Bone tissue, *34*, 49, *50*, **274**
  intramembranous formation of, 49, **283**
Bony labyrinth, 122, *123*, **274**
Borrowed (passive) immunity, 196
Bowel. See *Intestine.*
Bowman's capsule, 232, *232*, 233, *233*,
    234, **274**
Brachial artery, *179*
Brachialis muscle, *83*, *84*, 87(t)
Brachial plexus, *112*, 113
Brachial region, 13, *13*

Brachiocephalic artery, *17*, *160*, *174*,
    175(t)
Brachiocephalic vein(s), *160*, 176(t), 177
  left, *18*
  right, *177*
Brachioradialis muscle, *83*, *84*, 87(t)
Bradycardia, **164**, **274**
Brain, 7, *92*, 93–100, *94*, *95*, *103*, **274**
  arterial supply to, 175, *176*, 177
  complexity of, 93–94
  CT examination of, *20*, 104
  damage to, 95
  dependence of, on blood supply, 95
    on glucose, 139
  divisions of, 95, 96(t)
  gray matter of, 96(t), 97
  hemorrhage in, 104
  inflammation of, 103
  protective coverings of, *102*
  respiratory regulation by, 205
  venous drainage of, 102, *102*, 177, *177*
  ventricle(s) of, *20*, 95, *95*, **95**, 97, 99,
    103
  white matter of, 95, 96(t), 100
Brain stem, *94*, **95**, **274**
Branches, of aorta, *174*, 175(t)
  of spinal nerves, 113, *113*
Breast(s), *13*, 253, *253*
  adipose tissue of, 253, *253*
  cancer of, 253
  ducts of, 253, *253*
  glandular tissue of, 253, *253*
  lymphatics of, *182*
  nipple of, 253, *253*
    areola of, 253, *253*, **273**
Breast milk, 253
  antibodies in, 196
  stimulation of secretion of, 137
Breathing, 202–204, *203*
  mechanics of, 202–204, *203*
  muscles used in, 87(t)
  nose, 200
Brim, pelvic (pelvic inlet), 57(t), 65, *65*
Broca's area, 100, *101*, **274**
Brodmann's classification, of functional
    areas of cerebral cortex, 100, *101*
Bronchial artery, *174*, 175(t)
Bronchial tree, 201
Bronchiole(s), *199*, *200*, 202, **274**
Bronchitis, 206, **274**
Bronchus (bronchi), *8*, *199*, *200*, 201
  parasympathetic actions on, 116(t)
  primary, *200*
  right, *17*
  secondary, *200*
  sympathetic actions on, 116(t)
Buccal, **274**
Buccal region, 13
Buccinator muscle, *84*, *85*, 86(t)
Buds, taste, *124*, 125, 213
Buffer, **274**
Bulbourethral gland (Cowper's gland),
    248, 249, **274**
Bundle, atrioventricular, 163, *163*
Bursa, 71, **274**
Bursitis, **274**
Buttocks, *13*, **274**

Cage, thoracic, 56(t), 65
Calcaneal region, *13*

Calcaneus, 53, 57(t), *66*, *84*, **274**
Calcitonin, 133(t), 138, **274**
Calcium, 223(t)
  in blood, regulation of levels of, 134–
    135, *135*, 138
  in bone, 49
  in human body, 2(t)
Calcium ions, 244
Calf, *13*
Calorie, **274**
Calyx, 230, *231*, 232, **274**
cAMP (cyclic adenosine monophosphate),
    132
Canal(s), alimentary, **211**, **272**
    wall of, 211, *212*
  anal, 222, **272**
  carotid, *61*
  central, of spinal cord, *101*, 102, **275**
  haversian, 49, *50*
  hypoglossal, *60*
  inguinal, **282**
  optic, *60*
  root, 213–214, *214*, **291**
  semicircular, *122*, *123*, 123, **291**
  vertebral, *14*, 15, *62*, **295**
Cancer, **274**
  breast, 253
  cervical, 252
  colonic, 222
  prostate gland, 249
  thymosin for, 196
Canines, 214, *215*, **274**
Capillaries, 170, *170*, *171*, *172*, **274**
  glomerular, 232, 233, *233*
  in gas exchange, 204, *204*
  in inflammation, 190, *191*
  lymph, 183
  peritubular, *232*, 233
  resistance of, to blood flow, 180
  skin, 42, *43*
  walls of, 170–171
Capsule, Bowman's, 232, *232*, 233, *233*,
    234, **274**
  joint, 70–71
  renal, 230, *231*
Carbohydrate(s), 4, 222, **275**
  digestion of, 218, 219(t)
Carbon, in human body, 2(t)
Carbon dioxide, diffusion of, 204, *204*
  effects of increased production of, 205
  in exhaled air, 204, 205(t)
  in inhaled air, 205(t)
  transport of, 205
Cardiac, **275**. See also *Heart.*
Cardiac centers, 97
Cardiac cycle, 164, *165*, **275**
Cardiac muscle tissue, 35, 35(t), 160, 163–
    164, **275**
Cardiac output, **164**
  and blood pressure, 180, *180*
Cardiac sphincter, 216
Cardiopulmonary resuscitation (CPR),
    205
Cardiovascular system, 147
Carotid artery, 179
  common, *16*, *17*, *18*, 179
    left, *160*, *173*, *174*, 175(t)
    right, *173*, *174*, 175(t)
  external, left, *174*
  internal, 175
    left, *174*, *176*

Carotid canal, *61*
Carpal bones, *52, 53,* 56(t), *64,* 65
Carpal region, 13, *13*
Cartilage, *34,* **275**
    articular, *48, 49,* 70
    costal, *52,* **276**
Castration, 250, **275**
Catabolism, **5,** *9,* **275**
Catecholamine, **275**
Cation(s), 244, **275**
Caudad, 11
Cavernous bodies of penis, *248*
Cavernous sinus, *177*
Cavity (cavities), abdominal, *14, 16,* **271**
    abdominopelvic, *14, 15, 16,* **271**
        quadrants of, *15,* 16–17
        regions of, *15,* 17
    body, *14, 15,* 15–17, **274**
    bone marrow, 49
    cranial, *14, 15*
    dorsal, *14, 15*
    eye, *120,* 121
    marrow, 49
    nasal, *8,* 199, *200*
        mucous membrane lining, 201
        protective function of hairs in, 190
        receptors in, 123, *124*
    oral, *8,* 212–213
        starch digestion in, 218, 219(t)
    pelvic, *14, 16,* **288**
    pericardial, *14, 16,* **288**
    peritoneal, 211
    pleural, 202, **288**
    pulp, 213, *214,* **290**
    scrotal, *14*
    thoracic, *14, 15, 16,* 202, **294**
        in breathing, 202, 203, *203*
    ventral, *14, 15*
CBC (complete blood count), 152(t)
Cecum, *16, 17, 210,* 222, **275**
Celiac artery, *173,* 175(t)
Celiac region, 13, *13*
Celiac trunk, *174*
Cell(s), 4, 25–33, **275.** See also specific
    types of cells.
    division by, 29–31, *31,* 33
    ingestion by, 29, *30*
    life cycle of, 30–31, *31*
    nucleus of, *4,* **28, 286**
    organelles of, *4,* 27
    plasma membrane of, 27
        movement through, 28–29
    size and shape of, *26,* 26–27
    structure of, *27*
    tonicity of solutions and, 28, *29*
Cell body of neuron, 35, *36, 92, 93,*
    275
Cell cycle, 30–31, *31*
Cell-mediated immunity, *193,* 193–194,
    275
Cell membrane, 27
    movement through, 28–29
Cellular level of organization, in human
    body, *3,* 4
Cellular respiration, 204
Cellular sheath (neurilemma), *93, 93*
Cementum, *214,* **275**
Central canal of spinal cord, *101,* 102,
    275
Central incisor, *215*
Central lobe, 100

Central nervous system (CNS), 91–108,
    92, **275.** See also *Brain* and *Spinal
    cord.*
    nucleus (nuclei) in, 93, **286**
    protective coverings of, *102,* 102–104,
        103
    tracts in, 93, **294**
        ascending, 102
        descending, 102
Central sulcus of cerebrum, *94, 99, 100,
    101*
Centrioles, 30
Centrum vertebrae, *62, 63,* 64(t)
Cephalic, 11, **275**
Cephalic region, 13, *13*
Cerebellar artery, superior, left, *176*
Cerebellar cortex, 98–99
Cerebellum, *94, 95,* 96(t), *97,* 98–99,
    275
Cerebral aqueduct, *97, 103,* **275**
Cerebral arteries, *176*
Cerebral cortex, 96(t), 99, **275**
    functional areas of, 96(t), 100, *101*
Cerebral hemisphere(s), 96(t), *97, 99, 99*
Cerebral palsy, **275**
Cerebrospinal fluid (CSF), *103,* 103–104,
    275
Cerebrovascular accident (CVA), 95, **275**
Cerebrum, *94, 95,* 96(t), *99,* 99–100, **275**
    arteries of, *176*
    central sulcus of, *94*
    convolutions of, 99
    fissures of, 99, *99*
    fornix of, *95,* 100
    gyrus (gyri) of, *99,* 100, *101,* **281**
    hemispheres of, 96(t), *97, 99, 99*
    lobes of, *94,* 96(t), 99, *99,* 100, *100*
    sensory areas of, 96(t), 100, *101,* **291**
    sulci of, *94, 99, 99,* 100, *101*
Cerumen (earwax), 122
Ceruminous glands, 122
Cervical, **275**
Cervical curve, *62*
Cervical lymph nodes, *182*
Cervical nerves, *112,* 113
Cervical plexus, *112,* 113, **275**
Cervical region, 13, 14
Cervical vertebra(e), *52, 53,* 55(t), 61,
    62, 63
    inferior, 55(t), *63*
Cervix, **275**
    uterine, 250, *251,* 252
        cancer of, 252
        dilation of, in labor, 257
Chambers of heart, 160, *160, 161, 162,
    163*
    contraction and relaxation of, 164, *165*
Chemical compound(s), 4
Chemical element(s), 4
    in human body, 2(t), 4
Chemical level of organization, in human
    body, 2, *3,* 4
Chemical receptors, **290**
Chest, *13.* See also *Thoracic* entries.
Chewing muscles, 86(t)
Chiasma, **275**
    optic, *95,* 98
Childbirth, 257
Childhood, 258
    tooth eruption in, 214, *215*
Chloride ions, 244

Chlorine, 223(t)
    in human body, 2(t)
Cholecystokinin, 218
Cholesterol, **275**
Cholinergic fiber, **275**
Cholinesterase, 78, **275**
Chondrocyte, **275**
Chordae tendineae, *162, 165,* **275**
Chorionic gonadotropin, human, 255, **281**
Choroid, **120,** *120,* **275**
Choroid plexus, 103, *103,* **275**
Chromatin, 28
Chromosome(s), 28, 30, 31, **275–276**
    sex, **292**
Chronic, **276**
Chronic bronchitis, 206
Chyme, 216, 218, 221, **276**
Cilia, 27, **276**
Ciliary muscle, 121, **276**
Circle of Willis, 177, **276**
Circulating antibodies, 194
Circulation, of blood, 171–172, *172, 173*
    pulmonary, 171–172, *172,* **289–290**
    systemic, 171, 172, *172,* **293**
        resistance in, 180
    of lymph, 183
Circulatory shock, 180–181
Circulatory system, 5(t), 7, 147–187
    blood in, 147–157, 170–181
    heart in, 159–168
    lymph in, 181–184
    transport functions of, 147, 204–205
Circumcision, **276**
Circumduction, 69(t), **276**
Clavicle (collarbone), *16, 19, 52, 53,*
    56(t), *83*
Cleft, synaptic, **293**
Climax, **276**
Clitoris, *250, 252, 253,* **276**
Clot, **276**
Clotting, *151,* 151–152
Clotting factors, 151
CNS (central nervous system), 91–108,
    92, **275.** See also *Brain* and *Spinal
    cord.*
    nucleus (nuclei) in, 93, **286**
    protective coverings of, *102,* 102–104,
        103
    tracts in, 93, 102, **294**
Cobalt, 223(t)
Coccygeal nerves, 113
Coccygeal plexus, *112*
Coccyx, *19, 52, 53,* 55(t), 61, *62, 63,* **276**
Cochlea, *122,* **123,** *123,* **276**
Cochlear nerve, 111(t), *122,* 123, *123*
Coenzyme, **276**
Coitus, **276**
Collagen, 35, 43, **276**
Collagen fibers, *34,* 35
Collapsed lung, 204
Collarbone (clavicle), *16, 19, 52, 53,*
    56(t), *83*
Collateral ganglia, 115
Collecting duct, *232, 233, 234*
Colon, 222, **276**
    ascending, *16, 17, 210,* 222, **273**
    cancer of, 222
    CT appearance of, *20*
    descending, *16, 17, 18, 210, 213,* 222,
        277

Colon (*Continued*)
  sigmoid, *17, 18, 210, 213,* 222, **292**
  transverse, *16, 17, 210, 213,* 222, **294**
Color blindness, **276**
Colostrum, 253
Column(s), spinal. See *Vertebra(e)*;
  Vertebral column.
  spinal cord, *101,* 102
Comedo, 44
Commissure, **276**
Common bile duct, *217,* 218, **276**
Common carotid artery, *16, 17, 18,* 179
  left, *160, 173, 174,* 175(t)
  right, *173, 174,* 175(t)
Common iliac artery, *17, 173, 174,*
  175(t)
  left, *18*
Common iliac vein, *17, 173,* 176(t)
  left, *18*
Communicating arteries of cerebrum, *176*
Compact bone, *48, 49, 50,* **276**
Compartments, fluid, 241–242, *242*
Complement, **276**
Complement system, 196
Complete blood count (CBC), 152(t)
Complex, antigen-antibody, 194, 196
  Golgi, 27, **280**
Compound(s), 4, **276**
Computed tomography (CT), brain on,
  20, 104
  transverse sections on, *20*
Conception, **276**
Conchae (turbinates), *200,* 200–201, **276**
  inferior, 55(t), *58*
  middle, 54(t), *58, 124*
  superior, 54(t)
Conduction system, of heart, *163,* 163–
  164
Condyle(s), 51(t), **276**
  femoral, 57(t)
  mandibular, *59*
  occipital, 54(t), *61*
  tibial, 57(t)
Condyloid process, *59*
Cones, **121,** **276**
Congenital, **276**
Conjoined twins, 257
Conjunctiva, **120,** *120,* **276**
Connective tissue, *33, 34, 34,* 35, **276**
Connective tissue fibers, 34–35
Connective tissue membranes, 36
Contraction, of diaphragm, 202
  of heart, 164, *165*
  of intercostal muscles, 202
  of muscle, 78–79, *80*
    isometric, *79, 80,* **283**
    isotonic, *79, 80,* **283**
  of uterus, in labor, 257
Contraction phase, of cardiac cycle, 164,
  165
Contralateral, **276**
Convoluted tubules, *232, 233, 233,* 234
Convolutions, cerebral, 99
Copper, 223(t)
Cord, spermatic, *16,* 248, *249,* **292**
  spinal, *7, 92, 95, 97,* 100, *101,* 102,
    103, **292**
    central canal of, *101,* 102, **275**
    columns of, *101,* 102
    CT appearance of, *20*
    fissures of, 100, *101,* 102

Cord (*Continued*)
  gray matter of, *101,* 102, *113*
  nerves emerging from, 92, *92,* 111,
    112, 113, *113,* **292**
    dorsal root of, 113, *113*
    ventral (anterior) root of, 113,
      113, **272**
  white matter of, *101,* 102, *113*
  umbilical, 256, *256,* **295**
  vocal, 201, **296**
Cornea, **120,** *120,* **276**
Coronal (frontal) plane, **12,** *12,* **276,**
  280
Coronal suture, 51, *59*
Coronary, **276**
Coronary artery (arteries), *160, 161, 163,*
  175(t)
Coronary artery disease, **276**
Coronary sinus, *161, 163,* **276**
Coronary veins, 163
Coronoid process, of mandible, *59*
Corpus callosum, *95,* 100, **276**
Corpuscle, pacinian, **287**
  renal, 232
Corpus luteum, 251, 254, *254,* 255, **276**
Cortex, **276**
  adrenal, 134(t), *140,* 140–141, *142,*
    271
  cerebellar, 98–99
  cerebral, 96(t), 99, **275**
    functional areas of, 96(t), 100, *101*
    motor, 100
  renal, 230, *231*
Cortisol (hydrocortisone), 134(t), 141,
  142, **276**
Costal cartilage, *52,* **276**
Costal region, 14
Cowper's gland (bulbourethral gland),
  248, 249, **274**
Coxal bones, 56(t), 65, *65*
CPR (cardiopulmonary resuscitation), 205
Craniad, 11
Cranial bones, 54(t)
Cranial cavity, *14,* 15
Cranial nerves, 92, 97, *110,* 111, 111(t),
  277
Cranial region, *13,* 14
Cranium, 10, 51, **277**
Creatine phosphate, 79, **277**
Crest, 51(t)
  iliac, 57(t), *65*
Cretinism, 137, **277**
Cribriform plate of ethmoid bone, 54(t),
  60
Crista galli, 54(t), *60*
Cross (horizontal, transverse) plane, **12,**
  12, **281**
Crown of tooth, 213, *214*
CSF (cerebrospinal fluid), *103,* 103–104,
  275
CT (computed tomography), brain on, *20,*
  104
  transverse sections on, *20*
Cubital region, *13,* 14
Curve, of vertebral column, *62*
Cushing's syndrome, **277**
Cusps, of heart valves, *162*
  of venous valves, 170
Cutaneous, **277.** See also *Skin.*
Cutaneous region, 14
CVA (cerebrovascular accident), 95, **275**

C1 vertebra (atlas), *19,* 55(t), *63*
  anterior tubercle of, *63*
  posterior arch of, *63*
  posterior tubercle of, *63*
C2 vertebra (axis), 55(t), *63*
  odontoid process of (dens axis), 55(t),
    63
Cycle, cardiac, 164, *165,* **275**
  life, 257–258
  menstrual, 250, 254, *254,* **285**
Cyclic adenosine monophosphate (cAMP),
  132
Cytoplasm, 27

Deamination, **277**
Debt, oxygen, 79, **287**
Decibel, **277**
Deciduous teeth, 214, *215,* **277**
Deep, 12
Defecation, 222
Defense mechanisms, 189–198
  immune, 192(t), 192–196, *193, 195*
  inflammatory, 190, *191*
  macrophages in, *191,* 192
  nonspecific, 189, 190, *190,* 192
  specific, 189, *190,* 192–196
Dehydration, 235, 242, **277**
Deltoid muscle, *19, 83, 84, 85,* 87(t)
Dendrites, 35, *36,* 92, *93,* **277**
Dens axis (odontoid process of axis),
  55(t), *63*
Dental alveoli, *61,* 213
Dentin, 213, *214,* **277**
Deoxyribonucleic acid (DNA), 4, **277**
Depolarization, **277**
Depressions, bony, 51(t)
Dermatitis, vitamin deficiency and, 224(t)
Dermis, 42, *42, 43, 44, 125,* **277**
Descending aorta, *17, 160, 174*
Descending branch of left coronary
  artery, *160*
Descending colon, *16, 17, 18, 210, 213,*
  222, **277**
Descending tracts, in central nervous
  system, 102
Dextrin, **277**
Diabetes insipidus, 136, 235–236, **277**
Diabetes mellitus, 139, **277**
Dialysis, **277**
Diaphragm, *8, 14, 15, 16, 17,* 87(t), *200,*
  202, *217,* **277**
  contraction and relaxation of, in
    breathing, 202, 203, *203*
Diaphysis, *48, 49,* **277**
Diarthrosis (synovial joint), 66, *67,* 70,
  70–71, **277, 293**
Diastole, *164,* 179, **277**
Diastolic blood pressure, 181
Diencephalon, *95,* 96(t), **98,** **277**
Differential cell count, 153(t)
Diffusion, *28, 28,* **277**
  gas exchange by, 204, *204*
Digastric muscle, *85,* 86(t)
Digestion, **211,** 218, **277**
  and nutrient absorption, 220–221
  in duodenum, *217,* 218, 220
  in mouth, 218, 219(t)
  in small intestine, *217,* 219(t), 220(t)
  in stomach, 216, 220, 220(t)
  of carbohydrates, 218, 219(t)

Digestion (*Continued*)
of lipids (fats), 218, 219(t), 220
of proteins, 220, 220(t)
of starch, 218, 219(t)
Digestive enzymes, 215, 217, 218, 219(t), 220, 220(t)
Digestive glands, accessory, 211
Digestive system, 5(t), *8*, *210*, 211–228, **277**
food processing by, 211. See also *Food*.
support for organs in, 212, *213*
Digestive tract, **211**
wall of, 211, *212*
Directional terms, 10–12, *11*
Dirty air, 205–206
Disc(s), intercalated, 164
intervertebral, **61**, **283**
optic, **121**
Distal, 12, **277**
Distal convoluted tubule, *232*, *233*, *233*
Distal phalanges, of fingers, *64*
of toes, *66*
Diuretic, 236, **277**
Division, by cells, 29–31, *31*, 33
DNA (deoxyribonucleic acid), **4**, **277**
Donors, universal, 152
Dorsal, 11
Dorsal branch of spinal nerve, 113, *113*
Dorsal cavity, *14*, 15
Dorsalis pedis artery, *179*
Dorsal median fissure of spinal cord, *101*, 102
Dorsal root of spinal nerve, 113, *113*
Duct, bile, common, *217*, 218, **276**
CT appearance of, *20*
collecting, *232*, *233*, *234*
ejaculatory, *248*, 249, **277**
hepatic, right, *217*
lymphatic, right, *182*, 183, **290–291**
mammary, 253, *253*
pancreatic, *217*, **287**
semicircular, **291**
sperm (vas deferens), *9*, *18*, 249, *249*, **295**
thoracic, *8*, *182*, 183, **294**
Duodenum, *17*, *18*, *210*, *216*, 217, *217*, **277**
digestion in, 217, 218, 220
Dura mater, **102**, *102*, *103*, 104, **277**
venous sinuses of, 102, *102*, *103*, 177, *177*
Dwarfs, 137

Ear(s), 121–123, *122*, *123*
inner, 122–123, *123*, **282**
middle, 121, *122*
outer, 121–122
Ear bones, 55(t), 122, *122*
Eardrum (tympanic membrane), 122, *122*, **295**
Earwax (cerumen), 122
ECG (electrocardiogram), **277–278**
Edema, 190, **277**
EEG (electroencephalogram), **278**
Effectors, sympathetic and parasympathetic actions on, 116(t)
Efferent, **277**
Efferent arterioles, *232*, *232*, *233*, *233*, *234*, **277**

Efferent nerves. See *Motor nerve* entries.
Efferent neurons (motor neurons), 109, 111, 113, 115
in reflexes, 104, *104*, *114*
Ejaculation, 249, 250, **277**
Ejaculatory duct, *248*, 249, **277**
EKG (electrocardiogram), **277–278**
Elastic fibers, 35
Electrical nerve stimulation, trans-cutaneous, 126
Electrocardiogram (ECG, EKG), **277–278**
Electroencephalogram (EEG), **278**
Electrolyte(s), 241, **278**
Electrolyte balance, 244
Electron microscope, 26
Element(s), 4, **278**
in human body, 2(t), *4*
Elimination, **211**, 221–222, **278**
vs. excretion, 229
Embryo, 251, 255, *256*
Emphysema, 206, **278**
Emulsification, **278**
Enamel, 213, *214*, **278**
Encephalitis, 103
Endocardium, 160, **278**
Endochondral bone development, 49
Endocrine glands, 7, 33, 131–145, *132*, 133(t)–134(t), **278**
Endocrine system, 5(t), 7
Endocrinology, 132, **278**
Endogenous, **278**
Endolymph, 123, **278**
Endometrium, *251*, 252, 254, *255*, **278**
Endomysium, 77, *78*, **278**
Endoneurium, **278**
Endoplasmic reticulum, 27, **278**
Endorphin, 126, **278**
Endosteum, 49, **278**
Endothelium, 170, **278**
Energy, autonomic nervous system and, 115
Enkephalin, **278**
Enzyme(s), **4**, **278**
digestive, 215, 217, 218, 219(t), 220, 220(t)
Eosinophil, 150, *150*, **278**
Epicondyle, 51(t)
Epidermis, *42*, 42–43, *125*
Epididymis, *18*, 249, *249*, **278**
Epidural space, **278**
Epiglottis, *200*, 201, 215, **278**
Epimysium, 77, *78*, **278**
Epinephrine, 133(t), 140, *142*, **278**
Epineurium, **278**
Epiphyseal plate, **278**
Epiphysis, *48*, **49**, **278**
Epithelial cells, 26, 27
Epithelial membranes, 36
Epithelial tissue, *32*, 33, **278**
Epithelium, *32*, 33
digestive tract, 211, *212*
olfactory, 123, *124*
pseudostratified, **289**
squamous, **292**
Equilibrium, 123
Erection, 250, **278**
Eruption, of teeth, 214, *215*
Erythroblastosis fetalis, 155, *155*
Erythrocyte (red blood cell), *148*, 149–150, *150*
Erythrocyte (red blood cell) count, 153(t)

Erythropoiesis, **278**
Erythropoietin, 236, **278**
Esophageal artery, *174*, 175(t)
Esophagus, *8*, *17*, *18*, *200*, *210*, 215–216, *216*, **278**
pushing of bolus in, 216
Essential amino acids, **278**
Estradiol, **279**
Estrogens, 134(t), 141, 251, 253–254, **279**
Ethmoid bone, 54(t), *58*, *59*
cribriform plate of, 54(t), *60*
perpendicular plate of, *58*
Ethmoid sinuses, 54(t)
Eustachian tube (auditory tube), 122, *122*, **273**
Eversion, 70(t), **279**
Excretion, **229**, 230, **279**
Exercise, heart rate during, 166
isometric, *80*
isotonic, *80*
metabolism during, 79
Exhalation (expiration), 202, 203, *203*, 204, **279**
Exhaled air, carbon dioxide in, 204, 205(t)
nitrogen in, 205(t)
oxygen in, 205(t)
Exhaustion, 141
Exocrine glands, 33, **279**
Expiration (exhalation), 202, 203, *203*, 204, **279**
Extension, 68(t), **279**
External anal sphincter, 222
External auditory meatus, *59*, 121, *122*
External carotid artery, left, *174*
External iliac artery, *173*, *174*, 175(t)
External intercostal muscle, *19*, 87(t)
External jugular vein, *176*, *177*
External maxillary artery, *179*
External oblique muscle of abdomen, *19*, *83*, *84*, *85*, 86(t)
aponeurosis of, *85*
External urethral sphincter, 236
Exteroceptor, **279**
Extracellular, **279**
Extracellular fluid, 242, **279**
cations in, 244
Extracellular fluid compartment, 241, 242, *242*
Extrinsic eye muscles, **120**, *120*, 121
Eye(s), *13*, **120**, 120–121
parasympathetic actions on, 116(t)
sympathetic actions on, 116(t)
Eyeball, **279**

Face, **279**
Facet(s), **279**
of vertebrae, 51(t), *62*, *63*
Facial artery, *174*
Facial bones, 54(t)–55(t)
Facial muscles, 86(t)
Facial nerve, *110*, 111(t), 125
Facial region, *13*
Fallopian (uterine) tube, *9*, *17*, *250*, 251, *251*, **279**, **295**
False ribs, *52*, 56(t)
Falx cerebri, 102, *102*
Fascia, **279**
superficial, 43

Fascicles, 77, 78, **279**
Fat, 222, **279**
    digestion of, 218, 219(t), 220
    polyunsaturated, **289**
    saturated, **291**
Fatigue, muscle, 79
Fat (adipose) tissue, 34, 35, 43, **271**
    mammary, 253, 253
    sympathetic actions on, 116(t)
Feces, 222, **279**
Feedback, **279**
Feedback system(s), 10
    negative, 10
        endocrine regulation by, 134–135,
        135
    positive, 10
        endocrine regulation by, 135
Feet, 13, 66
    muscles of, 88(t)
Female pelvis, 65, 65
Female reproductive system, 9, 250, 250–
    255, 251
Femoral artery, 16, 18, 173, 174, 179
Femoral nerve, 112, 113
Femoral region, 13, 14
Femoral vein, 16, 18, 173
Femur, 19, 52, 53, 57(t), 65
    condyles of, 57(t)
    head of, 53, 57(t)
    trochanter of, 51(t)
        greater, 57(t)
        lesser, 57(t)
Fertilization, 251, 255, 255, **279**
Fetal membranes, 255
Fetus, 256, **279**
    effects of Rh incompatibility on, 155,
    155
Fever, 190, **279**
Fiber(s), cholinergic, **275**
    collagen, 34, 35
    connective tissue, 34–35
    elastic, 35
    muscle. See Muscle cells.
    nerve, 92
        motor, 78, 79
            crossing of, 97
        Purkinje, 163, **290**
        reticular, 35
Fibrillation, **279**
Fibrin, 151, 152, **279**
Fibrinogen, **279**
Fibroblast, **279**
Fibrocartilage, **279**
Fibula, 52, 53, 57(t), 66, 66
Filaments, actin, **78**
    myosin, **78**
Filtrate, 232, 233, 234
Filtration, **28**
    glomerular, 233–234, 234
Fimbriae, 251
Finger(s), phalanges of, 52, 53, 56(t), 64,
    65
Fingerprints, 43
First heart sound, 164
First messenger, 132
First molar, 215
First premolar, 215
Fissure(s), **279**
    bony, 51(t)
    cerebral, 99, 99
    orbital, superior, 58

Fissure(s) (Continued)
    spinal cord, 100, 101, 102
Fixator, 81, **279**
Flagellum, **279**
    of sperm cell, 26, 28
Flank, 13
Flexion, 68(t), **279**
Floating ribs, 52, 56(t)
Fluid, body, 241
    cerebrospinal, 103, 103–104, **275**
    extracellular, 242, **279**
        cations in, 244
    interstitial (tissue), 170, 170, 183, 242,
        283
    intracellular, 241, 242
        cations in, 244
    synovial, 71, **293**
Fluid balance, 241–246, 243
    hypothalamic function and, 98, 242–
    243
Fluid compartments, 241–242, 242
Fluid intake, 242, 243
Fluid output, 242–243, 243
Fluorine, 223(t)
Folds, peritoneal, 212, 213
Folic acid, 224(t)
Follicle, graafian, 251, **280**
    hair, 42, 44, 44, 125, **281**
    ovarian, 251, 254, 254
Follicle-stimulating hormone (FSH), 137,
    250, 251, 254, **279**
Fontanelle, 51, **279**
Food, 211, 222
    breaking down of, by teeth, 214
    conversion of, to bolus, 215
    digestion of, **211**, 218, **277**
        in duodenum, 217, 218, 220
        in mouth, 218, 219(t)
        in small intestine, 217, 219(t), 220(t)
        in stomach, 216, 220, 220(t)
        nutrient absorption following, 220–
        221
    esophageal pushing of, toward stomach,
    216
    ingestion of, **211**, **282**
        in oral cavity, 212–213
    mineral-rich, 223(t)
    processing of, 211
    swallowing of, 215
    vitamin-rich, 224(t)–225(t)
Foot, 13, 66
    muscles of, 88(t)
Foramen (foramina), 51(t), **280**
    incisive, 61
    infraorbital, 58, 59
    interventricular, 97, 103
    intervertebral, 62
    jugular, 60
    mental, 58, 59
    obturator, 57(t), 65
    supraorbital, 58
    transverse, 55(t), 63
    vertebral, 63, 64(t)
Foramen lacerum, 61
Foramen magnum, 54(t), 60, 61
Foramen ovale, 60, 61
Foramen rotundum, 60
Foramen spinosum, 60
Forearm, 13, 14, **280**
    muscles of, 87(t)
Forehead, 13

Foreskin, **280**
Fornix, of cerebrum, 95, 100
    of vagina, 252
Fossa, 51(t), **280**
    glenoid, 56(t)
    jugular, 61
Fourth ventricle of brain, 95, 95, 97, 103
Fovea of retina, **121**, **280**
Fraternal twins, 257
Frontal bone, 52, 54(t), 58, 59, 60
    squama of, 58
Frontalis muscle, 86(t)
Frontal lobe, 94, 99, 100, 101
Frontal (coronal) plane, 12, 12, **276**, **280**
Frontal region, 13, 14
Frontal sinus, 54(t), 124, 174
FSH (follicle-stimulating hormone), 137,
    250, 251, 254, **279**
Functional areas, of cerebral cortex,
    96(t), 100, 101
Functional muscle groups, 81, 86(t)–88(t)
Fundus, **280**
    uterine, 252

Gallbladder, 8, 16, 17, 210, 217, 218, **280**
Gamete, 248, **280**
Gamma globulin(s), 149, 190, 194, **280**
    for hepatitis, 196
Ganglion (ganglia), 93, **280**
    autonomic, **273**
    basal, 99, **273**
    collateral, 115
    prevertebral, **289**
    spinal, 113, 113, **292**
Gas exchange, 204, 204
Gas transportation, by circulatory system,
    204–205
Gastric artery, 174
Gastric glands, **280**
Gastric juice, 216
Gastrin, 218, **280**
Gastrocnemius muscle, 83, 84, 88(t)
Gastrointestinal tract, 211, **280**
Gene(s), **280**
    activation of, by steroid hormones, 132
General adaptation syndrome, 141
General senses, 125–126
General sensory area, 101
Genetics, **280**
Genitalia, **280**
    female, 9, 250–252, 250–255
    male, 9, 248, 248–250, 249
Giants, 137
Gigantism, **280**
Girdle, pectoral (shoulder), 56(t), 64–65
    pelvic, 56(t)–57(t), **65**
Glabella, 58
Gland(s), 33, **280**. See also specific
    glands.
    endocrine, 7, 33, 131–145, 132, 133(t)–
        134(t)
    exocrine, 33
Glandular breast tissue, 253, 253
Glans penis, 248, 249
Glenoid fossa, 56(t)
Glial cells, 35, 36, 92, **280**
Gliding joint, 67, 68(t), **280**
Globulin(s), **280**
    gamma, 149, 190, 194, **280**
    for hepatitis, 196

Glomerular filtration, 233–234, *234*
Glomerulus, 232, *232, 233, 234*, **280**
Glossopharyngeal nerve, *110*, 111(t), 125
Glottis, 201, **280**
Glucagon, 133(t), 138, 139, *139*, **280**
Glucocorticoid hormones, 134(t), 141, **280**
Glucose, 79, 218, **280**
   in blood, regulation of levels of, 138–139, *139*
Glucosuria, **280**
Gluteal region, *13*, 14
Gluteus maximus muscle, *19*, 84, 87(t)
Gluteus medius muscle, *19, 83, 84*, 87(t)
Gluteus minimus muscle, 87(t)
Glycogen, 79, **280**
   storage of, 218
Goblet cell, *33, 221*
Goiter, 137, **280**
Golgi complex, 27, **280**
Gonad(s), 248, **280**
Gonadotropic hormones, 133(t), 137, 250, **280**
Gonadotropin, human chorionic, 255, **281**
Graafian follicle, **280**
Gracilis muscle, *19, 83, 84*, 88(t)
Graft rejection, **281**
Granular leukocytes, 150, *150*
Granulations, arachnoid, *102, 103, 103*
Gravity, and resistance to blood flow, 181
Gray matter, **281**
   of brain, 96(t), 97
   of spinal cord, *101, 102, 113*
Greater omentum, *16*, 212, *213*, **281**
Greater trochanter, 57(t)
Greater vestibular glands, 253, **281**
Greater wing of sphenoid bone, *59, 60, 61*
Groin, *13*, 14, **281**
Growth hormone (somatotropin), 133(t), 137, **281**
Growth impairment, vitamin deficiency and, 224(t)
Guanine, **281**
Gum, *214*
Gustation, 125
Gustatory, **281**
Gustatory area, primary, *101*
Gyrus (gyri) of cerebrum, *99*, 100, *101*, **281**

Hair(s), *6, 42, 44, 44*, 125
Hair follicle, *42, 44, 44*, 125, **281**
Hair root, *44*
Hair shaft, *42, 44*
Hamstrings, **281**
Hand, *13*
   bones of, *52, 53*, 56(t), *64*, 65
Hard palate, *61*, 215, **281**
Haversian canals, 49, *50*
Haversian system (osteon), 49, *50*, **281**, **287**
hCG (human chorionic gonadotropin), 255, **281**
Head, *13*
   muscles of, 86(t)
Headache, 126
Head of bone, 51(t)
Hearing, 123

Heart, 7, *18*, 159–168, *160, 161, 170, 172*. See also *Cardiac* entries.
   atrium (atria) of, *160*, **273**
      auricle of, *160*, 162, **273**
      contraction and relaxation of, 164, *165*
      left, *161, 163, 173*
      right, *160, 161, 163, 173*
   blood vessels of, 162–163
   chambers of, 160, *160, 161*, 162, *163*
   conduction system of, *163*, 163–164
   contraction and relaxation of, 164, *165*
   disease of, coronary artery disease and, **276**
      ischemic, **283**
   innervation of, *115*
   muscle tissue of, 35, 35(t), 160, 163–164
   parasympathetic actions on, 116(t)
   regulation of, by nervous system, 164
   sympathetic actions on, 116(t)
   valve(s) of, *161*, 162, *162*
      opening and closing of, 164, *165*
   ventricle(s) of, 160
      contraction and relaxation of, 164, *165*
      left, *160, 161, 163, 173*
      right, *160, 161, 163, 173*
   wall of, 159–160
Heartburn, 216
Heart murmur, 164, **281**
Heart rate, 164, 166, **281**
Heart sounds, 164, **281**
Heel, *13*
Helper T cells, 194, **281**
Hematocrit, 153(t), **281**
Hemisphere(s), cerebral, 96(t), *97*, 99, *99*
Hemoglobin, 149, 152(t), **281**
   deficiency of, 150
   oxygen bond with, 149, 204–205
Hemolysis, 152, 154
   in Rh-positive fetus, 155
Hemorrhage, 180, **281**
   cerebral, 104
   splenic rupture and, 184
Hepatic, **281**. See also *Liver*.
Hepatic artery, *174, 178*
Hepatic duct, right, *217*
Hepatic portal system, **281**
Hepatic portal vein, *178, 179, 217*, 218
Hepatic vein, *173*, 176(t), *178*
Hepatitis, 196
Heredity, **281**
Hilus, of kidney, 230, *231*, **281**
   of lung, 202
Hinge joint, *67*, 68(t)
Hip, *13*
Histamine, **281**
Histology, **281**
HIV (human immunodeficiency virus), **281**
Holocrine gland, **281**
Homeostasis, **10**, *10*, 141, **281**
   fluid, 241–246, *243*
      hypothalamic function and, 98, 242–243
   renal function and, 236
Homeostatic mechanisms, 5, 10, *10*
Horizontal (cross, transverse) plane, **12**, *12*, **281**
Horizontal plate of palatine bone, *61*

Hormones, 132–144, 133(t)–134(t), **281**. See also specific hormones.
Hot flashes, 254
Human body. See *Body*.
Human chorionic gonadotropin (hCG), 255, **281**
Human immunodeficiency virus (HIV), **281**
Humerus, *19, 52, 53*, 56(t), 65
   head of, 56(t)
Hyaline, **281–282**
Hydrocephalus, 103–104
Hydrocortisone (cortisol), 134(t), 141, *142*, **276**
Hydrogen, in human body, 2(t)
Hydrogen bond, **282**
Hydrolysis, **282**
Hydrophilic, **282**
Hydrophobic, **282**
Hymen, *251, 252, 252*, **282**
Hyoid bone, 55(t)
Hyperglycemia, 139
Hypersecretion, 135
Hypertension, 181, **282**
Hypertonic, **282**
Hypertonic solution, 28, *29*
Hyperventilation, 205, **282**
Hypochondriac region, *15*
Hypogastric region, *15*
Hypoglossal canal, *60*
Hypoglossal nerve, *110*, 111(t)
Hypoglycemia, **282**
Hyposecretion, 135
Hypothalamus, 7, 95, 96(t), *98*, 132, 133(t), 135, *136*, **282**
   and adrenal function, 141, *142*
   and fluid balance, 98, 242–243
   and temperature regulation, 104
Hypothyroidism, 137, **282**
Hypotonic, **282**
Hypotonic solution, 28, *29*
Hypoxia, **282**

Identical twins, 257
Ileocecal valve, 221
Ileum, *17, 213*, 217, **282**
Iliac artery, common, *17, 173, 174*, 175(t)
   left, *18*
   external, *173, 174*, 175(t)
   internal, *173, 174*, 175(t)
Iliac crest, *53*, 57(t), 65
Iliac region, *15*
Iliac spine, anterior superior, 57(t)
Iliacus muscle, 87(t)
Iliac vein, common, *17, 173*, 176(t)
   left, *18*
Ilium, *19, 52*, 57(t), 65, *65*
Immune, 189, **282**
Immune responses, 189, 192(t)
Immunity, 192–196, **282**
   active, 196, **271**
   antibody-mediated, 194, *195*
   cell-mediated, *193*, 193–194, **275**
   passive (borrowed), 196
   thymus gland in, 184, 196
Immunization, 196, **282**
Immunodeficiency virus, human, **281**
Immunoglobulins, **282**. See also *Antibody* entries.

Immunology, 189, **282**
Immunosuppression, **282**
Implantation, 251, 255, *255*, **282**
Impotence, **282**
Impulse transmission, 93, **294**
 to muscle cells, 78, *79*
Incisive foramen, *61*
Incisors, 214, *215*
Incompatibility, Rh, 155, *155*
Incus, 55(t), 122, *122*
Infancy, 258, **282**
Infarct, **282**
Infection. See also *Pathogens*.
 bacterial, 194
  defenses against, 190
   macrophages in, *191,* 192
  vs. viral infection, 150, 151
 viral, 194
  defenses against, 192
  hepatitis due to, 196
  meningitis due to, 102
  vs. bacterial infection, 150, 151
Inferior, 11, **282**
Inferior articular process of vertebra, *63*, 64(t)
Inferior cervical vertebrae, 55(t); *63*
Inferior mesenteric artery, *173, 174,* 175(t)
Inferior mesenteric vein, *178*
Inferior nasal concha (inferior turbinate), 55(t), *58*
Inferior nuchal line, *61*
Inferior phrenic artery, *174,* 175(t)
Inferior sagittal sinus, *177*
Inferior turbinate (inferior nasal concha), 55(t), *58*
Inferior vena cava, *17, 18, 160, 161, 173,* 175, *178, 217, 231,* **282**
 veins draining into, 176(t)
Inflammation, 190, *191,* **282**
Infraorbital foramen, *58, 59*
Ingestion, **211, 282**
 by cells, 29, *30*
 in oral cavity, 212–213
Inguinal canal, **282**
Inguinal region, *13,* 14
Inhalation (inspiration), 202–203, *203,* **283**
Inhaled air, 205–206
 carbon dioxide in, 205(t)
 nitrogen in, 205(t)
 oxygen in, 205(t)
Inhibiting hormones, 133(t), 137
Inlet, pelvic, 57(t), 65, *65*
Inner ear, 122–123, *123,* **282**
Innominate bones, 56(t), 65, *65*
Inorganic compound(s), **4**
Insertion, muscle, **282**
 sites of, 81, 86(t)–88(t)
Inspiration (inhalation), 202–203, *203,* **283**
Insula, *94*
Insulin, 133(t), 138, 139, *139,* **283**
Insulin-dependent diabetes mellitus, 139
Intake, fluid, 242, *243*
Integration, 93, **283**
Integumentary system, 5(t), *6,* 41, **283**.
 See also *Skin.*
Interatrial septum, 162, **283**
Intercalated discs, 164
Intercellular, **283**

Intercellular substance, 33
Intercostal artery, *174*
 posterior, 175(t)
Intercostal muscle(s), contraction and relaxation of, in breathing, 202, 203
 external, *19,* 87(t)
 internal, 87(t)
Intercourse, 252
Interferons, 192, **283**
Interleukins, **283**
Internal anal sphincter, 222
Internal auditory meatus, *60*
Internal carotid artery, 175
 left, *174, 176*
Internal iliac artery, *173, 174,* 175(t)
Internal intercostal muscle, 87(t)
Internal jugular vein, *16, 18,* 176(t), *177, 177*
Internal oblique muscle of abdomen, *85*
Internal urethral sphincter, 236
Interneuron, **283**
Interoceptor, **283**
Interphase, 30, *31,* **283**
Interstitial, **283**
Interstitial cells, 250, **283**
Interstitial (tissue) fluid, 170, *170,* 183, 242, **283**
Interventricular foramen, 97, *103*
Interventricular septum, *161,* 162, **283**
Intervertebral disc, **61, 283**
Intervertebral foramen, *62*
Intervertebral joints, 67
Intestinal glands, *221*
Intestine, delivery of blood to, 179
 large, *8,* 211, 221–222. See also *Colon.*
 parasympathetic actions on, 116(t)
 small, *8, 16, 210,* 211, 217, **292**
  digestion in, 217, 219(t), 220(t)
  villi of, *212,* 217, 220–221, *221*
  wall of, *212*
 sympathetic actions on, 116(t)
Intracellular, **283**
Intracellular fluid, 241, 242
 cations in, 244
Intracellular fluid compartment, 241, 242, *242*
Intramembranous bone formation, 49, **283**
Inversion, 69(t), **283**
Involuntary muscles, 35, 35(t)
Iodine, 223(t)
 deficiency of, 137
 in human body, 2(t)
 protein-bound, 137
Ion, **4,** 244, **283**
Ionic bond, **283**
Ionization, **283**
Ipsilateral, **283**
Iris, 120, *120,* **283**
 parasympathetic actions on, 116(t)
 sympathetic actions on, 116(t)
Iron, 223(t)
 deficiency of, 150
 in human body, 2(t)
Ischemia, **283**
Ischemic heart disease, **283**
Ischial spine, 57(t), 65
Ischial tuberosity, 57(t)
Ischium, *52, 53,* 57(t), 65, *65,* **283**
Islets of Langerhans, 133(t), 138–139, **283**

Isometric contraction, **79,** *80,* **283**
Isotonic, **283**
Isotonic contraction, **79,** *80,* **283**
Isotonic solution, 28, *29*

Jejunum, *17, 213,* 217, **283**
Joint(s), 66, *67,* 68(t), 70–71, **283.** See also specific joints.
 movement at, 68(t)–70(t)
Joint capsule, 70–71
Jugular foramen, *60*
Jugular fossa, *61*
Jugular vein, external, 176(t), *177*
 internal, *16, 18,* 176(t), *177, 177*
 left, *173*
 right, *173*
Junction, neuromuscular (motor end plate), 78, *79*
Juxtaglomerular apparatus, 233, *233*
Juxtaglomerular cells, **283**

Keratin, 43, **283**
Ketone bodies, **283**
Ketosis, **283**
Kidney(s), *9, 17, 18, 19, 140, 173,* 230, *230, 231,* 232, **284.** See also *Renal* entries.
 CT appearance of, *20*
 delivery of blood to, 234
 function of, and homeostasis, 236
 hilus of, 230, *231,* **281**
 left, *231*
 location of, 230
 nephrons of, 232, *232*
 pyramids of, 230, *231,* **290**
 renin release by, 181, 236
Killer T cells, 192(t), 194
Kilocalorie, **284**
Kinesthetic sense, 126
Knee, *13,* 70
Knobs, synaptic, 92, **293**

Labia, *250, 251,* 252, 252–253, **284**
Labor, 251, 257, **284**
Labyrinth, **284**
 bony, 122, *123,* **274**
 membranous, 123, *123*
Lacrimal bone, 55(t), *58, 59*
Lacrimal glands, 120
Lactation, 137, **253**
Lacteal, 220, *221,* **284**
Lactic acid, 79, **284**
Lactose, 218, **284**
Lacunae, 49, 50, *50,* **284**
Lambdoidal suture, 51, *59*
Lamina, lateral, of pterygoid process, *61*
 medial, of pterygoid process, *61*
 of vertebra, *63,* 64(t)
Large intestine, *8,* 211, 221–222. See also *Colon.*
Laryngitis, 201
Laryngopharynx, 201, 215, **284**
Larynx (voice box), *8,* 199, *200,* 201, **284**
Lateral, 12, **284**

Lateral condyle of tibia, 57(t)
Lateral incisor, *215*
Lateral longitudinal arch of foot, *66*
Lateral malleolus, *53*, 57(t), *66*
Lateral pterygoid lamina, *61*
Lateral ventricles of brain, *97, 99, 103*
Latissimus dorsi muscle, *19, 83, 84,* 87(t)
Left atrium, *161, 163, 173*
  auricle of, *160*
Left brachiocephalic vein, *18*
Left cerebral hemisphere, *99, 99*
Left common carotid artery, *160, 173, 174,* 175(t)
Left common iliac artery, *18*
Left common iliac vein, *18*
Left coronary artery, descending branch of, *160*
Left external carotid artery, *174*
Left internal carotid artery, *174, 176*
Left jugular vein, *173*
Left kidney, *231*
Left lung, *16, 173, 200*
Left posterior communicating artery of cerebrum, *176*
Left pulmonary artery, *160, 173*
Left pulmonary vein, *160, 161, 173*
Left renal artery, *231*
Left subclavian artery, *17, 160,* 175(t)
Left subclavian vein, *173, 182*
Left superior cerebellar artery, *176*
Left ureter, *231*
Left ventricle, *160, 161, 163, 173*
Left vertebral artery, *174, 176*
Leg, *13, 14,* **284**
  muscles of, 88(t)
Length conversions, 270(t)
Lens, *120,* **121, 284**
Lesion, **284**
Lesser omentum, *17, 212,* **284**
Lesser pelvis, 57(t)
Lesser trochanter, 57(t)
Lesser vestibular glands, 253, **284**
Lesser wing of sphenoid bone, *60*
Leukemia, 150, **284**
Leukocyte (white blood cell), *26, 27, 148, 150,* 150–151
  agranular, 150, *150*
  granular, 150, *150*
Leukocyte (white blood cell) count, 153(t)
Levels of organization, in human body, 2, *3, 4*
LH (luteinizing hormone), 137, 250, 251, 254, **284**
Life cycle, 257–258
Ligament(s), *49,* **284**
  ovarian, *250, 251, 251,* **287**
  round, *251*
  suspensory, of lens, 121
Ligamentum arteriosum, *160*
Light microscope, 26
Limb(s), lower, *13,* 57(t)–58(t), 65–66
  superficial lymphatics of, *182*
  upper, *13,* 56(t), 65
    superficial lymphatics of, *182*
Limbic lobe, 100
Line(s), nuchal, *61*
Linea alba, *83*
Lingual tonsils, 183
Lipase, 218, 220
Lipid(s), 4, 222, **284**
  digestion of, 218, 219(t), 220

Liver, *8, 16, 17, 173, 210, 213,* 218. See also *Hepatic* entries.
  CT appearance of, *20*
  delivery of blood to, 179, 218
  excretory function of, 230, *230*
  right lobe of, *217,* 218
  sympathetic actions on, 116(t)
Lobe(s), **284**
  of cerebrum, *94,* 96(t), *99, 99,* 100, *100*
  of liver, *217,* 218
  of pituitary gland, anterior, 133(t), *136,* 136–137
    posterior, 133(t), 136, *136*
Local hormones, 134
Long bone, *48, 49*
Longitudinal arch of foot, *66*
Longitudinal fissure of cerebrum, *99, 99*
Loop of Henle, *232, 233*
Lower limb, *13,* 57(t)–58(t), 65–66
  superficial lymphatics of, *182*
Lumbar artery, *174,* 175(t)
Lumbar curve, *62*
Lumbar nerves, *112,* 113
Lumbar plexus, *112,* 113
Lumbar puncture, 104
Lumbar region, *13, 14, 15*
Lumbar vertebra(e), *52, 53,* 55(t), *61, 62, 63*
Lumen, **284**
Lumen(s), *8, 17,* 199, 201–202. See also *Pulmonary* entries.
  air movement into and out of, 202–204
  alveoli of, 199, 201, *202*
    in gas exchange, 204, *204*
  circulation to and from, 171–172, *172*
  collapsed, 204
  CT appearance of, *20*
  disease of, 206
  excretory function of, 230, *230*
  hilus of, 202
  protection of, from damage, 206
  surface area of, 203
Lunula, 44
Luteinizing hormone (LH), 137, 250, 251, 254, **284**
L1 vertebra, *112*
Lymph, 181, 183, **284**
Lymphatic, **284**
Lymphatic duct, right, *182,* 183, **290–291**
Lymphatic organs, 183–184
Lymphatics, *182,* 183, **284**
Lymphatic system, 7, 147, *170,* 181–184, *182,* 192
Lymphatic vessels, *8, 170, 182,* 183
  lacteal, 220, *221,* **284**
Lymph capillaries, 183
Lymph nodes, *8, 182,* 183, **284**
Lymph nodules, **284**
Lymphocytes, *26, 27,* 150, *150,* 183, **284**
  B (B cells), 192(t), 193, 194, *195,* **274**
    memory, 192(t), 194, **285**
  T (T cells), 192(t), *193,* 193–194, 196, **293**
    helper, 194, **281**
    killer, 192(t), 194
    memory, 192(t), 194
Lysosomes, 27, 192, **284**

Macrophages, *191,* 192, 192(t), 193, 206, **284**

Macrophages (*Continued*)
  sinusoid, 171
Magnesium, 223(t)
  in human body, 2(t)
Magnesium ions, 244
Malar (zygomatic) bone, 55(t), *58, 59, 61*
Male hormones, 250
Male pelvis, 65, *65*
Male reproductive system, 9, *248,* 248–250, *249*
Malleolus, lateral, *53,* 57(t), *66*
  medial, 57(t)
Malleus, 55(t), 122, *122*
Maltase, 218
Maltose, 218
Mammary ducts, 253, *253*
Mammary glands, 253, **284**
Mammary region, *13, 14*
Mammography, **285**
Mandible, *52, 53,* 54(t), *58, 59*
  coronoid process of, *59*
  ramus of, *59*
Mandibular condyle, *59*
Manganese, 223(t)
Manubrium of sternum, 56(t), **285**
Marrow, *48, 49*
  red, *48, 49,* 149
  yellow, *48, 49*
Marrow cavity, *49*
Masseter muscle, *84, 85,* 86(t)
Mast cell, **285**
Mastoid process, *19, 53,* 54(t), *59, 61, 122*
Maxilla, *52, 53,* 54(t), *58, 59*
  palatine process of, 54(t), *61*
  zygomatic process of, *61*
Maxillary artery, external, *179*
Maxillary sinus, 54(t), *174*
Measles, immunization against, 196
Meatus, 51(t), **285**
  auditory, external, *59, 121, 122*
  internal, *60*
Medial, 11–12, **285**
Medial condyle of tibia, 57(t)
Medial longitudinal arch of foot, *66*
Medial malleolus, 57(t)
Medial pterygoid lamina, *61*
Median fissure of spinal cord, *101,* 102
Median nuchal crest, *61*
Median plane, **285**
Mediastinum, *14, 16,* **285**
Medulla, **285**
  adrenal, 133(t), 140, *140, 142,* **271**
    sympathetic actions on, 116(t)
  renal, 230, *231*
Medulla oblongata, *94,* 95, *95,* 96(t), 97, *97,* **285**
  pyramids of, **290**
Meiosis, **285**
Melanin, 44, 45, **285**
Melatonin, 134(t), 143
Membrane(s), **36**
  arachnoid, *102,* **102,** *103,* 104, **273**
  connective tissue, 36
  epithelial, 36
  fetal, 255
  mucous. See *Mucosa.*
  parietal, 36
  plasma, 27, **288**
    movement through, 28–29
  pleural, 202
  serous, 36, 202
  synovial, 36

Membrane(s) (*Continued*)
    tympanic (eardrum), 122, *122*, **295**
    visceral, 36
Membrane bones, **285**
Membranous labyrinth, 123, *123*
Memory B cells, 192(t), 194, **285**
Memory T cells, 192(t), 194
Meninges, **102**, **285**
Meningitis, 102
Meniscus, **285**
Menopause, 254–255, **285**
Menstrual cycle, 250, 254, *254*, **285**
Menstruation, 252, 254, **285**
Mental foramen, *58*, *59*
Mesenteric artery, 179
    inferior, *173*, *174*, 175(t)
    superior, *173*, *174*, 175(t)
Mesenteric vein, inferior, *178*
    superior, *178*, 179
Mesentery, 17, 212, *212*, *213*, **285**
Mesocolon, 212, **285**
Messenger, first, 132
    second, 132
Metabolic rate, basal, **273**
Metabolic wastes, 229–230
Metabolism, 5, *9*, **285**
    anaerobic, 79
    exercise and, 79
Metacarpal bones, *52*, *53*, 56(t), *64*, 65
Metaphase, 31, *31*, **285**
Metaphysis, 49, **285**
Metastasis, **285**
Metatarsal bones, *52*, *53*, 58(t), 66, *66*
Metric system, 269(t)–270(t)
Microscopy, 26
Microtubules, 31
Microvilli, **285**
Micturition, 236, **285**
Midbrain, *95*, 96(t), 98, **285**
Middle age, 258
Middle cerebral artery, right, *176*
Middle ear, 121, 122
Middle nasal concha (middle turbinate),
    54(t), *58*, *124*
Middle phalanx of finger, *64*
Middle sacral artery, 175(t)
Middle turbinate (middle nasal concha),
    54(t), *58*, *124*
Midsagittal plane, **12**, *12*
Milk (breast milk), 253
    antibodies in, 196
    stimulation of secretion of, 137
Mineral(s), nutrient, 222, 223(t)
Mineralocorticoids, 134(t), 141, **285**
Mitochondria, 27, **285**
Mitosis, 29, **285**
Mitral (bicuspid) valve, *161*, 162, *162*,
    274
    stenosis of, 162
Molars, 214, *215*
Molecule, 4, **285**
Monocyte, 150, *150*, **285**
Monoglyceride, **285**
Mons pubis, 252, *252*
Motor area(s), 96(t), 100
    primary, *101*, **289**
Motor cortex, 100
Motor end plate (neuromuscular
    junction), 78, *79*
Motor nerve(s), 78, 92
Motor nerve fibers, 78, *79*
    crossing of, 97

Motor neurons (efferent neurons), 109,
    111, 113, 115
    in reflexes, 104, *104*, *114*
Mouth, *8*, 212–213
    starch digestion in, 218, 219(t)
Mouth region, *13*
Movement, at joints, 68(t)–70(t)
    coordination of, by cerebellum, 99
    of air, into and out of lungs, 202–204
    through plasma membrane, 28–29
Mucosa, 36, **285**
    in digestive tract, 211, *212*, *221*
    in nasal cavities, 201
Mucus, **285–286**
Multiple births, 257
Multiple sclerosis, 93
Murmur, heart, 164, **281**
Muscle, **286**
Muscle cells, 26, 27, 35, 77, 78, *78*
    impulse transmission to, 78, *79*
    smooth, *26*, *171*
Muscle fascicles, 77, *78*
Muscle fatigue, 79
Muscle fibers. See *Muscle cells.*
Muscle tissue, 33, 35, 35(t), 49, 77–90,
    286. See also specific muscles.
    actions of, 86(t)–88(t)
    agonist (prime mover), 81, *81*
    antagonist, 81, *81*, **272**
    cardiac, 35, 35(t), 160, 163–164, **275**
    contraction of, 78–79, *80*
        isometric, 79, *80*, **283**
        isotonic, 79, *80*, **283**
    CT appearance of, *20*
    digestive tract, 211, *212*, *221*
    fixator, 81, **279**
    functional groups of, 81, 86(t)–88(t)
    gastric, *216*
    insertion of, **282**
        sites of, 81, 86(t)–88(t)
    origin of, **287**
        sites of, 81, 86(t)–88(t)
    shapes of, *82*
    skeletal, 35, 35(t), 77–90, **292**
    smooth, 35, 35(t), **292**
    spasms of, 138
    striations in, 78
    synergist, 81
Muscle tone, 79, **286**
Muscular system, 5(t), *6*, 77–90
Mutation, **286**
Myelin, 93, **286**
Myelinated neurons, 100
Myelin sheath, 93, *93*
Myocardium, 160, **286**
Myofibril, **286**
Myofilament, **286**
Myosin, **286**
Myosin filaments, **78**

Nails, 6, 44, **286**
Nares, 200, **286**
Nasal bone, *52*, 55(t), *58*, *59*
Nasal cavity, *8*, 199, 200
    mucous membrane lining, 201
    protective function of hairs in, 190
    receptors in, 123, *124*
Nasal conchae (turbinates), 54(t), *58,
    124, 200*, 200–201, **276**

Nasal septum, 200
Nasopharynx, 201, 215, **286**
Natural killer cells (NK cells), 192(t),
    286
Navel, *13*
Neck, *13*
Neck of tooth, *214*
Needle insertion, into subarachnoid space,
    104
Negative feedback system, 10
    endocrine regulation by, 134–135, *135*
Neonatal period, 257–258
Neonate, 257, **286**
Neoplasm, **286**
Nephron(s), 232, *232*, **286**
Nerve(s), 7, 92, **93**, **286**. See also specific
    nerves.
Nerve cells (neurons), 26, 27, 35, *36*, **92**,
    93, *93*, **286**
    afferent (sensory), 109, 111, 113, **272**
        in reflexes, 104, *104*, *114*
    association, **273**
        in reflexes, 104, *104*, *114*
    efferent (motor), 109, 111, 113, 115
        in reflexes, 104, *104*, *114*
    in multiple sclerosis, 93
    myelinated, 100
    postganglionic, **289**
    postsynaptic, **289**
    preganglionic, **289**
    presynaptic, **289**
Nerve fibers, 92
    motor, 78, *79*
        crossing of, 97
Nerve stimulation, 126
Nervous system, 5(t), 7, 91–118
    autonomic, 92, 98, 113–116, **273**
        parasympathetic division of, *114*,
            115, **287**
            actions of, 116(t)
        sympathetic division of, *114*, 115,
            293
            actions of, 116(t)
    central, 91–108, *92*, **275**. See also
        Brain and *Spinal cord.*
        nucleus (nuclei) in, 93, **286**
        protective coverings of, *102*, 102–
            104, *103*
        tracts in, 93, **294**
            ascending, 102
            descending, 102
    peripheral, 92, *92*, 109–118, **288**
    regulation of heart by, 164
    somatic, 92, 109–113, **292**
Nervous tissue, 33, 35, *36*
Neural response, 104
Neurilemma (cellular sheath), 93, *93*
Neuromuscular junction (motor end
    plate), 78, *79*
Neurons (nerve cells), 26, 27, 35, *36*, **92**,
    93, *93*, **286**
    afferent (sensory), 109, 111, 113,
        272
        in reflexes, 104, *104*, *114*
    association, **273**
        in reflexes, 104, *104*, *114*
    efferent (motor), 109, 111, 113,
        115
        in reflexes, 104, *104*, *114*
    in multiple sclerosis, 93
    myelinated, 100
    postganglionic, **289**

Neurons (nerve cells) (*Continued*)
  postsynaptic, **289**
  preganglionic, **289**
  presynaptic, **289**
Neurotransmitters, **93**
Neutrophil, 150, *150*, **286**
Nicotinic acid (niacin), 224(t)
Nipple, 253, *253*
  areola of, 253, *253*, 273
Nitrogen, in exhaled air, 205(t)
  in human body, 2(t)
  in inhaled air, 205(t)
  in metabolic wastes, 229
NK cells (natural killer cells), 192(t), **286**
Node(s), atrioventricular, 163, *163*, 273
  lymph, 8, *182*, 183, **284**
  sinoatrial, 163, *163*, **292**
Nodule(s), lymph, **284**
Nonelectrolytes, 241
Non–insulin-dependent diabetes mellitus, 139
Nonself, vs. self, 189–190
Nonspecific defense mechanisms, 189, 190, *190*, 192
Norepinephrine, 133(t), 140, *142*, **286**
Nose. See *Nasal* entries.
Nostrils, 200
Nuchal lines, *61*
Nucleic acids, 4, **286**
Nucleolus, 28, **286**
Nucleotide, **286**
Nucleus (nuclei), atomic, **286**
  cellular, 4, 28, **286**
  central nervous system, 93, **286**
Nutrients, **211**, 222, **286**
  absorption of, 220–221
  mineral, 222, 223(t)
  vitamin, 222, 224(t)–225(t)
Nutrition, **286**

Obesity, **286**
Oblique muscle(s) of abdomen, external, 19, *83*, 84, 85, 86(t)
  aponeurosis of, *85*
  internal, *85*
    aponeurosis of, *85*
Obturator foramen, 57(t), *65*
Occipital bone, *53*, 54(t), *59*, *60*, *61*
Occipital condyle(s), 54(t), *61*
Occipital lobe, *94*, *99*, 100, *101*
Occipital region, *13*, 14
Oculomotor nerve, *110*, 111(t)
Odontoid process of axis (dens axis), 55(t), *63*
Old age, 258
Olfactory epithelium, 123, *124*
Olfactory nerve, *110*, 111(t), 125
Omentum, greater, *16*, 212, *213*, **281**
  lesser, *17*, 212, **284**
Oocyte, **286**
Openings, bony, 51(t)
Ophthalmic region, *13*, 14
Opposition, **286**
Optic, **286**
Optic canal, *60*
Optic chiasma, *95*, 98
Optic disc, **121**
Optic nerve, *110*, 111(t), *120*, 121
Optimum, **286**
Oral cavity, 8, 212–213
  starch digestion in, 218, 219(t)

Oral region, *13*, 14
Orbicularis oculi muscle, *83*, 84, 85, 86(t)
Orbicularis oris muscle, *83*, 85, 86(t)
Orbit, *52*, *59*, **286**
Orbital fissure, superior, *58*
Orbital region, *13*, 14
Organ(s), 4, **286**
  digestive, structures supporting, 212, *213*
  lymphatic, 183–184
  sensory, 119–129
  sex, 248–255
    female, *9*, 250–252, 250–255
    male, *9*, 248, 248–250, *249*
    parasympathetic actions on, 116(t)
    sympathetic actions on, 116(t)
  skeletal muscle as, 77
Organelle(s), 4, 27, **286**
Organic compound(s), **4**
Organism, *3*, 4
Organization levels, in human body, 2, *3*, 4
Organ level, in human body, *3*, 4
Organ of Corti, 123, **287**
Organ systems (body systems), *3*, 4–5, 5(t), *6–9*
Orgasm, **287**
Orifice, **287**
Origin, muscle, **287**
  sites of, 81, 86(t)–88(t)
Oropharynx, 201, 215, **287**
Osmosis, 28, *29*, **287**
Osmotic pressure, 28, 242, **287**
  and urine volume, 235, *235*
Osseous, **287**
Ossicles, **287**
  auditory, 55(t), 122, *122*, 273
Ossification, **49**, **287**
Osteoblast, **49**, 50, **287**
Osteoclast, 50, **287**
Osteocyte, 49, 50, *50*, **287**
Osteon (haversian system), 49, *50*, **281**, **287**
Osteoporosis, **287**
Outer ear, 121–122
Outlet, pelvic, 57(t), *65*
Output, cardiac, **164**
  and blood pressure, 180, *180*
  fluid, 242–243, *243*
Oval window of ear, 122, *122*, **287**
Ovarian artery, *174*, 175(t)
Ovarian follicle, 251, 254, *254*
Ovarian ligament, *250*, 251, *251*, **287**
Ovarian vein, 176(t)
Ovary, 7, *9*, *17*, *132*, 134(t), *250*, 251, *251*, 254, **287**
Ovulation, 251, 254, **287**
Ovum (ova), 26, *26*, 251, 255, **287**
Oxidation, **287**
Oxygen, diffusion of, 204, *204*
  in exhaled air, 205(t)
  in human body, 2(t)
  in inhaled air, 205(t)
  transport of, 149, 204–205
Oxygen debt, 79, **287**
Oxygen-poor blood, 160, 171, 172, *172*, *173*
Oxygen-rich blood, 160, 171, 172, *172*, *173*
Oxyhemoglobin, 149, 204–205, **287**
Oxytocin, 98, 133(t), 136, 253, **287**

Pacemaker of heart, 163, *163*
Pacinian corpuscle, **287**
Pain receptors, 104, 126
Palate, **287**
  hard, *61*, 215, **281**
  soft, 215, **292**
Palatine bone, 55(t)
  horizontal plate of, *61*
Palatine process, 54(t), *61*
Palatine tonsils, 183
Palmar region, *13*, 14
Palsy, cerebral, **275**
Pancreas, 7, *8*, *18*, *132*, 210, 217, **287**
  endocrine, 133(t), 138–139
  exocrine, 217
Pancreatic duct, 217, **287**
Pancreatic enzymes, 218, 219(t), 220, 220(t)
Pancreatitis, 217
Pantothenic acid, 224(t)
Papanicolaou test, 252
Papilla, **287**
  renal, 230, *231*
Papillary muscles, 161, 162, *162*, 165
Parasympathetic division, of autonomic nervous system, *114*, 115, **287**
  actions of, 116(t)
Parathyroid glands, 7, *132*, 133(t), 138, **287**
Parathyroid hormone (PTH), 133(t), 134–135, *135*, 138, **287**
Parietal, **287**
Parietal bone, *52*, *53*, 54(t), *58–61*
Parietal branches of aorta, 175(t)
Parietal lobe, *94*, *99*, 100, *101*
Parietal membrane, 36
Parietal peritoneum, 211
Parietal pleura, 202
Parotid glands, 214, **287**
Parturition, 257, **287**
Passive (borrowed) immunity, 196
Patella, *52*, 57(t), *65*
Patellar reflex, **287–288**
Patellar region, *13*, 14
Pathogens, **189**, **288**. See also *Infection*.
  defense mechanisms against, 189–196
    immune, 192(t), 192–196, *193*, *195*
    inflammatory, 190, *191*
    macrophages in, *191*, 192
    nonspecific, 189, 190, *190*, 192
    specific, 189, *190*, 192–196
Pectoral, **288**
Pectoral girdle (shoulder girdle), 56(t), 64–65
Pectoralis major muscle, *83*, 87(t), *253*
Pectoralis minor muscle, 87(t)
Pectoral region, 14
Pedal region, *13*, 14
Pellagra, 224(t)
Pelvic brim (pelvic inlet), 57(t), *65*, 65
Pelvic cavity, *14*, 16, **288**
Pelvic girdle, 56(t)–57(t), *65*
Pelvic inlet (pelvic brim), 57(t), 65, *65*
Pelvic nerves, 115
Pelvic outlet, 57(t), *65*
Pelvic region, *13*, 14
Pelvis, **288**
  female, 65, *65*
  male, 65, *65*
  true (lesser), 57(t)
Penis, *9*, *18*, 248, 249–250, **288**
Pepsin, 216, 220, **288**

Peptidases, 220
Peptide, **288**
Pericardial cavity, *14*, 16, **288**
Pericardial sac, *16*
Pericardium, 160, **288**
Perilymph, 123, **288**
Perimysium, 77, *78*, **288**
Perineal region, 15
Perineum, 253, **288**
Periosteum, *48, 49*, **288**
  layers of, *50*
Peripheral nervous system (PNS), 92, *92*,
  109–118, **288**
Peristalsis, 211, 216, **288**
Peritoneal cavity, 211
Peritoneum, **288**
  folds of, 212, *213*
  parietal, 211
  visceral, 211, *212*, **296**
Peritonitis, 211–212, **288**
Peritubular capillaries, *232*, 233
Permanent teeth, 214, *215*
Permeability, selective, 28
Peroneus muscle, *83, 84*, 88(t)
Perpendicular plate of ethmoid bone, *58*
PET (positron emission tomography), **289**
Petrous portion of temporal bone, *60*
PG (prostaglandin), 134, **289**
pH, **288**
Phagocytes, in protection against
  pathogens, *191*, 192
Phagocytosis, 29, *30*, 192, **288**
Phalanx (phalanges), **288**
  of fingers, *52, 53*, 56(t), *64*, 65
  of toes, *52, 53*, 58(t), 66, *66*
Pharyngeal tonsil, 183
Pharynx, *8*, 199, *200*, 201, *210*, 215, **288**
Phosphate ions, 244
Phosphorus, 223(t)
  in human body, 2(t)
Photoreceptor, **288**
Phrenic artery, inferior, *174*, 175(t)
Phrenic nerves, 113, 205
Physiology, *1*, **288**
Pia mater, *102*, *102, 103*, **288**
Pigment, bile, 230
Pigment cells, *42*, 44
Pineal gland, *7*, *95*, *132*, 134(t), 141, **288**
  CT appearance of, *20*
Pinna, 121, *122*, **288**
Pituitary dwarfs, 137
Pituitary gland, *7*, *95*, *132*, 133(t), 135–
  137, *136*, **288**
  and adrenal function, 141, *142*
Pivot joint, 68(t)
Placenta, 255, *256*, 257, **288**
Planes of body, 12, *12*
Plantar region, *13*, 15
Plasma, *148*, **149**, **288**
Plasma cell, 192(t), *194*, **288**
Plasma membrane, 27, **288**
  movement through, 28–29
Plate, cribriform, of ethmoid bone, 54(t),
  60
  epiphyseal, **278**
  horizontal, of palatine bone, *61*
  perpendicular, of ethmoid bone, *58*
Platelet (thrombocyte), *150*, 151, 183,
  288
Platelet (thrombocyte) count, 153(t)
Platysma muscle, *83*
Pleura, **288**

Pleural cavity, 202, **288**
Pleural membrane, 202
Pleural sacs, *14*, 16
Pleurisy, 202
Plexus, 113, **289**
  brachial, *112*, 113
  cervical, *112*, 113, **275**
  choroid, 103, *103*, **275**
  coccygeal, *112*
  lumbar, *112*, 113
  sacral, *112*, 113, **291**
PNS (peripheral nervous system), 92, *92*,
  109–118, **288**
Polypeptides, 220
Polysaccharides, **289**
Polyunsaturated fat, **289**
Polyuria, **289**
Pons, *95*, 96(t), *97*, 97–98, **289**
Popliteal artery, *179*
Popliteal region, *13*, 15
Portal system, hepatic, **281**
Portal vein, *179*
  hepatic, *178*, *179*, *217*, 218
Position, anatomical, 11, *11*, **272**
Position receptors, 126
Positive feedback system, 10
  endocrine regulation by, 135
Positron emission tomography (PET), **289**
Postcentral gyrus, *99*, 100, *101*
Posterior, 11, **289**
Posterior arch of atlas, *63*
Posterior cavity of eye, 121
Posterior cerebral artery, right, *176*
Posterior column of spinal cord, *101*, 102
Posterior communicating artery of
  cerebrum, left, *176*
Posterior intercostal arteries, 175(t)
Posterior lobe of pituitary gland, 133(t),
  136, 136
Posterior median fissure of spinal cord,
  101, 102
Posterior tubercle of atlas, *63*
Postganglionic neuron, **289**
Postsynaptic neuron, **289**
Potassium, 223(t)
  in human body, 2(t)
Potassium ions, 244
Potential, action, 78, **271**
  resting, **290**
Precapillary sphincter, *171*
Precentral gyrus, *99*, 100, *101*
Prefixes, 265–266
  in metric designations, 269(t)
Prefrontal area, *94*
Preganglionic neuron, **289**
Pregnancy, **289**
  preparation for, 254
  uterine contractions in, 257
Premolars, 214, *215*
Premotor area, *101*
Prenatal development, 256–257
Prepuce, *248*, 249, **289**
Presbyopia, 121
Pressure, blood, **179**, **274**
  diastolic, 181
  factors affecting, 179–181, *180*
  measurement of, 181
  systolic, 181, **293**
  osmotic, 28, 242, **287**
  and urine volume, 235, *235*
Pressure differences, in breathing, 202–
  204

Pressure points, 179
Pressure receptors, *125*
Presynaptic neuron, **289**
Prevertebral ganglion, **289**
Primary bronchus, *200*
Primary functional areas, of cerebral
  cortex, 100, *101*
Primary motor area, *101*, **289**
Primary sex characteristics, 250
Prime mover (agonist muscle), 81, *81*
Process(es), 51(t)
  acromion, *53*, 56(t)
  alveolar, 54(t), *214*
  articular, of vertebrae, *62, 63*, 64(t)
  condyloid, *59*
  coronoid, of mandible, *59*
  mastoid, *19*, *53*, 54(t), *59*, 61, *122*
  odontoid, of axis (dens axis), 55(t), *63*
  palatine, 54(t), *61*
  pterygoid, lateral lamina of, *61*
    medial lamina of, *61*
  spinous, of vertebrae, 55(t), *62, 63*,
    64(t)
  styloid, of temporal bone, 54(t), *59*, 61
    of ulna, 56(t)
  transverse, of vertebrae, *63*, 64(t)
    foramina of, 55(t), *63*
  xiphoid, *52*, 56(t)
  zygomatic, of maxilla, 61
    of temporal bone, 54(t), *59*
Progesterone, 134(t), 254, **289**
Prolactin, 133(t), 137, 253, **289**
Prolapse, **289**
Proliferation, **289**
Pronation, 69(t), **289**
Prophase, 30, *31*, **289**
Proprioceptors, 126, **289**
Prostaglandin (PG), 134, **289**
Prostate gland, *9*, *248*, 249, **289**
  cancer of, 249
Protein(s), 4, 222, **289**
  digestion of, 220, 220(t)
  stimulation of synthesis of, 137
Protein-bound iodine, 137
Prothrombin, 151–152, **289**
Prothrombin activator, 151
Prothrombin time (PT), 153(t)
Proximal, 12, **289**
Proximal convoluted tubule, *232*, 233
Proximal phalanges, of fingers, *64*
  of toes, *66*
Pseudostratified epithelium, **289**
PT (prothrombin time), 153(t)
Pterygoid process, lateral lamina of, *61*
  medial lamina of, *61*
PTH (parathyroid hormone), 133(t), 134–
  135, *135*, 138, **287**
Puberty, 250, **289**
Pubic arch, 65
Pubic region, *13*
Pubic symphysis (symphysis pubis), *16*,
  52, 57(t), 65, *65*, **293**
Pubis, *52*, 57(t), 65, *65*, *248*
Pudendum, **289**
Pulmonary, **289**. See also *Lung(s)*.
Pulmonary alveoli, 199, 201, *202*
Pulmonary artery (arteries), *18*, 160, *160*,
  161, *165*, 171, 172, *172*
  left, *160*, *173*
  right, *160*, *173*
Pulmonary circulation, 171–172, *172*,
  289–290

Pulmonary trunk, *173*
Pulmonary valve, *161*, 162
Pulmonary vein(s), *18*, 160, *161*, 171, 172, *172*
   left, *160*, *161*, *173*
   right, *160*, *161*, *173*
Pulmonary ventilation, 202
Pulp, 213, *214*
Pulp cavity, 213, *214*, **290**
Pulse, 179, *179*, **290**
Pump, sodium-potassium, **292**
Pupil, *120*, **121**, **290**
   parasympathetic actions on, 116(t)
   sympathetic actions on, 116(t)
Purkinje fibers, *163*, **290**
Pus, **290**
Pyloric sphincter, 216, **290**
Pylorus, *216*
Pyramid(s), **290**
   of kidney, 230, *231*, **290**
   of medulla oblongata, **290**
Pyramidal tracts, **290**
Pyridoxine (vitamin B₆), 224(t)

Quadrants, of abdominopelvic cavity, *15*, 16–17
Quadriceps femoris muscle, *19*, *83*, 88(t)
Quadruplets, 257

Radial artery, 179, *179*
Radius, *52*, *53*, 56(t), 65
Ramus, **290**
Ramus of mandible, *59*
Rapid eye movement (REM) sleep, **290**
RAS (reticular activating system), **290**
Reabsorption, renal tubular, 234, *234*, **295**
Reception, 93
Receptors, **290**
   beta, *274*
   blood pressure mediation by, 180, 181
   chemical, **290**
   hormone, 132
   olfactory, 123, *124*
   pain, 104, 126
   position, 126
   pressure, *125*
   sensory, 109, 110, 119–120, **290**
   sound, 123
   tactile, 125, *125*
   taste, *124*, 125
   temperature, 126
   touch, *125*
   vibration, *125*
   visual, 121
Rectum, *8*, *17*, *210*, 222, *248*, *250*, **290**
Rectus abdominis muscle, *83*, *85*, 86(t)
Red blood cell (erythrocyte), *148*, 149–150, *150*
Red blood cell (erythrocyte) count, 153(t)
Red marrow, *48*, *49*, 149
Referred pain, 126
Reflex(es), **104**, *114*, **290**
   bladder-emptying, 104
   patellar, **287–288**
   withdrawal, 104, *104*
Reflex centers, 96(t), 97, 98

Refractory period, **290**
Regions, of abdominopelvic cavity, *15*, 17
   of body, *13*, 13–15
Rejection, graft, **281**
Relaxation, of diaphragm, 203
   of heart, 164, *165*
   of intercostal muscles, 203
Relaxation phase, of cardiac cycle, 164, *165*
Releasing hormones, 98, 133(t), 137
REM (rapid eye movement) sleep, **290**
Renal, **290**. See also *Kidney(s)*.
Renal artery, *173*, *174*, 175(t), *231*
   left, *231*
Renal capsule, 230, *231*
Renal corpuscle, 232
Renal cortex, 230, *231*
Renal medulla, 230, *231*
Renal papilla, 230, *231*
Renal pelvis, *231*, 232, **290**
Renal pyramids, 230, *231*, **290**
Renal tubules, 232, *232*, 233, *233*, *234*
   reabsorption by, 234, *234*, **295**
   secretion by, 234, *234*, **295**
Renal vein, *173*, 176(t), *231*
   right, *231*
Renin, 181, 236, **290**
Reproductive system, 5(t), *9*, 247–261
   female, *9*, 250, 250–255, *251*
   male, *9*, *248*, 248–250, *249*
Resistance, to blood flow, *180*, 180–181
Resistance reaction, 141
Respiration, **199**, 205, **290**
   cellular, 204
Respiratory centers, 97, *200*, 205
Respiratory passageway, protective function of mucosa in, 190
Respiratory system, 5(t), *8*, 199–208, *200*
   protection of, from dirty air, 205–206
Response(s), actual, 93
   immune, 189, 192(t)
   neural, 104
Resting potential, **290**
Resuscitation, 205
Reticular activating system (RAS), **290**
Reticular fibers, 35
Reticular formation, 97
Reticulum, endoplasmic, **27**, *278*
Retina, *120*, **121**, **290**
   fovea of, **121**, *280*
Retinal arteries, *120*
Retinal veins, *120*
Retroperitoneal, 230, **290**
Rh incompatibility, 155, *155*
Rhodopsin, **290**
Rh system, 154, **290**
Rib(s), *19*, *52*, 56(t)
   CT appearance of, *20*
   false, *52*, 56(t)
   floating, *52*, 56(t)
   true, *52*, 56(t)
Riboflavin (vitamin B₂), 224(t)
Ribonucleic acid (RNA), **4**, **290**
Ribosome, 27, **290**
Rickets, **290**
Ridge, supraorbital, 54(t)
Right anterior cerebral artery, *176*
Right atrioventricular valve, *161*
Right atrium, *160*, *161*, *163*, *173*
   auricle of, *160*
Right brachiocephalic vein, *177*

Right bronchus, *17*
Right cerebral hemisphere, 99, *99*
Right common carotid artery, *173*, *174*, 175(t)
Right coronary artery, *160*, *161*
Right hepatic duct, *217*
Right jugular vein, *173*
Right lobe of liver, *217*, 218
Right lung, *18*, *173*, *200*
Right lymphatic duct, *182*, 183, **290–291**
Right middle cerebral artery, *176*
Right posterior cerebral artery, *176*
Right pulmonary artery, *160*, *173*
Right pulmonary vein, *160*, *161*, *173*
Right renal vein, *231*
Right subclavian artery, *17*, *173*, 175(t)
Right subclavian vein, *177*, *182*
Right ureter, *231*
Right ventricle, *160*, *161*, *163*, *173*
RNA (ribonucleic acid), **4**, **290**
Rods, **121**, **291**
Roentgenogram, **291**
Root(s), of hair, 44
   of spinal nerve, 113, *113*
     dorsal, 113, *113*
     ventral (anterior), 113, *113*, **272**
   of tooth, 213, *214*
Root canal, 213–214, *214*, **291**
Rotation, 69(t), **291**
Round ligament, *251*
Round window of ear, *122*
Rugae, of stomach, 216, *216*
   of vagina, 252
Rupture, of spleen, 184

Sac(s), air, pulmonary, 199, *201*, *202*
    in gas exchange, 204, *204*
   pericardial, *16*
   pleural, *14*, 16
Saccule, **291**
Sacral artery, middle, 175(t)
Sacral curve, *62*
Sacral nerves, *112*, 113
Sacral plexus, *112*, 113, **291**
Sacral region, *13*, 15
Sacroiliac joints, 65
Sacrum, *18*, *19*, *52*, *53*, 55(t), 61, *62*, *63*, 65
Saddle block, 104
Saddle joint, 68(t), **291**
Sagittal plane, **12**, *12*, **291**
Sagittal sinus, inferior, *177*
   superior, *102*, *103*, *177*
Sagittal suture, 51
Saliva, 214–215, **291**
Salivary amylase, 215, 218, 219(t), **291**
Salivary glands, *8*, *210*, 214, 218, 219(t), **291**
   parasympathetic actions on, 116(t)
   sympathetic actions on, 116(t)
Salt taste, *124*, 125
SA (sinoatrial) node, 163, *163*, **292**
Sarcolemma, **291**
Sarcomere, **291**
Sarcoplasm, **291**
Sartorius muscle, *83*, 88(t)
Saturated fat, **291**
Scapula, *19*, *52*, *53*, 56(t)
   spine of, *53*, 56(t)

Schwann cell, **291**
Sciatic nerve, *112*, 113
Sclera, **120**, *120*, **291**
Sclerosis, multiple, 93
Scrotal cavity, *14*
Scrotum, *18*, 248, *248,* **291**
Scurvy, 224(t)
Sebaceous glands, *42*, **43**, 44, **291**
Sebum, **43**, **291**
Secondary bronchus, *200*
Secondary sex characteristics, 250, **291**
Second heart sound, 164
Second messenger, 132
Second molar, *215*
Second premolar, *215*
Secretion, **291**
    abnormal, 135
    renal tubular, 234, *234*, **295**
Section, planes of, 12, *12*
Selective permeability, 28
Self, vs. nonself, 189–190
Sella turcica, 54(t), *60*, 135, **291**
Selye, H., on reactions to stress, 141
Semen, 249, **291**
Semicircular canals, *122*, 123, *123*, **291**
Semicircular ducts, **291**
Semilunar valve, *161*, 162, *162*, **291**
    opening and closing of, 164, *165*
Seminal vesicles, *248*, 249, **291**
Seminiferous tubules, 248, *249*, **291**
Sensation, **291**
Sense organs, 119–129
Sensory areas of cerebrum, 96(t), 100, *101*, **291**
Sensory nerves (afferent nerves), 92
Sensory neurons (afferent neurons), 109, 111, 113, **272**
    in reflexes, 104, *104*, *114*
Sensory receptors, 109, 110, 119–120, **290**
Septum, **291**
    interatrial, 162, **283**
    interventricular, *161*, 162, **283**
    nasal, 200
Serosa, 36, 202, **291**
Serratus anterior muscle, *83*, 87(t)
Serum, **149**, **291–292**
Sesamoid bone, **292**
Sex cells, 30
Sex characteristics, primary, 250
    secondary, 250, **291**
Sex chromosomes, **292**
Sex hormones, 141
Sex organs, 248–255
    female, *9*, *250–252*, 250–255
    male, *9*, *248*, 248–250, *249*
    parasympathetic actions on, 116(t)
    sympathetic actions on, 116(t)
Sexual intercourse, 252
Sheath, cellular (neurilemma), 93, *93*
    myelin, 93, *93*
Shock, circulatory, 180–181
Shoulder, *13*, 67
Shoulder girdle (pectoral girdle), 56(t), 64–65
Siamese twins, 257
Sigmoid colon, *17*, *18*, *210*, *213*, 222, **292**
Simple epithelium, 33
Sinoatrial (SA) node, 163, *163*, **292**
Sinus(es), **292**
    air-filled, 51, 51(t), 61, *200*, 201

Sinus(es) (*Continued*)
    cavernous, *177*
    coronary, *161*, *163*, **276**
    ethmoid, 54(t)
    frontal, 54(t), *124*, *174*
    maxillary, 54(t), *174*
    sagittal, inferior, *177*
        superior, *102*, *103*, *177*
    sphenoid, 54(t), *124*
    venous, **177**
        of dura mater, 102, *102*, *103*, 177, *177*
Sinusitis, 61, 201
Sinusoids, 171, 179, **292**
Skeletal muscle, 35, 35(t), 77–90, **292**
Skeletal system, 5(t), *6*, 47–75
    appendicular, 50
    axial, 50
    bones comprising, *52–53*, 54(t)–58(t)
        joints between, 66, 67, 68(t), 70–71
        movement at, 68(t)–70(t)
Skin, *6*, 41–46, **292**
    appendages of, 44
    color of, 44–45
    excretory function of, 230
    glands in, *42*, 43–44
    hair follicles in, *42*, 44, *44*, *125*
    layers of, *42*, 42–43, *125*
    microscopic structure of, *42*
    protective function of, 41–42, 190
    tactile receptors in, 125, *125*
Skull, 51, 61, 68–71, *103*, **292**
Skull suture(s), 51, *59*, 67, **293**
Sleep, rapid eye movement, **290**
Small intestine, *8*, *16*, *210*, 211, 217, **292**
    digestion in, 217, 219(t), 220(t)
    villi of, *212*, 217, 220–221, *221*
    wall of, *212*
Smell, 123, 125
Smooth muscle, 35, 35(t), **292**
Smooth muscle cells, *26*, *171*
Sockets, tooth, 61, 213
Sodium, 2(t), 223(t)
Sodium ions, 244
Sodium-potassium pump, **292**
Soft palate, 215, **292**
Soleus muscle, *83*, *84*, 88(t)
Solute, **292**
Solution(s), **292**
    effects of tonicity of, 28, *29*
Solvent, **292**
Somatic nervous system, 92, 109–113, **292**
Somatotropin (growth hormone), 133(t), 137, **281**
Somesthetic, **292**
Somesthetic association area, *101*
Sound receptors, 123
Sound waves, 122
Sour taste, *124*, 125
Spasms, muscle, 138
Specific defense mechanisms, 189, *190*, 192–196
Speech area, 100, *101*
Spermatic cord, *16*, 248, *249,* **292**
Sperm cell(s), 26, *26*, 248, 255, **292**
    flagellum of, *26*, 28
Sperm duct (vas deferens), *9*, *18*, 249, *249,* **295**
Sphenoid bone, 54(t), *58*, *61*
    greater wing of, *59*, *60*, *61*

Sphenoid bone (*Continued*)
    lesser wing of, *60*
Sphenoid sinus, 54(t), *124*
Sphincter, **292**
    anal, 222
    cardiac, 216
    precapillary, *171*
    pyloric, 216, **290**
    urethral, 236
Sphygmomanometer, 181, **292**
Spinal accessory nerve, *110*, 111(t)
Spinal artery, anterior, *176*
Spinal block, 104
Spinal column. See *Vertebra(e)*; *Vertebral column.*
Spinal cord, 7, *92*, *95*, *97*, 100, *101*, *102*, *103*, **292**
    central canal of, *101*, *102*, **275**
    columns of, *101*, *102*
    CT appearance of, *20*
    fissures of, 100, *101*, *102*
    gray matter of, *101*, *102*, *113*
    nerves emerging from, *92*, *92*, 111, *112*, 113, *113*, **292**
        dorsal root of, 113, *113*
        ventral (anterior) root of, 113, *113*, **272**
    white matter of, *101*, *102*, *113*
Spinal ganglion, 113, *113*, **292**
Spinal nerve(s), *92*, *92*, 111, *112*, 113, *113*, **292**
    dorsal root of, 113, *113*
    ventral (anterior) root of, 113, *113*, **272**
Spinal tap, 104
Spine(s), 51(t)
    of ilium, anterior superior, 57(t)
    of ischium, 57(t), 65
    of scapula, *53*, 56(t)
Spinous processes of vertebrae, 55(t), *62*, *63*, 64(t)
Spleen, *8*, *17*, *18*, *20*, *182*, 183–184, **292**
Splenectomy, 184
Splenic artery, *174*
Splenic vein, *178*
Spongy bone, *48*, *49*, *50*
Sprain, **292**
Squama, of frontal bone, *58*
    of temporal bone, *59*
Squamous epithelium, **292**
Squamous suture, *59*
Stages of labor, 257
Stapes, 55(t), 122, *122*
Starch, digestion of, 218, 219(t)
Steady state, 5, 10
Stem cells, 149
Stenosis, **292**
    mitral, 162
Sterile, **292**
Sterilization, **292**
Sternocleidomastoid muscle, *16*, *83*, *84*, *85*, 86(t)
Sternum, *52*, 56(t)
    body of, 56(t)
    manubrium of, 56(t), **285**
    xiphoid process of, *52*, 56(t)
Steroid hormones, 132, 140–141
Stethoscope, in detection of heart sounds, 164
    in measurement of blood pressure, 181
Stimulation, nerve, 126

Stimulus, **119**, **293**
Stomach, 8, 16, 17, *210*, 213, 216, *216*, *217*, **293**
  CT appearance of, *20*
  destruction of bacteria in, 190
  digestion in, 216, 220, 220(t)
  innervation of, *115*
  rugae of, 216, *216*
  structure and function of, 1–2, 216
Stratified epithelium, *32*, 33
Stratum, **293**
Stress, 10, 141, *142*
Stressor, 10, 141, **293**
Striations, in muscle tissue, 78
Stroke, 95
Stroke volume, **293**
Styloid process, of temporal bone, 54(t), *59*, *61*
  of ulna, 56(t)
Subarachnoid space, *102*, 103, *103*, **293**
  anesthetic injection into, 104
  needle insertion into, 104
Subclavian artery, 16, *174*
  left, *17*, *160*, 175(t)
  right, *17*, *173*, 175(t)
Subclavian vein, 176(t)
  left, *173*, *182*
  right, *177*, *182*
Subcostal artery, 175(t)
Subcutaneous, **293**
Subcutaneous layer, **293**
Subcutaneous tissue, 35, 42, *42*, *43*, *125*
Subdural space, *102*, **293**
Sublingual glands, 214, **293**
Submandibular glands, 214, **293**
Submucosa, **293**
  in digestive tract, 211, *212*, *221*
Substrate, **293**
Sucrose, 218
Suderiferous (sweat) glands, *42*, *43*, 230
  sympathetic actions on, 116(t)
Suffixes, 266
Sulcus (sulci), 51(t), **293**
  cerebral, 99
    central, *94*, *99*, 100, *101*
Sulfur, 223(t)
  in human body, 2(t)
Suntan, 45
Superciliary arch, *58*
Superficial, 12, **293**
Superficial fascia, 43
Superficial lymphatics, of lower limb, *182*
  of upper limb, *182*
Superior, 11, **293**
Superior articular process of vertebra, *62*, *63*, 64(t)
Superior cerebellar artery, left, *176*
Superior mesenteric artery, *173*, *174*, 175(t)
Superior mesenteric vein, *178*, *179*
Superior nasal concha (superior turbinate), 54(t)
Superior nuchal line, *61*
Superior orbital fissure, *58*
Superior sagittal sinus, *102*, *103*, *177*
Superior turbinate (superior nasal concha), 54(t)
Superior vena cava, *18*, *160*, *161*, *172*, *173*, 175, **293**
  veins draining into, 176(t)
Supination, 69(t), **293**

Supraorbital foramen, *58*
Supraorbital ridge, 54(t)
Suprarenal artery, 175(t)
Surfactant, 201
Suspensory ligament of lens, 121
Suture(s), 51, 67, **293**
  coronal, 51, *59*
  lambdoidal, 51, *59*
  sagittal, 51
  squamous, *59*
Swallowing, 215
Sweat, 230, **293**
Sweat (suderiferous) glands, *42*, **43**, 230
  sympathetic actions on, 116(t)
Sweet taste, *124*, 125
Swelling, of lymph nodes, 183
Symmetry, bilateral, 10
Sympathetic division, of autonomic nervous system, *114*, 115, **293**
  actions of, 116(t)
Symphysis, **293**
Symphysis pubis (pubic symphysis), *16*, *52*, 57(t), *65*, *65*, **293**
Symptom, **293**
Synapse, *93*, **293**
Synaptic cleft, **293**
Synaptic knobs, 92, **293**
Synaptic vesicles, **293**
Synarthrosis, 66, *67*, **293**
Syndrome, **293**
Synergist muscles, 81
Synovial fluid, 71, **293**
Synovial joint (diarthrosis), 66, *67*, *70*, 70–71, **277**, **293**
Synovial membrane, 36
Systemic, **293**
Systemic circulation, 171, 172, *172*, **293**
  resistance in, 180
Systole, *164*, **293**
Systolic blood pressure, 181, **293**

T₃ (triiodothyronine), 133(t), 137, **294**
T₄ (thyroxine), 133(t), 137, **294**
Tachycardia, **164**, **293–294**
Tactile, **294**
Tactile receptors, 125, *125*
Talus, *52*, *53*, 66
Tanning, 45
Target cell, **294**
Target tissues, 132, 133(t)–134(t)
Tarsal bones, 57(t), 66
Tarsal region, *13*, 15
Tarsus, **294**
Taste area, primary, *101*
Taste buds, *124*, 125, 213
T cells (T lymphocytes), 192(t), *193*, 193–194, 196, **293**
  helper, 194, **281**
  killer, 192(t), 194
  memory, 192(t), 194
Tears, 120
Teeth. See *Tooth* entries.
Telophase, 31, *31*, **294**
Temperature conversions, 270(t)
Temperature receptors, 126
Temperature regulation, 104
Temporal artery, *179*

Temporal bone, *52*, *53*, 54(t), *58–61*
  mastoid process of, *19*, *53*, 54(t), *59*, *61*, *122*
  petrous portion of, *60*
  squama of, *59*
  styloid process of, 54(t), *59*, *61*
  zygomatic process of, 54(t), *59*
Temporalis muscle, *85*, 86(t)
Temporal lobe, *94*, 100, *101*
Temporomandibular joints, 54(t)
Tendinitis, **294**
Tendon(s), 49, **294**
  Achilles, *84*, **271**
Tensor fasciae latae muscle, *85*
Teres major muscle, *84*, 87(t)
Testicular artery, *174*, 175(t), *249*
Testicular vein, 176(t), *249*
Testis, 7, *9*, *18*, *132*, 134(t), 248, *248*, *249*, **294**
Testosterone, 134(t), 250, **294**
Tetanus, **294**
Tetany, 138, **294**
Thalamus, *95*, 96(t), *98*, **294**
Thermoreceptor, **294**
Thiamine (vitamin B₁), 224(t)
Thigh, *13*, **294**
  muscles of, 87(t)–88(t)
Third molar, 214, *215*
Third ventricle of brain, *97*, *103*
Thirst center, *98*, 242
Thoracic aorta, 172, *174*, 175(t)
Thoracic cage, 56(t), 65
Thoracic cavity, *14*, 15, 16, 202, **294**
  in breathing, 202, 203, *203*
Thoracic curve, *62*
Thoracic duct, 8, *182*, 183, **294**
Thoracic nerves, *112*, 113
Thoracic region, *13*, 15
Thoracic vertebra(e), *53*, 55(t), 61, *62*, *63*
Thorax, **294**
Thrombin, 151, 152, **294**
Thrombocyte (platelet), 150, 151, 183, **288**
Thrombocyte (platelet) count, 153(t)
Thromboplastin, **294**
Thrombus, **294**
Thumb, *64*
Thymosin, 143, 196
Thymus gland, 7, 8, *132*, 143, *182*, **294**
  in immune function, 184, 196
Thyroid gland, 7, *16*, *132*, 133(t), 137, **294**
Thyroid hormones, 132, 133(t), 137
Thyroid-stimulating hormone (TSH), 133(t), 137, **294**
Thyroxine (T₄), 133(t), 137, **294**
Tibia, *52*, *53*, 57(t), *65*, 66, *83*
Tibialis anterior muscle, *83*, 88(t)
Tissue, 4, *33*, **294**
  bone, *34*, 49, *50*, **274**
    intramembranous formation of, 49, **283**
  circulation to, 172
  connective, 33, 34, *34*, 35, **276**
  epithelial, *32*, 33, **278**
  fat (adipose), *34*, 35, 43, **271**
    mammary, 253, *253*
  sympathetic actions on, 116(t)

Tissue (*Continued*)
 glandular, mammary, 253, *253*
 muscle. See *Muscle tissue.*
 nervous, 33, 35, *36*
 subcutaneous, 35, 42, *42*, 43, *125*
 target, 132, 133(t)–134(t)
Tissue (interstitial) fluid, 170, *170*, 183, 242, **283**
Tissue level of organization, in human body, *3*, 4
Toes, phalanges of, *52*, *53*, 58(t), 66, *66*
Tomography, computed, brain on, *20*, 104
 transverse sections on, *20*
 positron emission, **289**
Tone, muscle, 79, **286**
Tongue, 200, 212–213, **294**
Tonicity, of solutions, effects of, 28, *29*
Tonsillectomy, 183
Tonsils, **183**, **294**
Tooth (teeth), 213–214, *214*, *215*
 canine, 214, *215*, **274**
 deciduous, 214, *215*, **277**
 incisor, 214, *215*
 molar, 214, *215*
 premolar, 214, *215*
 wisdom, 214, *215*
Tooth sockets, *61*, 213
Torso, 13
Touch receptors, *125*
Toxic, **294**
Trachea (windpipe), *8*, *16*, *17*, 199, *200*, 201, **294**
Tract(s), central nervous system, 93, **294**
 ascending, 102
 descending, 102
 digestive, **211**
  wall of, 211, *212*
 gastrointestinal, 211, **280**
 pyramidal, **290**
Transcutaneous electrical nerve stimulation, 126
Transfusion, 152
Transmission, impulse, 93, **294**
 to muscle cells, 78, *79*
Transport, active, 29, **271**
 by circulatory system, 147, 204–205
 by red blood cells, 149
 carbon dioxide, 205
 oxygen, 149, 204–205
Transverse arch of foot, *66*
Transverse colon, *16*, *17*, 210, *213*, 222, **294**
Transverse fissure of cerebrum, 99
Transverse foramen, 55(t), *63*
Transverse (cross, horizontal) plane, **12**, *12*, **281**
Transverse processes of vertebrae, *63*, 64(t)
 foramina of, 55(t), *63*
Transversus abdominis muscle, 85, 86(t)
Trapezius muscle, *19*, *83*, *84*, 85, 86(t)
Trauma, **294**
 to spleen, 184
Triceps brachii muscle, *19*, 81, *81*, *83*, *84*, 87(t)
Tricuspid valve, 162, **294**
Trigeminal nerve, *110*, 111(t), 121
Triglycerides, 220
Triiodothyronine (T_3), 133(t), 137, **294**
Triplets, 257

Trochanter, 51(t)
 greater, 57(t)
 lesser, 57(t)
Trochlear nerve, *110*, 111(t)
Tropic hormone, 137, **295**
True pelvis, 57(t)
True ribs, *52*, 56(t)
Trunk, **295**
 celiac, *174*
 muscles of, 86(t)–87(t)
 pulmonary, *173*
Trypsin, 220
TSH (thyroid-stimulating hormone), 133(t), 137, **294**
T tubules, 78
Tube(s), auditory (eustachian), 122, *122*, **273**
 uterine (fallopian), *9*, *17*, 250, 251, *251*, **279**, **295**
Tubercle, anterior, of atlas, *63*
 posterior, of atlas, *63*
Tuberosity, 51(t)
 ischial, 57(t)
Tubule(s), convoluted, *234*
 renal, 232, *232*, 233, *233*, *234*
  reabsorption by, 234, *234*, **295**
  secretion by, 234, *234*, **295**
 seminiferous, 248, *249*, **291**
 T, 78
Tumor, **295**
Tunics, of blood vessels, 170, *171*
Turbinates (conchae), *200*, 200–201, **276**
 inferior, 55(t), *58*
 middle, 54(t), *58*, *124*
 superior, 54(t)
T1 vertebra, *112*
Twins, 257
Twitch, **295**
Tympanic membrane (eardrum), 122, *122*, **295**
Type A blood, 152, 154, *154*, 154(t)
Type AB blood, 152, 154, *154*, 154(t)
Type B blood, 152, 154, *154*, 154(t)
Type I diabetes mellitus, 139
Type II diabetes mellitus, 139
Type O blood, 152, 154, *154*, 154(t)
Typing (blood typing), 152, *154*, 154(t), 154–155

Ulcer, **295**
Ulna, *52*, *53*, 56(t), 65
Umbilical arteries, 256, *256*
Umbilical cord, 256, *256*, **295**
Umbilical region, *13*, 15, *15*
Umbilical vein, 256, *256*
Universal donors, 152
Upper limb, *13*, 56(t), 65
 superficial lymphatics of, *182*
Uremia, **295**
Ureter(s), *9*, *17*, *18*, *19*, 230, *231*, 236, **295**
 left, *231*
 right, *231*
Urethra, *9*, 230, *231*, 236, 248, *249*, 250, *252*, **295**
Urethral sphincter, 236
Urinalysis, **295**
Urinary bladder, *9*, *16*, *17*, *18*, 230, *231*, 236, *248*, *250*, **295**
 emptying of, 104, 236

Urinary system, 5(t), *9*, 229–239
Urination, 236
Urine, 234, **295**
 flow of, 230, 232, 236
 production of, 233–234, *234*
 regulation of volume of, 234–236, *235*
Uterine (fallopian) tube, *9*, *17*, 250, 251, *251*, **279**, **295**
Uterus, *9*, *17*, 250, *251*, 251–252, **295**
 body of, *250*, *251*, 252
 cervix of, *250*, *251*, 252
  cancer of, 252
  dilation of, in labor, 257
 contraction of, in labor, 257
 fundus of, 252
 wall of, *251*, 252
  implantation within, 251, 255, *255*, **282**
Utricle, **295**
Uvula, 215, **295**

Vaccines, 196
Vacuole, **295**
Vagina, *9*, 250, *251*, 252, *252*, **295**
 fornix of, 252
 rugae of, 252
 vestibule of, 253
Vagus nerve, *110*, 111(t), 125, **295**
Valve(s), aortic, *161*, 162
 atrioventricular, *161*, 162, **273**
  opening and closing of, 164, *165*
 cardiac, *161*, 162, *162*
  opening and closing of, 164, *165*
 ileocecal, 221
 mitral (bicuspid), *161*, 162, *162*, **274**
  stenosis of, 162
 pulmonary, *161*, 162
 semilunar, *161*, 162, *162*, **291**
  opening and closing of, 164, *165*
 tricuspid, 162, **294**
 venous, 170
Varicose veins, **295**
Vascular, **295**
Vas deferens (sperm duct), *9*, *18*, 249, *249*, **295**
Vasectomy, **295**
Vasoconstriction, **295**
Vasodilation, **295**
Vasomotor centers, 97
Veins, 7, 170, *170*, **295**. See also specific veins.
 resistance of, to blood flow, 180
 valves of, 170
 varicose, **295**
 walls of, 170, *171*
Vena cava, **295**
 CT appearance of, *20*
 inferior, *17*, *18*, *160*, *161*, *173*, 175, *178*, *217*, *231*, **282**
  veins draining into, 176(t)
 superior, *18*, *160*, *161*, *172*, *173*, 175, **293**
  veins draining into, 176(t)
Venous return, **166**
Venous sinuses, 177
 of dura mater, 102, *102*, *103*, 177, *177*
Ventilation, 202–204
Ventral, 11, **295**
Ventral branch of spinal nerves, 113, *113*

Ventral cavity, *14*, 15
Ventral root (anterior root) of spinal
    nerve, 113, *113*, **272**
Ventricle(s), **295**
    of brain, *95*, 97
        CT appearance of, *20*
        fourth, *95*, 95, 97, *103*
        lateral, 97, 99, *103*
        third, *97*, *103*
    of heart, 160
        contraction and relaxation of, 164,
            165
        left, *160*, *161*, *163*, *173*
        right, *160*, *161*, *163*, *173*
Venules, 170, *170*, *171*, **295**
Vermiform appendix, *210*, 222, **295**
Vertebra(e), 55(t), 61, *62*, *63*, 64(t)
    C1 (atlas), *19*, 55(t), *63*
        anterior tubercle of, *63*
        posterior arch of, *63*
        posterior tubercle of, *63*
    C2 (axis), 55(t), *63*
        odontoid process of (dens axis),
            55(t), *63*
    centrum of, *62*, *63*, 64(t)
    cervical, *52*, *53*, 55(t), 61, *62*, *63*
        inferior, 55(t), *63*
    coccygeal, *19*, *52*, *53*, 55(t), 61, *62*, *63*,
        276
    computed tomographic appearance of,
        20
    discs between, **61**, **283**
    facets of, 51(t), *62*, *63*
    foramen of, *63*, 64(t)
    joints between, 67
    L1, *112*
    lamina of, *63*, 64(t)
    lumbar, *52*, *53*, 55(t), 61, *62*, *63*
    processes of, *62*, *63*, 64(t)
        articular, *62*, *63*, 64(t)
        spinous, 55(t), *62*, *63*, 64(t)
        transverse, *63*, 64(t)
            foramina of, 55(t), *63*
    sacral, *18*, *19*, *52*, *53*, 55(t), 61, *62*, *63*,
        65
    T1, *112*
    thoracic, *53*, 55(t), 61, *62*, *63*
Vertebral artery, 177
    left, *174*, *176*
Vertebral canal, *14*, 15, *62*, **295**
Vertebral column, 10, 55(t), 61, *62*, **295**.
    See also *Vertebra(e)*.

Vertebral foramen, *63*, 64(t)
Vertebral vein, *177*
Vesicles, **295**
    seminal, *248*, 249, **291**
    synaptic, **293**
Vessels, blood, 170, *170*, **274**. See also
        specific types.
    in inflammation, 190, *191*
    resistance to flow in, 180
    sympathetic actions on, 116(t)
    walls of, 170–171, *171*
    lymphatic, 8, 170, *182*, 183
    lacteal, 220, *221*, **284**
Vestibular glands, greater, 253, **281**
    lesser, 253, **284**
Vestibular nerve, 111(t), *122*, 123, *123*
Vestibule, **295**
    of ear, *122*, 123, *123*
    of vagina, 253
Vestibulocochlear nerve, *110*, 111(t),
    123
Vibration receptors, *125*
Villus (villi), **296**
    of small intestine, *212*, 217, 220–221,
        221
Viral hepatitis, 196
Viral infection, 194
    defenses against, 192
    hepatitis due to, 196
    meningitis due to, 102
    vs. bacterial infection, 150, 151
Viscera, 15, **296**
Visceral, **296**
Visceral branches of aorta, 175(t)
Visceral membrane, 36
Visceral peritoneum, 211, *212*, **296**
Visceral pleura, 202
Vision, 121
Visual area, primary, 100, *101*
Visual association area, 100, *101*
Visual receptors, 121
Visual reflexes, 98
Vital centers, in medulla oblongata, 96(t),
    97
Vitamin(s), 222, 224(t)–225(t), **296**
Vitreous humor, *120*, **121**, **296**
Vocal cords, 201, **296**
Voice box (larynx), 8, 199, *200*, 201,
    284
Voluntary muscles, 35, 35(t)
Vomer, 55(t), *58*, *61*
Vulva, *252*, 252–253, **296**

Wall(s), of blood vessels, 170–171, *171*
    of digestive tract, 211, *212*
    of heart, 159–160
    of small intestine, *212*
    of uterus, *251*, 252
        implantation within, 251, 255, *255*,
            282
Wastes, disposal of, 221–222, 229–230,
    230
Water, consumption of, 234–235, 242
    requirement for, 222
White blood cell (leukocyte), 26, 27,
    148, 150, 150–151
    agranular, 150, *150*
    granular, 150, *150*
White blood cell (leukocyte) count,
    153(t)
White matter, **296**
    of brain, *95*, 96(t), 100
    of spinal cord, *101*, 102, *113*
Window, oval, of ear, *122*, 122, **287**
    round, of ear, *122*
Windpipe (trachea), 8, *16*, *17*, 199, *200*,
    201, **294**
Wing, greater, of sphenoid bone, 59, *60*,
    61
    lesser, of sphenoid bone, *60*
Wisdom tooth, 214, *215*
Withdrawal reflex, 104, *104*
Word roots, 267
Wound, **296**
Wrist, *13*

Xiphoid process, *52*, 56(t)

Yellow marrow, *48*, 49
Young adulthood, 258

Zinc, 223(t)
Zygomatic arch, *53*
Zygomatic (malar) bone, 55(t), *58*, 59,
    61
Zygomatic muscle, 83, 84, *85*, 86(t)
Zygomatic process, of maxilla, *61*
    of temporal bone, 54(t), *59*
Zygote, 251, **296**